# Schizophrenia

## 2nd edition

*Schizophrenia: A Scientific Delusion?*, first published in 1990, made a very significant contribution to the debates on the concepts of schizophrenia and mental illness. These concepts remain both influential and controversial and this new updated second edition provides an incisive critical analysis of the debates over the last decade. As well as providing updated versions of the historical and scientific arguments against the concept of schizophrenia which formed the basis of the first edition, Boyle covers significant new material relevant to today's debates, including:

- The development of DSM-IV's version of 'schizophrenia'
- Analysis of social, psychological and linguistic processes which construct 'schizophrenia' as a reasonable version of reality
- A detailed critical evaluation of recent alternatives to the concept of schizophrenia.

*Schizophrenia: A Scientific Delusion?* demonstrates that the need for analysis and debate on these issues is as great as ever and that we still need to question how we think about and manage what we call 'madness'.

**Mary Boyle** is Professor of Clinical Psychology, and Head of the Doctorate in Clinical Psychology at the University of East London. She has worked as an NHS Clinical Psychologist and her previous publications include the first edition of *Schizophrenia: A Scientific Delusion?* (1990) and *Rethinking Abortion: Psychology, Gender, Power and Law* (1997).

# Schizophrenia
## A Scientific Delusion?

## 2nd edition

# Mary Boyle

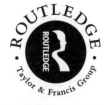

First published 1993 by Routledge
11 New Fetter Lane, London EC4P 4EE
Second edition 2002 by Routledge
27 Church Road, Hove, East Sussex BN3 2FA

Simultaneously published in the USA and Canada
by Taylor & Francis Inc
29 West 35th Street, New York, NY 10001

*Routledge is an imprint of the Taylor & Francis Group*

Typeset in Garamond by M Rules
Printed and bound in Great Britain by Biddles Ltd., Guildford
and King's Lynn
Cover design by Joyce Chester

*British Library Cataloguing in Publication Data*
A catalogue record for this book is available from the British Library

*Library of Congress Cataloging in Publication Data*
Boyle, Mary.
    Schizophrenia: a scientific delusion? / Mary Boyle – 2nd ed.
        p. cm.
    Includes bibliographical references and index.
    ISBN 0–415–22717–8 – ISBN 0–415–22718–6 (pbk)
    1. Schizophrenia – Diagnosis – History. I. Title.

    RC514 B65 2002
    616.89′82075–dc21

0–415–09700–2 (pbk)
Second edition ISBN 0–415–22717–8 (hbk)
Second edition ISBN 0–415–22718–6 (pbk)

# Contents

# Figures and tables

## Figure

## Tables

# Preface to the second edition

The opportunity to write a second edition of *Schizophrenia: A Scientific Delusion?* initially brought mixed feelings. In the decade or so since the publication of the first edition, the concept of schizophrenia has not only been subjected to increasing criticism, but there is now a significant literature on possible alternatives. Perhaps, then, there was no need for a second edition; perhaps the issue of 'schizophrenia's' status, and what should be put in its place, had been settled . . . or, perhaps not. Even a cursory study of recent theory and practice surrounding 'schizophrenia' and its alternatives would show that the situation is far more complex than that, and it was this complexity which both encouraged me to see a second edition as appropriate and made the writing of it such a challenging and fascinating task.

Four points in particular are worth highlighting. First, 'schizophrenia' and the assumptions which surround it are still simply taken for granted. The publication of DSM-IV in 1994, and its text revision in 2000, reinforced the diagnosis; each year, hundreds of papers are published which use the diagnosis of schizophrenia as an independent variable and which purport to tell us something of its underlying causes; researchers (e.g. Zakzanis and Hansen, 1998) still talk of 'the schizophrenic brain'; claims that schizophrenia is a genetic disorder are still frequently made; Schultz and Andreasen (1999) characterised current research as 'seek[ing] to detect causal mechanisms in schizophrenia through studies of neural connectivity and function, as well as models of genetic transmission, such as polygenic models of inheritance in genetic research' (1425); the US National Institute of Mental Health (Hyman, 2000) highlighted genetics, neuroimaging, post-mortem studies and developmental neurobiology as research priorities for schizophrenia, and suggested that 'perhaps no area has more promise for producing an understanding of what goes wrong in the brain in schizophrenia than does genetics' (2); Goldberg (2000), looking to the future, claimed that 'the greatest changes to our knowledge of mental disorders can be expected from a combination of [brain] imaging with other technologies – for example, electrophysiological data or neuropsychological data' (649). There is little here to suggest that criticisms of 'schizophrenia' and the theoretical models on which it is based, have had any impact at all. This raises the important issue of how and why 'schizophrenia' persists in the face of criticism and how it accommodates and responds to it. As criticism becomes more widespread and intense, then this issue assumes greater importance in any analysis.

The second point worth highlighting is that 'schizophrenia's' claimed relationship to science has always encouraged the belief that what matters is 'the latest research' and that historical analysis is a marginal, if worthy, pursuit. My experience with students and others suggests that fear of not knowing 'the latest research' is a very effective silencing mechanism; as each new generation of students and professionals becomes involved with madness, and as 'schizophrenia's' early history recedes, this mechanism becomes ever more effective. Both the first and second editions of this book take a very different view and see a fundamental conceptual analysis – including a historical analysis – of 'schizophrenia' and its associated assumptions as vital to our understanding of the problems 'schizophrenia' faces today; such analyses are also vital to resisting attempts to refashion the concept and to the development of constructive alternatives.

Third, the development of alternatives to 'schizophrenia' is proving to be a far from straightforward process. The literature represents a rich and imaginative range of ideas and practices but it also alerts us to the sheer persistence of 'schizophrenia', to the depth and pervasiveness of its surrounding assumptions, and to the ever-present danger of ending up, albeit in a new guise, more or less back where we started. Discussion of this process therefore seems just as important as discussion of 'schizophrenia' itself. Finally, I hesitated over writing a second edition partly because my research and clinical focus had shifted since I wrote the first and it might have seemed presumptuous to comment critically on the work of those more closely involved. But I believe strongly that how we think about and manage whatever we call madness – and, crucially, how our thinking about madness is managed – is an issue for all of us. And as the literature surrounding schizophrenia becomes more and more technical and obscure, the power of the diagnosis to silence becomes greater. This silencing can only be countered by open analysis and debate, with contributions from as many people as possible.

The structure of the second edition is similar to the first. The early chapters, which set out the theoretical framework for evaluating the validity of 'schizophrenia', and provide a historical analysis, have changed least and have been updated where necessary. Chapter 5, on the DSM, has been extended with a detailed discussion of the development of DSM-IV's concept of schizophrenia and of the efforts made to obscure its deficiencies and to present it as conceptually and empirically robust. This discussion is closely linked to the discussion of DSM-III, through an analysis of the DSM's attempts to manage its failure to fulfil the considerable hopes invested in it in relation to 'schizophrenia'. Chapter 6 has been updated to include recent adoption and genetic linkage research and to emphasise the importance of the way in which 'genetic' research is presented and misrepresented to professionals and the public. The latter part of the book, however, has been completely rewritten. In line with the increasing importance of the issue of how 'schizophrenia' accommodates criticism and persists in spite of it, Chapter 7 analyses this issue more extensively than in the first edition, and within a theoretical framework which acknowledges the importance of seeing 'schizophrenia' and its assumptions as 'truths' or 'knowledge' which are socially produced and managed. The final chapter, on alternatives to 'schizophrenia', has inevitably been enlarged to accommodate the welcome growth in this literature; this chapter, however, also focuses on the conceptual and practical problems raised by these developments and, in looking to the future, makes links to the book's earlier historical analysis in perhaps rather surprising ways.

The book as a whole is mainly concerned with how we think about or conceptualise those extreme forms of distress and deviance we call schizophrenia. Writing recently about the user/survivor movement, Campbell (1999) suggested that it had not yet impinged on *thinking* about distress. This comment, together with the persistence of the concept of schizophrenia in many quarters, suggests that the need for analysis and debate on this issue has not lessened in the last decade; I hope that this book will be seen as a constructive contribution to a vital public debate.

# Preface to the first edition

It is now almost a hundred years since Kraepelin introduced his concept of dementia praecox, the direct forerunner of Bleuler's and the modern concepts of schizophrenia. Criticising these concepts has been a popular sport for almost the same length of time, although the criticism has perhaps become more pointed, and more radical, over the last twenty years. A variety of responses has been made to the critics, with one of the most popular recent themes being 'We're getting there': given enough time and complex measuring equipment, diagnosis will be made more rigorous and the causes of schizophrenia will be better understood. There seems, too, to be little doubt amongst supporters of the concept that the route to progress will be via the laboratories of neuro-chemists, geneticists and molecular biologists. (See, for example, the Medical Research Council's 1987 Report on *Research into Schizophrenia*.)

The major aim of this book is to show that such answers will simply not do, because they ignore fundamental problems of the concept of schizophrenia and of variants such as the 'schizophrenia spectrum'. The book has four more specific aims. The first is to set out the claims made for 'schizophrenia' and, more importantly, what must be achieved for these to be accepted. It is my impression that this latter question is often glossed over, if not misrepresented, in much of the literature, so that it is difficult for readers to assess the strength of the claims. The second aim is to evaluate the extent to which the claims made for 'schizophrenia' are justified and the third (having concluded that they are not) is to discuss alternatives to the concept, both in terms of research design and theories of bizarre behaviour. Finally, by setting out in some detail the story of the introduction, development and use of 'schizophrenia' as well as some of the fallacious arguments used to support it, I hope to make understandable some of the reasons for the chaos and controversy which have so often surrounded the concept, for its persistence in spite of these, and to make clear why no amount of tinkering with it will bestow scientific respectability.

If the book can be said to adopt an approach, it is that of Social Constructionism. It has been said of this approach that it has the 'annoying feature of turning attention away from a problem and onto those who are trying

to deal with the problem' (Heise, 1988: 259). This book certainly has that feature: it concentrates not on 'schizophrenics' but on those who diagnose
schizophrenia. It will, therefore, probably annoy many people. I hope, however,
that for others it will be thought-provoking, and will encourage them seriously
to question traditional interpretations of bizarre behaviour and to make more
central the social and ethical issues involved both in theorising about, and
responding to, such behaviour.

# Acknowledgements

The impetus to study the concept of schizophrenia originally came from my experience of working with people who were diagnosed as schizophrenic and from the research and writing of, particularly, Ted Sarbin. I am especially grateful to Ted for his interest and encouragement over the years. I have also benefited greatly from discussions with Dick Hallam (to whom thanks also for the title!), Dave Harper and Ernie Govier. Discussions with service users have helped maintain my faith that in this area at least, ideas and concepts *matter*. Thanks, too, to Colin Berry for his meticulous translations of German manuscripts. Finally, special thanks to Clive Gabriel who has lived through both editions of this book and whose emotional, intellectual and practical support has been simply invaluable.

# Evaluating the validity of 'schizophrenia'

Two major claims have been made about the concept of schizophrenia: first, that it is a scientific concept or, at least, that those who use it work within a scientific framework (for example, Gottesman and Shields, 1982; Wing, 1988; APA, 1994; Sartorius, 1994; Ross and Pam, 1995) and, second, that the term refers to a particular kind of medical pattern known as a syndrome (Gottesman and Shields, 1982; Kendell, 1991; APA, 1994). These claims imply that the concept has been developed and is used in a manner similar to that of other concepts which claim scientific status *and* that the phenomena to which it refers are similar to those usually denoted by the medical term 'syndrome'. This chapter will describe in detail what is meant by these claims, not least because their meaning is rarely spelt out and is often misrepresented in the literature, but also as a necessary prelude to evaluating whether the introduction, development and use of the concept of schizophrenia actually conforms to the claims made about it.

## 'Schizophrenia' as a scientific concept

As Medawar (1984) and Chalmers (1990) have pointed out, attempts to define 'science', to give the term some absolute meaning, have always ended in failure. With this in mind, all that will be attempted here is a description of some of the ways in which those who call themselves scientists – particularly natural and medical scientists, with whom supporters of 'schizophrenia have identified themselves – tend to proceed. This rather pragmatic stance, however, should not be thought of as second best: the crucial issue is that, given the claims made about 'schizophrenia', then the ways it has been developed and used ought at least to be recognisable to philosophers and practitioners of natural and medical science. Kendell (1991), a supporter of 'schizophrenia', concurs, claiming that '[the concept of schizophrenia] can only be judged by the same criteria as other explanatory concepts' (60).

The search for patterns and attempts to describe relationships between phenomena are fundamental to scientific activity. They are central, too, to much non-scientific activity; of particular interest here is that they are central to lay or everyday attempts to understand behaviour and other events. What perhaps distinguishes the two is the scientist's persistent demand for the provision of certain types of evidence that a pattern has been observed and the imposition of various publicly demonstrable criteria for evaluating it. This demand for evidence, and its public evaluation, is crucial in view of our apparent propensity to claim that certain events 'go together', in the absence of any direct evidence that this is the case (see, for example, Shweder, 1977; Chapman and Chapman, 1982).

### Observables and unobservables in scientific theory

Scientific theories contain both observables and unobservables. The term 'observable' can give the misleading impression of referring to some outside reality, but I am using it here simply to mean readily agreed statements about sense data with a minimum of interpretation. In scientific research, simple statements about putative relationships between observables (when certain metals are brought close together, one moves towards the other) are used to justify inferring unobservables (magnetic force); as we shall see, these unobservables are then used to aid the construction of more elaborate theoretical statements.

It is readily agreed that 'schizophrenia' is an unobservable, an abstract concept inferred from overt behaviour or from verbal reports of behaviour and experience (Kendell, 1991; APA, 1994). Scientific theories, however, may contain different types of unobservables and it is important to distinguish them in assessing the validity of 'schizophrenia'. Beck (1953) has distinguished two types of unobservables by applying the concepts of *systemic* and *real* 'existence' and the language of logic to differentiate them. The first, he says, is that 'mode of existence of an (unobserved) entity all descriptions of which are analytical within a system of propositions', while real existence 'is the mode of existence attributed to an entity if there is any true synthetic proposition that can be made about it' (369). In other words, statements about an unobservable said to have real existence will contain words which are not reducible to the empirical relationships from which it is inferred and will imply hypotheses about the antecedents of these empirical relationships.

Benjamin (1937) has made the same distinction by contrasting what he calls abstractive and hypothetical methods in scientific activity. In the abstractive method, phenomena are grouped by a restrictive set of properties into classes whose relationship can be discovered empirically; nothing is added to what is observed. By contrast, the hypothetical method relates observations by 'inventing a fictitious substance or process or idea in terms of which the experiences can be expressed. It correlates observations by adding something to them' (184). Constructs formed by Benjamin's abstractive method (e.g. solubility, resistance, temperature, habit strength; hunger as X hours of food deprivation, and so on) would be said by Beck to have systemic existence, while those formed by the hypothetical method (electricity; proton; intelligence; diabetes) would be said to have real existence. MacCorquodale and Meehl (1948) have suggested the terms 'intervening variables' and 'hypothetical constructs' to distinguish these two types of unobservables, and these terms (with 'construct' and 'concept' used interchangeably) will be adopted here. Other names have, however, been suggested: Beck uses constructions and inferred entities, while Carnap (1937) uses the term 'dispositional concepts' rather than 'intervening variables'. Although all hypothetical concepts refer to unobservables, it is worth noting a distinction between two different types. The first is that which becomes, in Beck's phrase, an 'object of search' and which is postulated by scientists to show certain characteristics. The constructs of atom or proton are examples of this type; although unobserved at the moment, they are claimed to exist as a result of certain observations and mathematical calculations and may be observed at some future point, given appropriate technology. The second type of unobservable remains for ever an abstraction, which cannot be postulated to exist except in the most abstract sense. 'Intelligence', 'memory', 'diabetes' and 'multiple sclerosis' are examples of this type of hypothetical construct.

Which kind of concept is 'schizophrenia'? Kraepelin clearly did not see his concept of dementia praecox, from which the modern concept of schizophrenia is derived, as being reducible to a statement about correlations between behaviours. Instead, he postulated a 'metabolic disorder' to *account for* the putative correlations. Similarly, statements made today about the concept contain terms not reducible to statements about behavioural correlations. 'Schizophrenia' is said to be an illness; a biochemical disorder; a genetic disorder. What is implied by statements like these is not always specified but it is clear that something is being added to a statement about behavioural correlations. 'Schizophrenia' therefore functions as a hypothetical construct rather than an intervening variable; and, as an abstraction from observables, rather than an 'entity' postulated to exist as a result of observations, it also functions as one of the second type of hypothetical construct – no one ever expects to 'see' schizophrenia, any more than they expect to 'see' diabetes, regardless of how advanced technology becomes. It must be emphasised that this status as an eternal abstraction is perfectly respectable and has nothing to do with the present lack of a clear relationship between biochemical events and behaviour said to be symptomatic of schizophrenia. Even if such events were to be observed in the future, the concept of schizophrenia would remain an abstraction because there is no identity between it and any biological, genetic or behavioural event, any more than there is identity between the concept of diabetes and a specific biological event.

The most important distinction between hypothetical constructs (of both types) and intervening variables lies in the predictive function of hypothetical constructs (Benjamin, 1937; MacCorquodale and Meehl, 1948; Beck, 1953; Carnap, 1974). They have, or should have, the power to generate predictions about events which have not yet been observed. This power derives partly from the fact that hypothetical constructs, unlike intervening variables, are not reducible to statements about what has already been observed, but imply hypotheses about the antecedents of what has been observed. This distinction has important implications for evaluating the validity of the two types of construct. The validity of an intervening variable can be questioned only by denying the observations from which it was originally inferred, i.e. by claiming that such and such did not actually happen. The concept of solubility, for example, requires only that substances be observed to dissolve at different rates and to different extents in water or other liquids; it implies nothing about the variables which control this. These observations are therefore said to be both *necessary* and *sufficient* conditions for asserting the validity of the concept. For a hypothetical construct, the actual occurrence of the empirical relationships from which it was inferred is, of course, a necessary condition for asserting its validity, but it is not sufficient. The demonstration of predictive power is central to assertions of the validity of hypothetical constructs and is the sufficient condition for inferring them.

## The correspondence rules of hypothetical constructs

To say that a construct has predictive power is to say that it is capable of predicting events which, though observable in principle, have not yet been observed. Thus, the concept of intelligence may be capable of predicting performance differences in a laboratory task. It is possible to use unobservables to make and investigate statements about observables because of what are variously called correspondence rules (Carnap, 1974), operational rules (Bridgman, 1927) and The Dictionary (Campbell, 1920; cited in Carnap, 1974). These rules, which may be very simple or highly complex, specify what must be observed before a concept can be inferred and may specify quantitatively the relationship between variation in what is observed and variation in the inferred construct. The correspondence rules for the concept of intelligence, for example, specify the relationship between observable responses to items on a standardised test and 'amounts' of the unobservable concept, intelligence. Any investigation of the predictive power of a hypothetical construct therefore involves examining the relationship between two sets of observables.

## The process of change of correspondence rules

Inferred constructs usually start as relatively vague concepts associated with certain observations. It is then discovered, by empirical investigation, that these observations vary systematically with another observation which can be made more reliably and is more strongly correlated with relevant experimental changes. The concept of temperature, for example, was originally associated with global, subjective judgements of hot and cold. It was later shown that these judgements *and* a range of other phenomena were reliably correlated with measurable changes in the height of a mercury column. The correspondence rules for inferred constructs (i.e. what must be observed before the construct is inferred) therefore change over time as a result of increasing specification and elaboration of events which can be shown to be associated with the original set of observations from which the construct was inferred. That correspondence rules do change in this way may of course demonstrate a construct's predictive power.

This process of change in correspondence rules is well illustrated by the development of the medical concept of diabetes mellitus. The construct of diabetes was originally inferred by the Greeks from observations of the co-occurrence of inordinate thirst and urine production, lethargy and emaciation. These observations therefore constituted the first set of correspondence rules for the hypothetical construct of diabetes. In the seventeenth century it was noted that this cluster was frequently and reliably associated with sweet-tasting urine. Thus, a new correspondence rule could be set up between an observable event and the unobservable 'diabetes'. Later, it was discovered that sweet-tasting urine contained glucose which could be detected independently of the original observation of inordinate thirst, and so on, or judgements about the sweetness of urine. Yet another set of correspondence rules could therefore be set up. These, in turn, were superseded by rules specifying that diabetes mellitus was to be inferred when a certain relationship between intake of glucose and its level in the blood at certain time intervals was observed. (The 'division' of the concept of diabetes into mellitus and insipidus was necessitated by the observations that inordinate thirst and urine production were not always associated with sweet-tasting urine and, later, that they could be associated with low levels of anti-diuretic hormone.)

Every attempt to examine the fate of predictions from a hypothetical construct involves the use of its correspondence rules. Each attempt to show that the *sufficient* conditions for inferring the construct are fulfilled therefore involves invoking the *necessary* conditions for inferring its existence. In the very early stages of a construct's development, the necessary conditions – the putative regularities from which the construct was originally inferred – will also be the correspondence rules. Later, the necessary conditions will be invoked indirectly as the correspondence rules change. But it would be quite wrong to depict this process of change in correspondence rules as one of finding out what a hypothetical construct 'is'. Young (1951) and Carnap (1974) have noted how often the question, 'What is X?', where X is a hypothetical construct, is put to scientists by lay people. They point out that the question is unanswerable and is based on a misunderstanding of the function of hypothetical constructs. These concepts can only be described in terms of the observed events from which they are inferred and the predictions which have been made from them, in terms, that is, of the theoretical network in which they are embedded. The question 'What is diabetes?' would be answered (and attempts, however misguided, are often made to answer such questions) very differently in classical Greece and in the modern Western world and will, no doubt, be answered very differently again in the twenty-second century as the theoretical network is further elaborated. Each answer is 'true' but misleading; to pose the question at all is to reify the construct and to imply that there is a final, concrete answer.

## Deriving predictions from hypothetical constructs

The correspondence rules which tie unobservable to observable events provide the general means for examining predictions from a construct. The *content* of these predictions can be specified only by examining the whole theoretical network which surrounds the concept, the assumptions on which it is based, indeed, everything that is asserted about it (Cronbach and Meehl, 1955). The statements which make up this network may relate observables to each other, unobservables to observables, and/or unobservables to one another. But it is axiomatic that any construct which claims scientific status be embedded in a network in which at least some of its statements contain observables. The ease with which researchers can derive predictions from this network, and then investigate them, depends not on its simplicity but on its specificity. One obvious result of a lack of specificity is disagreement over the content of predictions; another is disagreement over the results of attempts to test an agreed prediction. There is no question of a concept's validity depending on a particular number of the predictions derived from it being upheld; there is certainly no quantitative answer to the question, 'How valid is construct X?' Rather, validity is usually assessed from a utilitarian stance by asking in what ways and for what purposes the construct has proved useful. The term 'utility' is therefore often used instead of 'validity' to reflect the fact that, as a rule, a hypothetical construct has no claim to validity unless it can be used to predict events which, without the construct, would probably have gone undetected. If the same events are predicted by different constructs, then that which carries fewest assumptions is usually preferred.

It may happen, however, that research fails to detect events predicted from a construct. The question then arises of whether the 'fault' lies with the construct, and its theoretical network, or with the method of inquiry. As will be seen in Chapter 2, the nineteenth-century medical profession sought to retain the concept of mental disease even though they were unable to detect the predicted differences between the brains of those said to be mentally diseased and the brains of those who were not. It was argued that existing methods of measuring brain function were not sufficiently advanced to detect the postulated differences. This may well have been true, but such a *post hoc* argument could be used indefinitely to justify the continued use of a concept, one of whose major predictions had no empirical support. It can be argued instead that if a construct has already led to the detection of previously unobserved events and if it predicts specific events observable in principle but undetectable by existing methods, then the failure to detect such an event might well indicate that a more sophisticated methodology is required and not that the construct is invalid. But if a concept is in the early stages of development, if it lacks a history of 'successful' predictions or is embedded in a loose theoretical network which cannot be used to predict specific events, then the 'failure' of a major prediction should direct attention to the concept itself. In particular, such failures should direct our attention to the fundamental question of whether the necessary condition for inferring the concept has been fulfilled; that is, was a set of regularities which would justify bringing the concept into existence ever observed? The question is crucial, as this necessary condition is invoked, directly or indirectly, every time a prediction is 'tested'. This failure to make reliable predictions to new observations, being embedded in a loose and ever-changing theoretical network and failing to specify what *would* be observed were technology to improve, is precisely the problem which besets the concept of schizophrenia (Bentall, 1990b; Boyle, 1994; British Psychological Society, 2000). The question, then, of whether the necessary conditions for inferring schizophrenia have been fulfilled – of whether anyone has ever observed a pattern of regularities which would justify the original and continued existence of the concept – will be central to this book.

## Lay and scientific concepts

These methods of developing and investigating constructs can be compared with the development and use of what are often called 'lay' or 'folk' concepts. Our language is rich in terms, particularly those referring to people, which are superficially similar to hypothetical constructs. Some of them (deep; hard) are obviously metaphorical and others (anxious; normal) less obviously so. There are some major differences between these concepts and those whose claims to scientific status are rarely disputed; two of these are of particular interest here. The first is that the correspondence rules of lay concepts are often many and varied, and vary from user to user. They also tend to change in idiosyncratic ways over time: the referents of the concept 'nice', for example, used to be very similar, when applied to women, to those of later concepts like 'fast'. The second difference is that, although these terms may appear to be derived from patterns of behaviour, no systematic attempts are usually made to check this; or, when they have been made (for example, Shweder, 1977; Kahneman *et al.*, 1982) the apparent patterns have been shown to be more closely related to cultural beliefs about 'what goes with what' than to reliable observations. It must be emphasised that attempts to demonstrate that lay concepts are not necessarily 'messy' (e.g. Cantor and Mischel, 1977; Cantor *et al.*, 1980) do not affect their status as lay constructs but at most can be said to demonstrate the orderliness of cultural beliefs and stereotypes.

None of this implies criticism of lay concepts or demonstrates their inferiority. They are not intended to serve the functions of scientific concepts but to be used in day-to-day discourse. It would place an intolerable burden on our interaction if we had to assess the reliability and validity of every concept before we could use it. Problems arise only when lay concepts are used *as if* they had been derived in a way quite different from they actually were (see, for example, Sarbin's 1968 discussion of 'anxiety' and Warburton's 1985 discussion of 'addiction'). I am making these points in some detail here because they may be important in understanding some of the problems encountered by 'schizophrenia' — not least because our sheer familiarity with lay concepts, in all their 'looseness', may blunt our critical faculties when it comes to assessing 'schizophrenia'.

## 'Schizophrenia' as a syndrome

The claim that 'schizophrenia' is a scientific concept implies that it was derived from the observation of a pattern of regularities. The claim that the term refers to a syndrome implies that it was derived from, and now refers to, a particular type of pattern. The nature of this pattern, and the ways in which it differs from that originally envisaged by Kraepelin, can perhaps best be clarified by describing some of the historical background to modern medical ideas about pattern description.

The aim of medicine, as of all branches of science, is to describe patterns and relationships. In medicine, however, ideas about pattern identification, about the grouping of phenomena, are inseparable from ideas about the concept of disease. Engle (1963) has described two important and contrasting views on diseases which can be traced to classical Greece. The Platonic tradition taught that reality was universal and unchanging, unlike perceptions received through the senses, which were relative and imperfect. Applied to medicine, these ideas led to a search for unvarying universals — individual diseases 'out there' and separable from the person. The Aristotelian tradition, by contrast, did not scorn sense data and encouraged the detailed study, for its own sake, of what were assumed to be the manifestations of disease in individuals, rather than the search for abstract (or metaphysical?) universals.

In practice, of course, it was not always easy to distinguish those who claimed adherence to one school or the other. The theories were expressed in a way which made their implications for research and practice less than clear, and in any case adherents to the Platonic school, their distrust of the senses notwithstanding, were forced to work with phenomena as they presented to the senses. They did this to such an extent that it seemed that every phenomenon they observed was classified as a disease — skin rashes, swellings, fevers, etc. Indeed, de Sauvages was able, in 1763, to list 2,400 diseases, most of which would now be considered to be individual symptoms (Zilboorg, 1941). It would therefore be naive to expect the Platonic and Aristotelian views to be clearly distinguishable in the actual activities of medical men (as distinct from what they said they were doing); nevertheless, two distinct themes, roughly corresponding to the two ancient traditions, can be discerned in the writings of philosophers and physicians on 'disease'. These have been variously characterised as ontological (disease-entity) versus biographical; qualitative versus quantitative; discontinuous versus continuous (Kendell, 1975b). Thomas Sydenham was one of the most articulate proponents of the ontological view of disease. Writing at the end of the seventeenth century, he reiterated the belief in the existence of natural and unvarying disease entities, separable from the person, and whose presentation was uniform across sufferers. These entities, he maintained, must be separated because each required a different treatment. Sydenham's ideas, which were heavily influenced by the classification systems of botanists and by the 'disease' of malaria, were extremely popular because, as Kräupl-Taylor (1979) suggests, they encouraged medical men to participate fully, via clinical observations, in the search for clinical data on which to base a classificatory system. Indeed, this was done with such enthusiasm that for almost every physician there was a classificatory system. These efforts were seriously hampered not only by tenuous acquaintance with the principles of classification (Zilboorg, 1941) but also by the fact that observations were subjective and limited to what could be observed 'at the bedside'.

Sydenham's ontological theories were strongly challenged in the late eighteenth century and the early nineteenth. In particular, critics attacked his view of disease entities as having a separate existence and suggested that disease was a quantitative and not a qualitative deviation from the norm, and that the course might vary from individual to individual. In 1847, Virchow declared that 'Diseases have no independent or isolated existence; they are not autonomous organisms, nor beings invading a body, nor parasites growing on it; they are only the manifestations of life process under altered conditions' (Kräupl-Taylor, 1979: 11). But later in the century Virchow was to alter his views to the extent that he was able, in 1895, to call himself a 'thoroughgoing ontologist'. His concept of disease entity was, however, very different from Sydenham's. The introduction of the microscope and the practice of histology in the late nineteenth century allowed the detailed investigation of the various bodily derangements which accompanied overt symptoms. For Virchow, a disease entity was a particular pathological abnormality. A disease entity therefore became an altered body part, a significant change which avoided the metaphysical overtones of Sydenham's theory. Classification consisted of descriptions of the various types of change which could be observed in different body organs; diagnosis was the matching of these to the changes observed in a particular patient.

Virchow's views in turn were challenged by bacteriologists at the end of the nineteenth century. The nature of their dispute is clearly illustrated by an example given by Kräupl-Taylor (1979). Virchow began from the premise that a pathological abnormality constituted a disease entity and that the diagnosis had to name the abnormality, no matter how it was caused. Diphtheria, for example, would be diagnosed whenever surface necrosis and membrane formation were observed in an organ. That these changes could have causes other than the presence of the diphtheria bacilli was not important to Virchow. To the bacteriologists, diagnosis consisted in identifying the kind of organism which had invaded the body, regardless of the nature of the pathological changes it might produce in any individual. The bacteriologists' views won the day because they proved more useful than those of Virchow. But the debate between them and Virchow was between one kind of ontological theory and another; there is no doubt that the bacteriologists' findings served to strengthen the already popular ontological theories to an extent never achieved by Sydenham and his many followers. Once again, a disease entity had become a discrete and separate unit, with its own distinctive cause, symptoms, course and outcome.

It is interesting to note the strength of ontological theories in popular discourse about physical ailments. As Kräupl-Taylor (1979) has pointed out, much of the language surrounding disease implies an ontological theory – we talk of 'catching' or 'getting rid of a disease'; we are 'attacked by diseases'; we 'carry diseases' which we 'pass on' to our children or to others. It is also notable that ontological theories seem to offer a reassuringly simple solution to the apparent chaos of physical suffering: a number of seemingly disparate phenomena can be accounted for and perhaps abolished by reference to one underlying cause.

### From disease entity to syndrome

Kraepelin's ideas about the phenomena with which he was confronted in asylums were derived from a Platonic view of the world. His belief in natural disease entities with an independent existence was, of course, strengthened by progress in understanding the so-called infectious diseases: the finding that single micro-organisms, with an independent existence, were responsible for certain clusters of phenomena with their own, apparently natural, course and outcome. Kraepelin accepted unquestioningly that the behaviour of asylum inmates was a manifestation of biological events, just as were the fevers, rashes and at times odd behaviours of those infected with various micro-organisms. He therefore assumed that the inmates' behaviour would be found to fall into natural clusters, representing qualitative deviations from whatever he thought of as normality and that each cluster would have its own distinct antecedent, both necessary and sufficient to produce the cluster.

But as I noted earlier, there were conflicting views as to the nature of these entities. Some said the entity was the observed cluster; others that it was the antecedent of the cluster; still others that it was the anatomical pathology which accompanied the overt cluster. Indeed, as Kräupl-Taylor (1982) has pointed out, Sydenham himself appears to have used the term 'disease entity' in two quite different ways – to refer both to an independent, God-given species and to the body's reaction to invasion by external agents. Kraepelin was well aware of the fact that any attempt to postulate antecedents for putative clusters of behaviour was pure speculation; similarly, it made no sense to suggest that the term 'disease entity' be applied to morbid anatomy when none could be found in many asylum inmates. However, as Jaspers (1963) has remarked, Kraepelin 'embarked on a new approach which hoped to arrive at disease entities in spite of everything' (566). This approach consisted in observing inmates' behaviour in an attempt to discover similarities amongst the most frequently appearing behaviours and similarities in the ways they changed over time. Charting behaviour changes over time (called 'the whole course of the illness') presented considerable problems as asylum doctors had direct access to inmates' behaviour only from the time of their incarceration. Attempts were made, however, to reconstruct the past from discussion with inmates or their relatives. Strictly speaking, Kraepelin's approach was not new; followers of both the Platonic and the Aristotelian traditions had stressed the importance of careful observation of morbid manifestations, although attempts to describe similarities amongst these phenomena in different individuals, and the view that a disease entity accounted for them, were largely confined to the Platonic school. The novelty of Kraepelin's approach lay in its emphasis on investigating the 'whole course of the illness' in an attempt to discover natural groupings, entities or patterns. Kraepelin believed that the behavioural clusters he hoped to discover would be found to have distinctive biological antecedents and cerebral pathology as well as course and outcome. The totality of this pattern would be called a natural disease entity.

It is well documented that Kraepelin's hopes of finding such patterns were never realised, either by him or by any of his successors (Jaspers, 1963; Wing, 1978a; Gottesman and Shields, 1982; Kendell, 1991). Instead, as I noted earlier, the term 'schizophrenia' is now said to refer to a syndrome, which is usually described as a clustering of symptoms and signs (Morris, 1978). More generally, the term 'syndrome' refers to the very basic fact that certain phenomena appear to cluster at greater than chance level. It is not assumed that the clusters of events denoted by the syndrome name are distinctive natural groupings, and people who display the cluster might vary widely in the way it changes over time. The antecedents of the cluster are generally unknown.

The connection between the medical idea of syndrome and more general scientific research – a connection which is crucial in evaluating 'schizophrenia' – can be seen in the fact that most syndrome names (e.g. rheumatoid arthritis) refer to hypothetical constructs: they are abstractions inferred from the observation of patterns of regularities. They should therefore fulfil the functions of summarising a pattern of observations and of allowing predictions to as yet unobserved events. Syndrome names are thus theoretical abstractions which are thought to be useful in research but which may be abandoned if and when they cease to fulfil this function. The construct of Down's syndrome, for example, has proved extremely useful in that it allowed predictions to previously unobserved features of chromosomes. The idea of a syndrome, unlike that of a disease entity, can encompass both qualitative and quantitative deviations from a norm: possessing certain characteristics which represent a quantitative deviation from some standard can still have implications which are different in important ways from those associated with the possession of a standard set of characteristics.

## The identification of syndrome patterns

One function of the construct denoted by a syndrome name is to summarise a meaningful cluster of phenomena; that is, a cluster unlikely to have occurred by chance and therefore likely to signify other, as yet unknown, events. But whereas it is easy to imagine that certain occurrences form a pattern (Shweder, 1977; Chapman and Chapman, 1982), it is much more difficult to determine whether a pattern actually has been observed. The method favoured by Kraepelin – that of charting the progress and outcome of a postulated cluster – has a number of problems associated with it, whether or not it involves ideas about disease entities. The use of the term 'outcome' in this context implies, erroneously, that a specific end-point can be identified. In practice, however, the term usually refers to a complex series of events or processes with no obvious end-point. Given the problems of deciding which variables to measure and when to end the process, and the finding that most of the clusters which are the source of syndrome names show considerable variability over time, it would be unproductive to rely on outcome as a criterion of meaningfulness for any postulated cluster. The problem is compounded by the fact that identification of possible new instances of the cluster (diagnosis) is impossible until their progress is charted, to check that it matches that of the earlier instances. A reliance on 'outcome' is apt to lead to *post hoc* diagnosis (and, as will be shown, Kraepelin himself fell into this trap) where a diagnostic label may be changed several times, depending on the progress of the phenomena from which it was inferred. For these reasons, reliance on progress or outcome to identify meaningful patterns has generally been rejected by medical researchers. A much less problematic and more productive method of judging whether a postulated cluster is meaningful – and the one usually adopted in medicine – is to search for a phenomenon which is reliably associated with the cluster and which has two other important characteristics: first, it can be measured reliably and independently of the cluster it is associated with and, second, it can be shown or reasonably assumed to be an antecedent of the cluster. In turn, this phenomenon may later be found to be associated with another reliably and independently measurable event, and so on along an assumed 'causal' chain. It is in this way, of course, that correspondence rules for an unobservable may become more reliable and more specific and its theoretical network more elaborate, as was described earlier for the concept of diabetes mellitus.

The identification of patterns known as syndromes is therefore a two-stage process: a researcher or clinician first identifies a cluster of features which they believe 'hang together'. They, or someone else, then needs to show that this cluster is reliably associated with another feature which can be measured independently. The importance of this two-stage process can be seen by examining the type of bodily features usually involved at each stage. Those features which make up the cluster at the first stage are usually those most easily and directly perceptible to an observer or to the person themselves (for example, pallor, sweating, rashes, vomiting, pain, and so on). Such phenomena are usually called symptoms and share a number of characteristics. First, they are often not directly observable to an onlooker (e.g. nausea) but are made available by verbal report. Second, the reliability with which they can be observed may be low. Third, they are overdetermined in that each may have many antecedents. The clustering of any of these events in an individual might therefore be a chance occurrence; worse, if the reliability of reports of their occurrence is low, then reports of their co-occurrence may be false. It is therefore very unwise to assume that any reported co-occurrence of events like these is meaningful or to infer from it the existence of an unobserved process. Instead, it is necessary to go to the second stage and to demonstrate that any supposed cluster of symptoms is reliably associated with another independently measurable event. In medicine, such events are called 'signs' and they differ from symptoms in a number of important ways. First, they can be observed with a much higher degree of reliability. Second, they are directly available to an observer, rather than being available only through introspection and verbal report or by inference from, for example, shaking or moaning. Third, although signs are also overdetermined, the number of antecedents is thought to be fewer than for symptoms. An unselected population will therefore show signs far less often than symptoms. Fourth, there should be plausible, even if speculative, theoretical links between those signs and symptoms whose co-occurrence is said to be meaningful, to justify the assumption that the signs are antecedents of the symptoms.

The distinction between signs and symptoms can be clarified using the example of glucose in the urine (Kräupl-Taylor, 1979). This is called a sign because it can be reliably measured by an external observer, its frequency of occurrence is less than is the individual frequency of events with which it may be associated (excess urine production, thirst, tiredness, and so on) and because there are plausible grounds for assuming that it is not a consequence of these. The term 'sign' suggests that an event signifies, or is indicative of, another event which can be independently observed. The presence of glucose in the urine may signify high blood-glucose (itself an overdetermined event) or diminished glucose reabsorption in the renal tubes. Because hyperglycaemia fulfils the criteria listed above, it too is a sign, in this case perhaps of pancreatic abnormalities. Signs, however, are often mistakenly said to be indicative of a syndrome name as, for example, when high blood-glucose levels are said to be a sign of diabetes. Statements like these are obviously tautological because syndrome names are concepts inferred from clusters of signs and symptoms; they are not observable events which can be measured independently of the sign.

People who receive the same syndrome name as a diagnostic label will usually be homogeneous for at least one sign in the cluster from which the syndrome name is inferred. They will, however, be heterogeneous for symptoms because the same sign may be associated with a variety of symptoms. This heterogeneity suggests that unknown mediating variables are operating in the chain from sign to symptoms. Similarly, because signs are overdetermined, people who show the same sign may be given different diagnostic labels to reflect the fact that the antecedents of the sign they share – probably unknown in the case of those given the syndrome name as a diagnostic label – appear to be different. These people are also likely to share a number of symptoms. But even those who do not share signs, and who receive different diagnostic labels, may share symptoms because different signs can be associated with the same symptoms (for example, nausea, abdominal pain, fever, and so on).

In spite of the heterogeneity amongst those given the same diagnostic label and the overlap amongst those given different labels, it seems useful to maintain the separation between some groups who share signs and symptoms because they do not seem to share antecedents. Only some of those who show glucose in the urine, for example, will show hyperglycaemia, and those who do will, in turn, show a variety of pancreatic abnormalities. It is therefore assumed that different processes led to the appearance of the signs in the various groups. This assumption may be supported by the observations that between-group variability in progress over time is considerably greater than within-group variance; that the groups, without intervention, reach obviously different endpoints; for example, early death versus average lifespan, or that response to the same intervention is quite different between groups. Taken together, these differences provide good grounds for separating the groups for research purposes. Even if such differences are not observed, the separation of the groups for the present can be justified if the proximal antecedents of the sign they share seem to be different.

## Evaluating the validity of 'schizophrenia'

If we return to the claims made about 'schizophrenia' with which the chapter began – that it is a scientific concept and a syndrome – then the claims can now be restated in this way: 'schizophrenia' is a hypothetical construct. It is inferred from a pattern, a set of regularities which conform to a syndrome (i.e. a meaningful cluster of signs and symptoms). These claims can be specified further in terms of the *necessary* and *sufficient* conditions for inferring hypothetical constructs.

## The necessary conditions

I noted earlier that the necessary condition for inferring a hypothetical construct is the observation of a pattern of regularities. Kraepelin's original inference of dementia praecox and then Bleuler's of schizophrenia therefore imply that such a pattern was observed in the behaviour of asylum inmates. And, because 'schizophrenia' is said to be a syndrome, the claim is implicitly made that this original cluster or, at least, the cluster which is the source of the modern concept of schizophrenia, conforms to a meaningful pattern of events which can reasonably be called signs and events which can reasonably be called symptoms.

One of the problems of discussing the status of the necessary conditions for inferring schizophrenia is that various sets of regularities have been put forward as the source of the construct. But because it is generally accepted that Kraepelin's construct of dementia praecox marked the beginning of the modern construct of schizophrenia (for example, Gottesman and Shields, 1982; M. Bleuler, 1991; Kendell, 1991; APA, 1994) – indeed the terms 'dementia praecox' and 'schizophrenia' were often used interchangeably at least until the 1930s – the regularities in the behaviour of asylum inmates allegedly observed by Kraepelin will be taken here as the first set of necessary conditions for inferring schizophrenia. These, together with the clusters suggested by Bleuler and Schneider, will be examined in Chapter 3 to assess how far they justify the claim that 'schizophrenia' came into existence through the observation of a meaningful pattern which could reasonably be described as a syndrome.

## The sufficient conditions

The sufficient condition for inferring a hypothetical construct is that it can be used to predict new observations. But it can hardly be overemphasised that if the necessary conditions for inferring a hypothetical construct have not been fulfilled, then the sufficient conditions cannot be either; you cannot, after all, expect to make new observations about the antecedents of a non-existent pattern. It must be said, however, that if the cluster from which schizophrenia was and is inferred *did* conform to the pattern denoted by 'syndrome', it would amount to the fulfilment of the necessary and just sufficient conditions for inferring it, because an originally postulated cluster of symptoms would have been shown to be reliably associated with an independently and reliably measurable event (a sign) and thus to have some predictive power.

But considerably more than this is claimed for 'schizophrenia'. A number of predictions have been derived from the construct but it is admitted that data relating to many of them, for example, that particular patterns of cognitive or psychophysiological or biochemical functioning will be observed, are in some disarray (for example, Wing, 1988; Chua and McKenna, 1995; McGrath and Emmerson, 1999). What users of 'schizophrenia' claim not to be in disarray are data relating to predictions about genetic inheritance. It has been claimed, for example, that this hypothesis has been 'proven' (APA, 1980), and that the evidence is 'incontrovertible' and 'beyond challenge' (Kendell, 1991). These claims will be examined in Chapter 6. They will be examined in some detail: first, because of their strength and near unanimity; second, because 'genetic' data may be used to justify both the continuing search for supporting biochemical data and the retention of a particular theoretical model, and third, because the presentation of this literature could offer examples of the ways in which the presentation of data in secondary sources might function to maintain the concept of schizophrenia.

Another way of implying that the sufficient conditions for inferring a construct have been met is by changing the correspondence rules. I noted earlier that the regularities from which a hypothetical construct is originally inferred form the first set of correspondence rules which tie the construct to observable events. I also noted that these rules may change as the initial set of events is shown to be reliably associated with other, reliably and independently measurable phenomena (i.e. the construct is shown to predict new observations). The correspondence rules for inferring schizophrenia have been changed a number of times since the concept was introduced (these are usually called diagnostic criteria, but the term 'correspondence rules' will be used here to help keep in mind the fact that the validity of 'schizophrenia' is to be evaluated by applying criteria used by the scientific community in general). These changes in correspondence rules will be examined in Chapters 4 and 5 in order to assess how far they reflect the processes described earlier. It is of course the case that the use of any set of correspondence rules implies that these refer to a pattern of phenomena. In other words, the publication of diagnostic criteria amounts to a public claim that these represent a pattern of regularities which justify inferring 'schizophrenia'. The correspondence rules/diagnostic criteria set out in DSM-III, DSM-IIIR and DSM-IV will therefore be examined, in Chapter 5, to assess the extent to which this is the case. This chapter will therefore be examining both the necessary and sufficient conditions for inferring 'schizophrenia'.

But before these criteria for assessing validity are applied to 'schizophrenia', it is important to set the introduction and use of the concept in their historical and social context. It is particularly important that this should have been done if the concept is found wanting, so as better to understand not only the problems it presents but why these should have happened in the first place. The next chapter will therefore consider the historical background to the introduction of the concepts of dementia praecox and schizophrenia.

# Chapter 2

# The background

## Events leading up to the introduction of 'schizophrenia'

The question which this chapter focuses on can be put like this: what made it seem reasonable to introduce the concept of dementia praecox/schizophrenia as a specific mental disease around the end of the nineteenth century? Or, to put it another way, how was it possible for the concept of schizophrenia to emerge, and to be accepted, at that time? Within a traditional account of schizophrenia as a scientific concept, albeit an imperfect one, these questions are rather perplexing. Schizophrenia, surely, was introduced and accepted because it *was* a reasonable (if imperfect) way of thinking about bizarre behaviour. It emerged because Kraepelin 'discovered' it; it emerged as the result of a gradual process of more scientific, enlightened and humane treatment of the 'mentally ill' (cf. Jones, 1972). In this framework, the historical background to the introduction of 'schizophrenia', while interesting in itself, is not seen as central to the current study and alleviation of 'mental illness'. But if we see the concept or idea of schizophrenia as a problem *in the present*, then it is not simply that conventional answers to questions about its emergence are problematic; we need also to pose different questions which may make little sense within the traditional account.

This approach to history, from the vantage point of a problem in the present, owes much to Michel Foucault (1971, 1972). It is an approach which stresses the dynamic nature of history in which the present 'situation' (in this case the claimed scientific, medical concept of schizophrenia) emerges from a complex and shifting interplay amongst language, historical events, sources of authority, social institutions and regulatory practices. The result is the production of a particular version of 'the truth'; the task of historical analysis is to make that process of production intelligible. The aim of this chapter, then, is to make intelligible the emergence of the version of 'truth' represented by the concept of schizophrenia.

In Western Europe and the United States, the period between the middle of the eighteenth century and the beginning of the twentieth saw a number of important changes in theories of and methods of dealing with the problem of deviant behaviour. Scull (1979) describes one of these changes as a shift in responsibility for social deviance from the family and local community to a formal and centralised authority. This transition, however, involved much more than the compulsory construction of state asylums. It was accompanied by the transformation of the term 'insanity' from a 'vague, culturally defined phenomenon afflicting an unknown but probably small, proportion of the population into a condition which could only be authoritatively diagnosed, certified and dealt with by a group of legalised experts' (Scull, 1975: 218). The segregation of those labelled insane from society in general and other deviants in particular was therefore contemporaneous with the growth of medical influence over this population and with the emergence of the new speciality of psychiatry.

A third major change, which post-dated the others by several decades, was the importance attached to the activities of classification and differential diagnosis of what were claimed to be distinct varieties of insanity. There had certainly been attempts to bring order to the heterogeneity of strange behaviour (i.e. behaviour which observers could not understand) throughout the seventeenth, eighteenth and early nineteenth centuries, but these were armchair, academic exercises conducted by writers, philosophers and physicians with no consensus – and little discussion – of the principles on which such an endeavour might be based. The classification systems had little effect on practice, even that of their creators. This state of affairs contrasts with the central role assigned to classification systems by Brill (1974) who states that he 'know[s] of no psychiatry that can get along without one' (1121). The continued importance of classification is also evident from the regular publication and increasing popularity (Kirk and Kutchins, 1992) of official classification systems via the *Diagnostic and Statistical Manual of Mental Disorders*.

The most comprehensive account of the first two of these processes in relation to the English asylum system – the centralisation of responsibility for mad people and the transformation of the concept of insanity – has been provided by Andrew Scull (1975, 1979). Like Foucault (1971), Scull has been concerned to demonstrate that the development of a state asylum system and the growth of medical influence over deviant behaviour cannot be seen as twin processes in a progression towards more humane and scientific treatment of the 'mentally ill'. A major part of the account which will be presented here draws on Scull's work. The account will necessarily be briefer than the topic merits, but as I said earlier it is intended to help make intelligible the introduction and development of 'schizophrenia' rather than provide an exhaustive account of the development of the asylum system. Although many of the details which will be given apply to England, there was a remarkable similarity in the nature of the changes in the remainder of Western Europe and in the United States. (See, e.g., Zilboorg, 1941; Bockoven, 1956a, 1956b; Foucault, 1971.) This was in part attributable to exchange of ideas and to similarities in economic structure. Where differences *are* apparent, they are in the timing rather than the nature of events and can in part be traced to the degree of reluctance to accept control from central government (Castel *et al.*, 1982).

## The development of institutions

The building of state institutions for one category of deviant was a relatively late development from a trend towards an institutional response to deviance in general. Attempts to authorise institutions for those who could not or would not support themselves began in England and the remainder of Western Europe around the time of the Reformation when the Catholic Church's tradition of almsgiving was destroyed. In England, these attempts collapsed with the outbreak of the Civil War but were more successful in the rest of Europe with its tradition of absolute monarchy and where the threat deviants presented to the social order was perhaps felt more acutely. The English response – and later that of the United States – to deviant behaviour amongst the poor was therefore local and idiosyncratic, and included almshouses, houses of correction, charity hospitals and workhouses, each of which accepted a heterogeneous group of people. It was during this period that private madhouses first appeared. These developed out of the practice of some parishes of boarding out non-violent people who showed bizarre behaviour and the habit of relatives of giving over such people into the care of others, usually clergymen or physicians. The social and economic changes brought about by the first stages of the Agrarian and Industrial Revolutions transformed the problem of dealing with those who, for whatever reason, did not support themselves. From the middle of the eighteenth century the numbers in receipt of Poor Relief escalated and it was easy to assume that the locally based and somewhat idiosyncratic systems of Poor Relief were laxly administered and encouraged, rather than relieved, poverty and idleness.

The idea that relief should go only to those who deserved it was not new; the distinction, however, had never been very carefully applied in practice, possibly because the numbers involved were relatively small and, in any case, work could easily be forced from those who did not conform. At the beginning of the nineteenth century the distinction was re-emphasised, partly because of the large increase in numbers in receipt of Poor Relief and the fact that the force used by absolute monarchs could no longer be applied. Scull has also suggested that the distinction was crucial to the operation of the modern wage system, whose beginnings can be traced to this period. Institutions, in the form of workhouses, came to be seen as the ideal solution. Their unattractiveness would deter the able bodied, while a disciplined regime within them would prepare those not so deterred for a life of industrial labour. If this was clearly out of the question, then the discipline would do no harm. The gathering together of indigents in one place would also make more efficient the administration of the Poor Law.

The construction of institutions at this time and the growing practice of seg-regating deviants lacked some important features which were later to typify Western society's response to those who failed to conform to its norms. First, the segregation was on a relatively small scale in contrast with that achieved in the last quarter of the nineteenth century. Second, little attempt was made to dis-tinguish different types of deviant, except in terms of deserving or non-deserving. Third, medical interest in institutional populations was insignif-icant. Scull has suggested that the great stress which was laid on correctly distinguishing the able bodied from the non-able bodied unemployed pre-pared the ground for the later separation of what was called insanity 'from the previous inchoate mass of deviant behaviours so that it was seen as a distinct problem requiring specialised treatment in an institution of its own' (1979: 36).

One result of failing to separate out different classes of deviant within the workhouse quickly became apparent. By definition, the label 'mad' is applied to those whose behaviour is incomprehensible, who violate social norms in ways which inspire at least bewilderment, if not fear. Some of these people would continue to break rules within the institution. But the government of the day could hardly be expected to be interested in the management problems of workhouse keepers to the extent of passing a law forcing the construction in every county of institutions for the particularly troublesome. The end of the eighteenth century and the beginning of the nineteenth therefore saw a marked increase in the number of private madhouses, some of which were a result of parishes contracting with individuals to provide care for some of those in receipt of Poor Relief. There was virtually no restriction on entry into the madhouse trade and these establishments were run for profit, or in the hope of profit, by interested laymen (and women), clergymen and physicians. This free trade in lunacy was to pave the way for the controversy over who should be given the status of expert in this area. The trade was, however, on a comparatively small scale. In 1816, for example, there were thirty-six mad-houses in London, one-quarter of which were licensed for fewer than ten people. There was, of course, great disparity in conditions within these madhouses; as would be expected, conditions were worst in those which took in pauper lunatics. The inevitable abuses which occurred were to prove fertile ground for those active in the Reform Movement. To claim, however, that the reformers improved the lot of those labelled insane by showing that 'cruelty and neglect play no part except a shameful one, in the care of the mentally ill' (Lewis, 1966: 581) is, at best, an oversimplification of events.

### Lunacy and the Reform Movement

The early Reformers' cause was made easier by the fact that the issue of the management and disposal of 'lunatics' had been brought to public attention by the now disputed madness of George III and by Hadfield's attempt on the king's life. In 1800, Hadfield was found not guilty by reason of insanity, thus

raising the thorny problem of what was to be done with him, as no legal provision existed for detaining him. A retroactive piece of legislation was speedily
put on the statute authorising detention of such people, for the duration of the
king's pleasure, in the county gaol or other suitable receptacle. This legislation
brought with it the paradox that a man technically innocent was to be locked
up; it also raised the question of what constituted another suitable receptacle.
There were no obviously acceptable answers to these questions, but they did
ensure that government and the general public were disposed to view lunacy
as a problem in its own right. At the same time, a number of English magistrates began to agitate for changes in the quality of care provided in
madhouses. They did not base their suggestions on an ideology of madness,
but they were charged with the inspection of madhouses and were unhappy
about conditions there.

Scull has suggested that the Reform Movement was influenced by two competing philosophical systems – Benthamism and Evangelicalism. The latter
emphasised humanitarianism and discipline; it also contained, although rarely
made explicit, a large element of paternalism and moral control. Benthamism
emphasised the virtues of expertise and efficiency and the need for a science of
government. These ideas were to dictate the Reformers' goals – a reduction in
the cruelty and neglect which typified madhouses and a country-wide system
of centrally controlled asylums, regularly and thoroughly inspected by government agents or county officials. These goals – humanitarianism and
efficient, central control – were not, of course, confined to the problem of madhouses but were part of a much wider social and political movement.

In 1807, in England, a Commons Select Committee published the first
national report on private madhouses. Although the Committee was mainly
concerned with recording the number of inmates it did consider the plight of
criminal and pauper inmates, and in 1808 an Act was passed recommending
the building of asylums for pauper lunatics, with public money. The vast
majority of local magistrates simply ignored the recommendations and those
few asylums which were built did not provide appreciably better living conditions than had their predecessors. Scull has suggested that before any real
change could take place, either in support for a system of public asylums or in
conditions within them, there had to exist a cultural view of madness which
was radically different from that generally held in the early nineteenth century,
a point which highlights the crucial interdependence of language and social
practice. Bynum (1964), for example, has argued that the way in which those
labelled mad were treated at this time cannot simply be interpreted as a result
of cruelty and indifference. Rather, it must be seen as in part deriving from the
popular view which linked loss of reason to loss of humanity. The Aristotelian
and Elizabethan views of madness which linked it to genius and sensibility had
been largely lost sight of by the end of the eighteenth century, to be replaced
by the idea of the madman as a brute (Skultans, 1979). It was a short step to
the idea that madmen must be tamed, if necessary by force.

The unhappy position of Lunacy Reformers at the beginning of the nine-teenth century has been summarised by Scull:

> the desire to protect society, to simplify life for those charged with admin-istering local poorhouses and gaols and an unfocused, unsystematic feeling that the insane deserved more 'humane' treatment, did not amount to a coherent alternative vision of what could or should be done.
>
> (Scull, 1979: 64)

The Reformers were therefore unable to provide strong justification for the vast expenditure and interference in local affairs which the realisation of their aims would involve.

The new view of madness which was to provide this alternative vision was embodied in the work of the moral managers – moral in this case being closer in meaning to 'psychological' than to its modern connotations of virtue or ethics. The first attempt at systematic practice of these ideas can be traced to William Tuke, a layman, who in 1792 opened the York Retreat as an alterna-tive to the York Asylum which had a reputation for gross mistreatment of inmates. The rationale of the Retreat represented a move away from the idea of the mad as animals to be tamed to the view that they were merely lacking in powers of self-restraint; the task of the asylum was to re-establish these, using ideas of behaviour–consequence relationships remarkably similar to those underlying the token economy system developed 150 years later by Ayllon and Azrin. This view of the mad as essentially human but as exhibit-ing a defect in self-control did not, of course, develop in a cultural vacuum. Grange (1962) sees its counterpart in the romantic movement in literature, which saw the cultivation and analysis of emotion as a necessary part of exis-tence, rather than as something to be feared and avoided. In turn, as Skultans (1979) has pointed out, the moral managers emphasised the balance of passions rather than opposition to them. Asylum inmates were therefore to be taught the regulation of emotion.

Scull has suggested complementary reasons to account not only for changing cultural views of insanity in the nineteenth century but also for the fact that they were to become so influential in social policy. As he points out, supernat-ural accounts of events are favoured when people's control over important features of their environment is limited, as was the case in pre-industrial soci-ety. The Agrarian and Industrial Revolutions vastly increased the potential for control and brought with them – or, we might say, made necessary – new con-structions of human nature which emphasised change through training and internalisation of social norms, rather than control by external agents. Thus, the changing concept of insanity is seen as developing in parallel with changing ideas about people and their relationship with the environment. These ideas, however, not only reflected real events, they also served to justify the demands made on the new industrial working force to adapt to an alien environment.

Equally, the idea that man could strive to improve himself – whether in the asylum or out of it – was a basic tenet of the upwardly mobile middle classes and was in direct opposition to the medieval idea of a predestined social order.

The concept of rehabilitation was inherent in the new view of insanity. Moreover, the cure was to be effected not by esoteric medical means but by kindness and instruction through manipulation of the environment. While not denying the humanitarian motives of the reformers, Scull has pointed out that one of the major attractions of moral management was that it promised to transform into free, rational, self-determining and economically useful individuals, that part of the population which deviated most markedly from these ideals. US accounts (see, e.g., Bockoven, 1956b) also emphasise the important roles played by manual labour and religious worship in the attainment of discipline; indeed Castel (1994) has called moral management the 'therapeutic equivalent of work and prayer' (247).

But whatever their ideological base, Tuke's innovations at the Retreat quickly attracted attention. A French physician, de la Rive, imported the ideas to Continental Europe where they were to become, if anything, even more popular than in England. Phillipe Pinel, director of the Bicêtre hospital in Paris, was exploring a similar set of ideas, while in the United States moral management was popularised by the physicians Benjamin Rush and Eli Todd and was later used by Dorothea Dix as a justification for her energetic campaign for the building of state asylums.

The years between the setting up of the first Parliamentary Select Committee on Lunacy in 1805 and the second in 1815 therefore saw radical and well-publicised changes in ideas, not only on the nature of insanity but also in methods of dealing with those labelled insane. The Reformers had been active during this period, gathering facts on conditions in asylums and madhouses. A particularly horrific, even by nineteenth-century standards, catalogue of abuses uncovered in the York and Bethlem Asylums resulted in private inquiries and in pressure to review the situation on a national scale. The result was the setting up of the 1815 Parliamentary Committee. The Reformers came to this Committee with a very different and much stronger set of arguments with which to convince the government of the need for a network of humanely run county asylums than they had had at their disposal in 1805. It was not their intention that these asylums should be run by doctors; on the contrary, Wakefield, one of the Committee's witnesses, declared that he considered doctors to be 'the most unfit of any class of persons' to control asylums. (Bynum, 1964: 326). The Reformers were able to argue that practices within existing asylums not only constituted a morale outrage but were also theoretically unsound. They further argued that because there now existed a remedy for insanity, then the segregation of the insane from other indigents, with less potential, was essential. The Committee was presented with a vast amount of evidence of cruelty and neglect within asylums *and* with details of the alternatives which were available at the York Retreat. These could be

made available to all asylum inmates, it was argued, only through the construction of well-planned public asylums in every county and by the operation
of a stringent system of inspection.

The evidence presented to the Committee, and its subsequent report, represented a humiliating critique of the medical profession's handling of the
lunacy problem. As a result of the Committee report, a bill was introduced in
1816 directing the compulsory construction of county asylums with an extensive system of inspection. The bill was passed by the Commons but rejected by
the Lords. The rejection of this, and of two following bills in 1818 and 1819,
resulted partly (in the case of the 1816 bill) from a clause authorising the stringent inspection of the conditions under which 'single lunatics' in private homes
were kept, as well as (in the case of all three bills) from fierce opposition on the
part of proprietors of private madhouses and the medical profession. But one of
the most important reasons for the defeat of the bills, Scull suggests, was the
localist basis of English politics. A similar bill was to succeed only after parliamentary reform had seriously weakened the power of the rural aristocracy and
the issue of central versus local Poor Law administration had been resolved.

In 1827, yet another Parliamentary inquiry was set up into the condition of
pauper lunatics, resulting in a bill, in 1828, so wary of offending the Lords that
its provisions made little difference to the existing state of affairs. But, as Scull
has pointed out, the Metropolitan Commission, which by design included the
leading Parliamentary Reformers, was to become a most effective pressure
group for the Reformers' aims. In 1842, the chairman of the Commission
introduced a bill to extend the powers of the Commission for three years so
that it could produce a detailed report on all madhouses in the country. The
report, which appeared in 1844, was the most comprehensive ever produced.
It not only reiterated the merits of moral management but also provided an
elaborate justification for its implementation via the provision of purpose-built
public asylums. Asylums were necessary in the first place, the report suggested, because lunatics must be treated by experts in buildings designed to
optimise the effects of such treatment. But treatment must also be given by
strangers, in an environment other than that which had induced the problem
in the first place. More asylums were necessary because early admission was
essential if a cure was to be effected, and existing asylums were already over-
filled. This inconvenient fact, which suggested that a cure was not readily
available, was easily dealt with by the assertion that the inmates had not been
admitted early enough. The report served its purpose: in 1845 the Lunatics
Act made compulsory the building of county asylums for pauper lunatics, and
their regular inspection. A similar Act had been passed in France in 1838, with
relatively little opposition. Castel et al. (1982) attribute this to the greater
acceptance of centralised authority in Europe; in contrast, by 1890, only one
North American State – New York – had passed such an Act.

As Scull (1979) and Skultans (1979) have pointed out, the provision of
public asylums in the nineteenth century cannot be separated from the general

issue of the management of the poor and in particular from the issues of local versus central Poor Law administration and indoor versus outdoor Poor Relief. Similarly, the kind of regime to which the asylums aspired, and their goals for the inmates, cannot be separated from the view of human nature engendered partly by the Agrarian and Industrial Revolutions. To depict the provision of asylums and its underlying ideology as an enlightened, humanitarian move is to minimise both this and the fact that the purely humanitarian motives of the Reformers could have been satisfied simply by pressing for an end to cruelty and neglect. They might also have argued that because so many abuses took place in institutions, then the obvious answer was fewer of them. That they argued the opposite reflects the fact that their ideas were inextricably connected with prevailing economic and political concerns. The idea that those who are called mad should be treated with kindness may well be more in accord with modern ideals than is the idea that they should be chained and whipped. But this does not make the first idea, and the elaborate theoretical justification which surrounded it, any more rational or scientific than the second. Both were derived from prevailing lay theories of human nature which in turn shaped and were shaped by social, political and economic concerns.

The development of moral management might have encouraged the emergence of a group of people with some training in the management of the specific problem of lunacy, but it was a long way from the recognition of a specific group of people as having the right to speak authoritatively on the subject. Foucault (1971, 1979) has emphasised the importance of claims to and recognition of the 'right to speak' on a particular topic in shaping both what is said – and accepted – about the topic and the social practices which surround it. The next section will therefore examine the process by which the medical profession came to claim this right to speak authoritatively on insanity and to have the claim at least partly accepted.

## The growth of medical influence

Medical interest in bizarre behaviour (i.e. that which cannot readily be understood by reference to social norms) has a long history. The Ancient Greeks, for example, incorporated such behaviour into their humoral pathology, which was to be directly influential in Western thought until at least the seventeenth century and is still indirectly influential in theories of chemical and hormonal imbalances. The physician's interest, however, was shared by philosophers, theologians and writers, each of whom felt competent to construct theories of the nature and causes of whatever was viewed as madness. Inevitably, writings on the subject reflect this diversity of views. Physicians and philosophers did not write from opposing stances; rather, both managed to combine, often incoherently, philosophical, psychological and medical ideas. The mingling of the physical and the psychological reflects, of course, a preoccupation with the relationship between mind and body; this, and the fact that medical, philosophical and literary writings on insanity were often indistinguishable, was later to prove important in facilitating public acceptance of insanity as a medical problem. On a practical level, medical interest in insanity was also shared by other groups. But the co-occurrence of disturbing behaviour and bodily disease (if only by chance), and the traditional designation of physicians as helpers, gave them something of an advantage, regardless of expertise. Scull has pointed out that until about the middle of the eighteenth century physicians made little attempt to further their interest or to secure public recognition as experts in insanity, The first piece of English legislation to make separate mention of lunacy was the 1744 Vagrancy Act, which defined one category of vagrant as any persons 'who by lunacy or otherwise are so far disordered in their Senses that they may be dangerous to be permitted to go Abroad' (Bynum, 1964: 321). The Act authorised any person to detain such a vagrant, and two Justices of the Peace would then decide whether confinement in some secure place was necessary. The wording of the Act emphasises the fact that lunacy, however defined, was not regarded as a medical problem nor defined in law as an attribute of the person; it was defined in terms of behaviour which might prove harmful to others.

The years between 1744 and the next Act which dealt with lunacy – in 1774 – saw a marked increase in medical interest in the subject. A small number of institutions, called hospitals, were founded for the care of lunatics. Scull attributes medicine's growing interest in lunacy to the much larger number of private madhouses which appeared during this period and which provided a new source of potential status and profit for medical men, in competition with interested laypeople. The 1774 Act was, in fact, aimed at controlling these establishments. It confirmed that anyone who could obtain a licence could open a madhouse, but put inspection in the hands of the Royal College of Physicians and ruled that a medical certificate had to be obtained before anyone could be confined. Bynum (1964) has suggested that these provisions amounted to a public recognition of medical jurisdiction in insanity. Whether this is the case is, however, debatable. As Scull points out, the final decision about confinement rested in legal hands; the power of the Royal College of Physicians to inspect madhouses did not extend beyond the metropolitan area; elsewhere, it remained the duty of magistrates. And although the Act required a medical certificate prior to confinement, it said nothing about the qualifications of those into whose care the lunatic was assigned. It hardly makes sense to recognise lunacy as a medical problem but to continue to allow anyone who could obtain a licence to be responsible for the care of lunatics. Nevertheless, in the latter part of the eighteenth century and the beginning of the nineteenth, the medical profession had begun to take a far greater *practical* interest in the management of those labelled insane. In addition, the medical teacher William Cullen had begun to include the topic of insanity in his curriculum, thus allowing his pupils to lay claim to some specialist knowledge, an essential prerequisite for public recognition as an expert.

## Medicine and moral management

These first attempts to secure acceptance of the claim that lunacy was a medical problem were seriously threatened by the advent of moral management which, in both theory and practice, owed nothing to medicine. On the contrary, it explicitly denied the usefulness of medicine in managing the insane. In England, the threat was increased by the findings of the 1815 Select Committee, and by the bills which followed, which explicitly sought to remove medical powers of inspection granted under the 1774 Act. Not surprisingly, physicians were amongst the most vociferous opponents. As Bynum has noted, the implications of moral management 'for both medical theory and medical practice were not lost on the physicians of the early nineteenth century who attempted to assess its true significance . . . their income, prestige and medical theories were all threatened' (1964: 324–325).

The threat which moral management presented must be seen in the context of the structure of the medical profession in the early nineteenth century. There was then no such body as the medical profession as the term is understood today; instead, medical treatment was offered by three distinct groups: physicians, the elite, drawn mainly from the upper and upper-middle classes; surgeons, regarded as craftsmen and who in England had severed their links with barbers as recently as 1745; and apothecaries, the lowest status group. In practice, it is unlikely that the quality of care offered by these groups matched their professional standing. Except in Scotland, where medical education was controlled by the universities, the training received by physicians was in many ways inferior to that of surgeons and apothecaries. The clientele treated by the three groups did, however, broadly match their social standing.

The Royal College of Physicians, formed in 1518, had been for some time engaged in a battle to keep surgeons and apothecaries, who were seeking to improve their status, in an inferior position. Medical proprietors of madhouses were drawn from all three groups, but the most vociferous and articulate defenders of medicine's interest in this area were the physicians. Already much preoccupied with status, the physicians therefore found themselves in an invidious position in the first decades of the nineteenth century. If they supported the Reformers' attempts to introduce legislation compelling the building of public asylums, they ran the risk that the new institutions would be put in the hands of laypeople and that physicians would find themselves adopting a subordinate role. On the other hand, if they opposed the proposals, then the madhouse trade would presumably flourish and be open to all comers. Neither option augured well for physicians. Faced with this dilemma, the profession had a number of choices. First, they could present convincing evidence that those behaviours labelled insanity were caused by disease and could be cured by medical means. This they were unable to do. Second, they could agree to share the field with others and accept that moral management did not require any medical expertise. There is no evidence that this option was ever seriously considered. Third, they could attempt to persuade government and the public of their expertise by means of non-empirical argument, thus avoiding the awkward issue of their failure to provide empirical evidence in support of their claims.

In choosing the third option, physicians and their colleagues were committed to supporting the expansion of the public asylum system. As Scull has pointed out, however, government support for increasing the number of asylums had been won on the basis that moral management, not medical intervention, could restore sanity. The medical profession must therefore incorporate it into their scheme of things, either by arguing convincingly that they were best suited to administer asylums and organise such care and/or that intervention by non-medical means did not invalidate the proposition that insanity was a disease and therefore a medical matter. It is not immediately obvious which set of arguments would lead, however illogically, to such conclusions. Possibly as a result, initial attempts by physicians to defend their interests consisted mainly of rhetorical repetitions of the superiority of a medical approach. Such claims continued to be made throughout the century but were gradually joined by a more subtle set of arguments. These were of two sorts: the first suggested that a *combination* of medical and moral management would be more efficacious than either alone. William Neale, for example, declared in 1836 that:

> To those acquainted with the workings of the malady and its peculiar characteristics, it will be easy to perceive the errors and partial views of such as profess to apply a medicinal agent only, as a specific, or those who advocate a course of moral treatment only as a cure. There is no doubt that a co-operation of medical and moral means is requisite to effect a thorough cure.
> (Scull, 1979: 161–162)

But as Scull has pointed out, this concession to moral management was a harmless one. It could, after all, be administered by anyone, whereas medical treatment, it was claimed, required special training. Clearly, the medical profession could administer both but lay moral managers could not administer medical treatments. Thus, the medical position was not threatened.

The second set of arguments was derived from the long-standing debate on the nature of 'mind' and 'mental events'. Most Western physicians of the nineteenth century adhered to the dualist position put forward by Descartes and Hartley in which the concepts of mind and soul were virtually identical. The idea of physical disease presented no problems; when disease was said to be mental, however, or curable by non-physical means, then taxing philosophical and theological problems were raised. The moral managers appeared to be putting forward just such a view. Pinel, for example, had stated explicitly that insanity was not an organic disease and that what was psychological (mental) was best dealt with by psychological means. Samuel Tuke adopted a more pragmatic position. If insanity was a disease of the mind, then therapy should be aimed at the mind. If, on the other hand, it was a disease of the brain, as yet undetected, moral management was indicated by the reciprocal action of mind on brain.

These arguments, however, failed to tackle the (apparently) central issue of what exactly happened to the mind in a case of insanity. Traditional theological and philosophical theory held that the mind (or soul) was an immaterial essence, incapable of destruction by mortal means and thus, unlike the brain, protected from disease and decay. To argue otherwise was to challenge Christian belief in an immortal soul. The mind was seen as operating through a material object, the brain. Taken separately or together these premises seemed to lead to the conclusion that insanity *must* be seen as a disease of the brain, albeit one amenable in part to non-physical intervention. A corollary to these arguments was that the only alternative to viewing insanity as a brain disease was to see it as a spiritual matter, to be dealt with by the clergy. Forbes Wimslow, for example, stated that the contrary view to that which saw insanity as a medical problem was that it was:

> a spiritual malady . . . an affectation of the immaterial essence . . . a disorder of the soul and not simply the result of the derangement of the material instrument of the mind interfering with the healthy action of its manifestations.
>
> (Scull, 1979: 167)

These arguments had particular force in an increasingly secular society where even the clergy were loath to view deviant behaviour as a spiritual malady; the reformers, too, had been anxious to distance themselves from the idea of insanity as divine retribution and of the insane as deserving of punishment. The arguments put forward by medical men appeared happily to solve the dilemma of admitting to the efficacy of moral management while protecting the status of the soul and, of course, justified a humane approach to the lunatic. The appeal of such arguments must be seen not only in the context of a strongly Christian society but also of one which lacked, first, the idea that it is possible systematically to study and modify *behaviour* (which is, after all what was being discussed) without reference to the concepts of mind or brain and, second, the notion of certain behaviours as deviations from a particular set of cultural norms, rather than as phenomena which logically required the positing of some underlying disorder. But in spite of the appeal of these arguments, there remained the awkward fact that if insanity was a brain disease it was one which frequently could not be detected. Two explanations were put forward to account for this. First, the instruments and methods available to physicians were said not to be sophisticated enough to detect what were probably subtle changes in the brain. Second, structural changes were said probably to occur only in the later stages of insanity; in effect, lunatics died too soon for these to be observed. Bynum (1964) has noted that the very absence of brain pathology was taken by a few physicians as evidence that even in insanity the mind is not subject to decay.

By the middle of the nineteenth century the medical profession had assumed control of a large majority of public asylums in England, in Continental Europe and in the United States. Vacant posts which had been filled by lay superintendents were now almost invariably given to physicians. Although the arguments discussed above almost certainly contributed to this process, a number of other factors may have facilitated medical dominance. Scull has noted that many aspects of moral management worked against its being developed as a coherent *professional* ideology. The moral managers in general, and the Tukes in particular, had adopted an essentially pragmatic approach to intervention and had eschewed both premature theory building and the idea that moral treatment could only be carried out by a group of specially trained experts. This rendered the moral managers vulnerable to those less cautious in their theorising and in their claims. In addition, the language of moral managers was similar to that of medicine: they too spoke of afflictions, diseases, and treatments. Like medicine, they saw bizarre behaviour in dispositional terms. The conceptual gulf which separated moral and medical management was therefore not as wide as it might at first glance have appeared.

Physicians were therefore able to construct socially acceptable theories of insanity which incorporated moral management without compromising their professional status. Indeed, it could be argued that they enhanced it by appearing to be broad minded and open to new ideas. Physicians also possessed the important advantage of having already formed a profession of sorts; they were thus able to argue that the best way of ensuring that asylum superintendents were conscientious, reliable and properly motivated was to choose them from an already existing profession, rather than encouraging a free-for-all which might allow disreputable elements to enter the business. In England, the originator of moral management was a layman; in the remainder of Europe and in the United States its strongest advocates were physicians. This may have encouraged, or at least made less contentious, the idea that doctors should have charge of asylums. Each asylum must, in any case, employ a physician to deal with bodily ailments. Those responsible for the appointment of asylum superintendents increasingly came to see it as more efficient and economical to employ one person to do both jobs.

## The decline of moral management and the rise of somatic theories

The large-scale construction of asylums was overtly justified by the assertion that lunacy could be cured by moral management. By the end of the nineteenth century, however, this approach had become little more than a hazy recollection in the minds of asylum superintendents and had been replaced by a wholly somatic view of lunacy, both in theory and in practice.

A number of reasons have been put forward for the demise of moral management. Bockoven (1956a) suggests that one of the most important was the failure of the innovators to train enough people to staff the growing number of asylums. To this was added an enormous increase in the numbers committed to asylums, a factor widely cited in accounts of the decline of moral management (e.g. Bockoven, 1956a, 1956b; Leigh, 1961; Jones, 1972). It has been suggested that the ever-increasing number of asylum inmates made impossible the practice of moral management, with its emphasis on a detailed knowledge of the individual and its de-emphasis of regimented, custodial approaches. Bockoven (1956a) notes that the situation in the United States was further complicated by the fact that immigrants made the greatest contribution to the increase.

These two factors – lack of trained personnel and the vast increase in the number of inmates – might at first glance seem adequate as explanations of the decline of moral management, particularly as the pioneers of the approach had placed so much emphasis on asylums run as 'family' units. But closer examination shows the explanations to be unsatisfactory, or, at least, incomplete. First, one of the hallmarks of moral management was that it was essentially a pragmatic approach which, according to its proponents, did not require extensive training. It was this fact which, it was suggested earlier, partly contributed to the failure of lay moral managers to provide effective opposition to physicians in the competition for influence in asylums. In any case, the innovators had written extensively on the subject, giving details of what was thought to be the essence of the approach, so that any interested physician could easily acquaint himself with the few principles. Second, the citing of increased numbers of inmates as a cause of the decline of moral management can be shown to carry with it the assumption that the increase was relatively simple to explain and was one which the medical profession was powerless to prevent. Third, neither explanation can account for the vigour with which somatic theories were espoused in theory and practice.

It will be argued, instead, that the decline of moral and the growing influence of somatic theories cannot be understood separately from the increased numbers of asylum inmates, the problematic concept of insanity and the ambiguous professional position of mad-doctors in the second half of the nineteenth century.

## The rising population of asylum inmates

Throughout the nineteenth century, but particularly in the latter part, the number of people confined to asylums increased dramatically. In England and Wales, for example, the average number of inmates per asylum was 116 in 1827; by 1890 it was 802 (Scull, 1979). In addition, the estimated prevalence of insanity (a category made up of 'lunacy' and 'idiocy') in England and Wales increased from one in 802 in 1844 to one in 432 in 1868 and to one in 266 in

1914 (Hare, 1983). The increases were paralleled by a growing reluctance on the part of the state and local authorities to spend money on asylums, particularly as there seemed to be no limit to the numbers who needed to be contained within them. What had begun as purpose-built buildings for relatively small numbers gradually grew, in a haphazard fashion, into vast custodial receptacles where, not surprisingly, the emphasis on cure was replaced with concern with keeping the inmates under control. It is certainly true that moral management as practised by Tuke, Pinel and Rush would have been impossible under such circumstances; what is less clear is why the number of inmates should have increased at such a rate.

Both Scull and Hare have provided detailed evaluations of the nineteenth-century records of the numbers of the insane and of the sometimes fierce debate which surrounded their interpretation. The major question of concern was that of whether the increase in numbers was an administrative artefact or whether insanity really was, to use Hare's phrase, 'on the increase'. Both Hare and Scull are agreed that the rising population of the insane cannot be accounted for by more accurate registration in the second half of the nineteenth century, i.e. by the idea that a pool of hitherto unrecognised cases would now be included in official statistics. But thereafter they reach opposing conclusions: Hare argues that the evidence supports the view that there was a real increase in what would now be called the functional psychoses, and in particular in schizophrenia, in the second half of the nineteenth century; Scull concludes that the increase was more apparent than real. There is some reason for supposing that Hare may, in a roundabout way, be partly correct in his suggestion of a real increase in 'schizophrenia' at this time; the rather complicated issues surrounding this argument will be taken up at the end of the next chapter. Nevertheless, Scull's arguments remain relevant to the discussion of the demise of moral management. The first of these concerns nineteenth-century definitions of insanity; the second, the professional status of mad-doctors.

In the nineteenth century there were almost as many definitions of insanity as there were medical men who cared to write on the subject. But the definitions were as vague as they were numerous, so that it was extremely difficult to see how such a phenomenon might be recognised in practice. The public were reassured that this was possible, however, via the now familiar appeals to 'clinical judgement'. Mayo, for example, claimed in 1817 that:

> It must be borne in mind, that a great unanimity may exist among experienced observers as to the presence of certain mental states, characterised by certain generally accepted names, which states, at the same time, it would be very difficult to describe in any form of words, insomuch that the indefined name, in the use of which all experienced men are agreed respecting these states, will convey to all a more clear and distinct impression than any attempt at definition or even description.
>
> (Scull, 1979: 237–238)

Vague definitions of insanity, based on subjective judgements could, of course, be narrowly applied; their vagueness did not necessitate a rise in the number of asylum inmates. There are, however, good reasons for expecting a broad rather than a narrow application of the term in the nineteenth century. First, the perceived size and importance of a problem is likely to be directly related to the status of those who claim to be able to deal with it. The professional position of mad-doctors in the late nineteenth century will be discussed in more detail in the next section; it is worth noting, however, that it was not in medicine's professional interests to minimise the apparent size of the lunacy problem. The second factor which may have facilitated the use of a broad definition of insanity was the very existence of asylums designed to cure it. In assessing the importance of this factor, it should be borne in mind that the initial judgement of insanity was – and still is – made not by a doctor but by the lay public, on the basis of unwanted behaviour. Clearly, what is unwanted varies with time, place and the person making the judgement. It would be remarkable if such judgements were not influenced by the availability of a system for dealing with those labelled insane, on the apparently humanitarian grounds that they could be restored to health. Scull has therefore argued that the elastic concept of insanity was able to include a wider range of deviant behaviour than had hitherto been the case and that this could in part account for the rising population of the insane.

Hare has offered two arguments against this conclusion. First, the prognosis of asylum inmates apparently worsened during the last decades of the nineteenth century; contemporary observers attributed this to the admission of greater numbers of less favourable cases. Second, the 1909–13 statistics for England and Wales indicated that 'the group of conditions which we would now include in the term "functional psychoses" – mania, melancholia, delusional insanity and secondary dementia – formed at least 75 per cent of the total' (1983: 449). Hare, however, does not consider the possibility that the decline in prognosis could have been due not to less favourable cases but to less favourable conditions, including overcrowding and an increasing reliance on physical methods, than had prevailed in the heyday of moral management. The major problem with his second argument is that we have no way of knowing whether, or in what ways, the referents of terms like 'melancholia' or 'delusional insanity' changed over the years, so that the idea that they applied consistently to a particular type of person is very problematic. Both Scull and Hare are well aware that historical epidemiology of this sort is a very hazardous business. Nevertheless, the complete absence of any data on the reliability and validity of mad-doctors' diagnoses does mean that a widening of the vague concept of insanity remains a serious possible explanation for the apparent increase in the prevalence of insanity in the nineteenth century.

## The professional status of mad-doctors and the development of somatic theories

It may have been the case that, by the middle of the nineteenth century, the superintendents of almost all public asylums in England were medical men; this administrative superiority, however, did not amount to an ideal of professional autonomy and recognition as experts. The final decision as to whether an individual should be confined remained in legal hands, although a medical certificate was needed. There remained also the theoretical and practical difficulties faced by medicine in relation to deviant behaviour. It was recognised by the public and medical men alike that, rhetoric notwithstanding, the behaviour of asylum inmates could not in many cases be shown to be accompanied by brain or any other lesions nor to be responsive to the plethora of medical interventions available. Asylum doctors were uneasily aware of the fact that the existence of asylums had been justified by the claim that the inmates could be cured by purely non-medical means which they, trained in medicine, were supposed to administer. Worse, they did not appear to be making a very good job of it, as witness the rising number of admissions and the falling number in the category of discharged cured.

In the second half of the nineteenth century the medical profession therefore sought in a number of ways to enhance its status *vis-à-vis* deviant behaviour. As Zilboorg (1941) has pointed out, one of the more obvious ways of doing so is by forming professional organisations and by publishing specialist literature not easily available to nor comprehensible to lay people. In 1844, the newly formed Association for Medical Superintendents of American Institutions for the Insane began publication of *The American Journal of Insanity*. A similar organisation had been founded in Britain in 1841, called The Association of Medical Officers of Asylums and Hospitals for the Insane. Its journal, *The Asylum Journal*, appeared in 1853 but the title was soon altered to the more prestigious sounding *Journal of Mental Science*. The editorial of the second volume declared that 'Insanity is purely a disease of the brain. The physician is now the responsible guardian of the lunatic and must ever remain so.' In 1855 John Gray, one of the most vociferous proponents of a somatic theory of bizarre behaviour, became editor of *The American Journal of Insanity*. Not surprisingly, the number of papers on moral management declined, and the number on pathology increased, during his thirty years of editorship (Dunton, 1944).

There was, in addition, a considerable literature, aimed at both the specialist and the general reader, attempting to prove that the treatment of insanity, whatever it might entail, must remain in medical hands. John Millar, for example, argued in 1856 that:

> The shower bath is used as a corrective discipline. The matron uses the shower bath for swearing, bad language and filthy habits . . . the whole

question of its use I consider to be entirely within the province of the Superintendent as much as any other medical treatment he may think it necessary to employ.

(Scull, 1979: 202–203)

As Scull points out, this kind of argument neatly illustrates one paradox faced by the medical superintendents: if asylum inmates were suffering from brain disease they could not be held responsible for their behaviour and therefore punishment was pointless. Somehow or other, however, their behaviour had to be controlled and, of course, the time-honoured methods of reward and punishment were used. But this implied that the inmates *were* responsible for their behaviour. The only solution to this paradox was to incorporate everything that was done to the inmates into 'medical treatment'.

The mind(soul)–body question continued to preoccupy mad-doctors. The strength of feeling on this matter is illustrated by Pliny Earle's remark that:

Were the arguments for the hypothesis that in insanity the mind itself is diseased ten-fold more numerous than they are, and more weighty, I could not accept them. My ideas of the human mind are such that I cannot hold for a moment that it can be diseased, as we understand disease. This implies death as a final consequence, but Mind is eternal. In its very essence and structure (to use the term we apply to matter), in its elemental composition and its organisation, it was created for immortality, beyond the scope of the wear and tear and disorganisation and final destruction of the mortal part of our being.

(Bockoven, 1956a: 193)

Given this context, both professional and theoretical, it would be naive to expect mad-doctors to give their wholehearted support to moral management, regardless of the ease or difficulty with which it could be applied. Rather, we would expect them to do everything they could to advance the notion that the behaviour of asylum inmates was a manifestation of brain disease and was amenable only, or mainly, to purely medical remedies. The difficult and ambiguous position of medical superintendents is well illustrated by their response to the increase in the number of asylum inmates. The 1845 Act, requiring the building of county asylums, had specifically recommended that these be for curable cases only and that wherever possible separate receptacles be constructed for the incurables. The distinction between the two was made simply by assuming, in general, that an inmate of more than two years' standing was incurable. Retaining asylums for curable cases would, it was supposed, allow the concentration of skills on those most likely to derive benefit. It might be expected that asylum superintendents would be only too pleased to see the implementation of these recommendations which would, among other things, allow them to concentrate on perfecting the cure in whose name the asylums had been built. But, as Scull illustrates, the medical profession strongly resisted the idea of moving 'incurables' to a separate place. The apparently plausible justifications were that such a system would foster the very abuses reform was supposed to halt and that there was always the hope of a cure, regardless of the length of the inmates' confinement. The seemingly humanitarian basis of these arguments should not obscure the fact that any attempt to provide separate refuges for the 'incurables' could be seen as presenting a threat to asylum doctors. It was not envisaged that these places, which would be cheaper to run than asylums, would be under the control of doctors; the decreasing discharged cured figures suggested that the vast majority of lunatics would soon pass out of the profession's hands. This prospect was obviously unwelcome to an embryonic profession whose status was already precarious. Instead, asylum doctors were able to continue to justify their failure to cure by citing the huge number of inmates which made the task impossible. A few individual doctors protested about the situation and demanded action, but the profession as a whole took no concerted action, in marked contrast with their vigorous attempts to secure the construction of asylums. Scull (1979), reviewing the Reports of the Lunacy Commissioners (which included a large number of doctors), has noted that the distinction between praiseworthy and blameworthy asylums gradually came to be seen in terms of cleanliness, order and comfort, rather than in terms of numbers discharged cured. Local magistrates had suggested another solution to the problems faced by asylum doctors which would have freed them to concentrate on curing the inmates. This was the appointment of a lay administrator who would relieve the physician of the burden of paperwork and allow him to spend more time with the inmates. But asylum doctors vigorously opposed such suggestions to the point in two cases, at Hanwell hospital, of the medical superintendents' resigning in protest. Thus the relationship between the decline in moral management and the rising number of asylum inmates was not quite as straightforward as it might appear.

During the second half of the nineteenth century, asylum doctors increasingly behaved as if the inmates were literally sick. Microscopes became a standard part of asylum equipment; post-mortems were regularly performed to find the hypothesised brain lesions which were the cause of the inmates' strange behaviour; it became commonplace for asylums to have their own laboratories and to emphasise the importance of histopathological investigations; drugs were increasingly used to sedate the inmates. Bockoven (1956a) has linked this behaviour on the part of asylum doctors to the fact that the vast size of asylums made it impossible for the superintendents to become acquainted with the inmates and their problems. But while it is true that superintendents could not easily get to know all the inmates, this hardly necessitated their acting as if the inmates were sick to the point of examining their brains under a microscope. It is reasonable to suggest that what did necessitate such behaviour was the ambiguous professional status of mad-doctors. In order to convince the public and government that insanity was a medical matter, mad-doctors had to behave in the same fashion as their more secure colleagues who enjoyed the luxury of never, at least in recent history, having had to convince people that bodily ailments were a medical matter. And it was not only the public who must be convinced. Asylum doctors occupied the lowest rung of the professional ladder and were, as their title 'alienist' might suggest, as sep-arate from the rest of medicine as were their charges from the rest of society. Thus, every innovation in medicine was faithfully reproduced in the asylum, at the expense of the non-medical moral management.

For the most part, these imitations of medical practice were conspicuously unsuccessful either in discovering the causes of the inmates' behaviour or in altering it. It might therefore seem that it was only a matter of time until the professional pretensions of mad-doctors collapsed. The perceived, and actual, relationships between medicine and deviant behaviour were, however, radically altered by two processes. The first was the increasing interest in deviance shown by the new (and prestigious) medical speciality of neurology; the second the mounting evidence of a link between syphilis and the well-known cluster of features called, among other things, dementia paralytica.

## Neurology and insanity

By the seventh decade of the nineteenth century, public asylums, and partic-ularly those in the United States, had become huge, custodial receptacles with low standards of care. The necessary emphasis on the inmates' supposed sick-ness, plus the obviously unsuccessful attempts of the asylum doctors to discover either cause or cure, had induced a profound pessimism amongst them. They dealt mainly with poorer people, had few funds or facilities for research and lacked professional status. The situation did not, of course, go unnoticed, and in 1879 the American Neurological Association launched a series of attacks on mad-doctors and their asylums. The Association, repre-senting the new and growing specialism which dealt with disorders of the brain and nervous system, had been formed in 1875, although their *Journal of Nervous and Mental Disease* had first been published in 1874. The Association specifically excluded asylum doctors from its membership. They sought via various speeches and publications to gain acceptance for the view that asylums were damaging to the insane.

There are some interesting similarities and differences between the atti-tudes of neurologists at the end of the nineteenth century and those of the lunacy reformers at the beginning. Both groups were intent on exposing abuses in asylums; both were intent on showing that asylum inmates and anyone labelled mad should be dealt with in a manner quite different from the tradi-tional way. But there the similarities end. For the lunacy reformers, the answer was *more* asylums, an increase in custodial care; for the neurologists the answer was *fewer* asylums, a decrease in custodial care. The two opposing solutions probably reflect the mixed motives of the two groups. The lunacy reformers' efforts to increase institutional provision were inseparable from their desire to establish an efficient system of centrally controlled indoor Poor Relief; the neurologists' efforts to discredit asylums were almost certainly linked to their desire for professional advancement. It appeared that neurologists wanted the insane to be *their* customers and not those of asylum doctors. As neurologists came in general from fairly high-status backgrounds, and worked mostly in prestigious urban teaching hospitals, they were naturally disinclined to go where the insane were; instead they sought to bring the insane to them. To this end, Hammond, in 1879, declared that 'the medical profession (outside the hospital) is, as a body, fully as capable of treating cases of insanity as cases of any other disease . . . in many instances, sequestration is not only unnecessary, but positively injurious' (Bockoven, 1956a: 182). Obviously, neurologists must uphold the idea that those labelled insane were suffering from brain disease and they did this as vociferously as had mad-doctors.

Around the turn of the nineteenth century there appeared in the cities of the United States a new type of medical institution called a psychopathic hospital, which combined treatment with teaching and research and where out-patient clinics were first opened in 1912. A number of 'psychiatric institutes' were opened, as were 'psychiatric' wards in general hospitals. The ease and speed with which these developments took place is partly a reflection of the professional aspirations of neurologists but also of the US distaste for a unified, centrally controlled response to the lunacy problem. One important consequence of these developments was that people brought to the attention of neurologists those relatives who displayed behaviours which were less deviant, and which disturbed fewer people than did those of asylum inmates. The opening of out-patient clinics encouraged this trend, because neurologists declared themselves happy to see what they called milder cases. The already elastic criteria for applying the label insane or mentally disordered were thus widened still further.

It is notable that the relationship between mad-doctors and neurologists in Germany – from where Kraepelin's concept of dementia praecox was to emerge – was quite different from that in the United States or Britain. An institutional response to the problem of deviant behaviour and a system of non-restraint had been established there far more quickly and without the bureaucratic wrangling which had characterised the process in England and the United States. In Germany, the main proponents of asylums and of non-restraint had been doctors, and the number of them who specialised in insanity increased rapidly in the first decades of the nineteenth century. Zilboorg has commented that:

> The whole system of life in Germany reflected the tempo of rapid industrialisation and the ever increasing sense of communal relationship and these were in turn reflected in the psychiatric profession. The individual

worker, no matter how gifted, became part of a whole; the total accomplishment began to count more than the performance of any individual. As a result, a certain uniformity spread itself across German psychiatry. There was little strife. The rift between somatologists and the psychologists was well-nigh forgotten. German psychiatrists were almost without exception good neurologists and good neuroanatomists who in fact if not in spirit followed Griesinger's postulate and equated mental and nervous disease.

(Zilboorg, 1941: 446–447)

This may have meant that German neurologists and mad-doctors, who were in any case often the same people, did not waste time attacking each other; it also meant that the idea that the behaviour of most asylum inmates was caused by brain disease had been a virtually unchallenged article of faith in Germany for longer than in England and the United States. Moral management as an ideology had never had much impact in Germany, but was quickly transformed to an ideal of strict order and discipline.

Thus, by the end of the nineteenth century, the links between medicine and disturbing behaviour were firmly forged. The links were to be strengthened further by the results of research into the infectious diseases.

## Psychiatry and syphilis

The French physician Esquirol had noted as early as 1814 that some asylum inmates showed a consistent pattern of behaviour and physical features: the expression of beliefs which were clearly false, incoherent and inarticulate talk, tremors and loss of muscle power, followed by almost complete loss of the use of limbs and death. By the third decade of the nineteenth century this pattern had been described frequently by French physicians and, later, by physicians in other parts of Europe and the United States. It was also observed that the brains of these people showed various pathological changes at post-mortem, but the relationship between earlier syphilitic infection and these changes was not to be unambiguously demonstrated until the beginning of the twentieth century.

The fact that the link between the bizarre behaviour of these people, the physical changes observed before death and the brain pathology found afterwards, *and* the link between all of these and syphilis, was not fully appreciated during the nineteenth century was partly a result of the then current ideas about insanity. Hare (1959) has pointed out that the nineteenth-century physician was unhappily aware of the fact that while some of the inmates who expressed strange beliefs or spoke incoherently showed pathological brain changes at post-mortem, an equal (or greater) number did not. Similarly, a great many inmates (who might now be diagnosed as having, say, Parkinson's disease or Huntington's chorea) showed marked changes in motor behaviour.

To add to the confusion, the term 'paralysis' and its related term 'paresis', had a number of different referents. The physicians of the early nineteenth century therefore did not fully appreciate the significance of the co-occurrence of features called dementia paralytica, nor did they regard those displaying them as a distinct and homogeneous group for research purposes. Nor was the nature of the relationship between bizarre behaviour, the motor changes and the brain pathology easily grasped. A paralytic disorder might be seen as both a cause and an effect of strange behaviour, rather than both being seen as products of pathological brain changes. The cerebral changes noted in asylum inmates were so varied, or completely absent, that some physicians, including Pinel, despaired of relating them in any systematic way to the inmates' behaviour. A number of physicians did grasp the possible implications of the co-occurrence of features called dementia paralytica but, lacking conceptual and methodological sophistication and technical expertise, were unable to provide more than indirect – and often ignored – evidence for their theories. It was not until 1912, following significant technical innovations and conceptual advances which were both antecedent and the result of work on the infectious diseases, that the debate was closed by the finding of syphilitic spirochetes in the brains of those who had displayed the dementia paralytica cluster. The diagnosis of dementia paralytica had become objective in the 1890s when specific reactions of cerebro-spinal fluid were demonstrated and the indirect evidence linking dementia paralytica and syphilis had been mounting for some time before Noguchi's convincing direct evidence emerged in 1912. It is interesting to note that Kraepelin was one of those convinced by the indirect evidence.

Szasz (1976) has placed strong emphasis on the role of the dementia paralytica–syphilis link in fostering somatic theories of bizarre behaviour. Skultans disagrees and suggests that:

> the consequences which Szasz draws do not necessarily follow: the elaboration and proliferation of nomenclature did not take place. Early diagnosis and careful classification as preconditions for successful treatment were emphasised by the moral managers in the first half of the nineteenth century . . . With the increase in the size of asylums and the asylum population, the general standard of care deteriorated. Since cure was no longer a goal, classification was neglected.
>
> (Skultans, 1979: 7)

Skultan's argument, however, is based on a misunderstanding not only of developments in classification around the turn of the nineteenth century but also of the crucial differences between these and the earlier classificatory attempts of the moral managers.

# Syphilis and the classification of deviant behaviour

Medical men had always striven to accommodate strange behaviour into whatever theoretical framework was then being employed to study physical
ailments. They did this partly because they knew of no other way to think
about the matter; later, of course, it was to become a practical necessity to
maintain their professional claim that deviant behaviour was a medical matter.
Theories of physical suffering, however, were so firmly rooted in general theories of man and nature that to include behaviour seemed a perfectly reasonable
way to proceed. Thus, as I pointed out earlier, philosophical, medical and literary writings on madness were often indistinguishable. Medical ideas about
the nature of diseases and how or whether they should be classified were therefore faithfully reflected in writings about deviant behaviour. Ontological
theories, with their emphasis on the qualitative separateness of diseases and on
careful classification, were more popular in medicine than was the idea of disease as a quantitative deviation from some norm. Transferred to behaviour they
resulted, during the eighteenth and nineteenth centuries, in a plethora of
classification systems, no two of which appeared to agree on either the number
or nature of what were claimed to be types of insanity. One problem was the
lack of consensus as to the principles on which the endeavour should be based.
Some insisted that classification should be by the most prominent symptom (it
was apparently assumed that it would be obvious to an observer which behaviour merited this label); others claimed that groups of symptoms should be the
basis of a classificatory system. Henry Maudsley insisted that the only good
classificatory system was one based on aetiology. To add to the confusion,
words and deeds did not always match. As Zilboorg (1941) has pointed out,
Skae and de Sauvages, who insisted on a classification based on symptoms,
slipped, apparently unnoticed by themselves, into classifying on the basis of
assumed cause.

There was also the problem of the uses to which these various systems
might be put. It is difficult to avoid the conclusion that one of the systems'
major functions was to convince medical men and the public of the complexity of insanity and of the detailed and expert knowledge needed to deal with
it. Certainly, when it came to intervention, the niceties of classification seemed
to be forgotten. Until relatively recently, medicine possessed a small number
of cure-alls and when these were discussed in the context of bizarre behaviour
the writers reverted to general terms such as cerebral irritation or more usually,
insanity. They had, of course, little option because the precise connections
between the behaviour of those labelled insane, the various interventions and
the abstract groups named in the classification systems were, to say the least,
tenuous.

The moral managers, by contrast, adopted their usual pragmatic approach to
the business of classification. For them, it must serve practice. Tuke (1813)
suggested that 'the general comfort of the patients ought to be considered; and

those who are violent require to be separated from the more tranquil, and to be prevented, by some means, from offensive conduct towards their fellow sufferers'. Thus, inmates should be 'arranged into classes, as much as may be, according to the degree to which they approach to rational and orderly conduct' (141). This separation was also designed to teach inmates that 'good' behaviour earned different consequences from 'bad'.

In the more abstract world of the physicians the chaos of classification systems for insanity was such that more than one recommended abandoning the whole business. Neumann, for example, suggested in 1859 that:

> We shall never be able to believe that psychiatry will make a step forward until we decide to throw overboard the whole business of classification . . . There is but one type of mental disturbance and we call it insanity.
>
> (Zilboorg, 1941: 438)

The problem for psychiatrists was that as long as their medical colleagues continued to emphasise the importance of grouping phenomena in particular ways, they must follow suit or risk creating professionally damaging gaps in theory and practice. In any case, as psychiatrists were trained as doctors, it is hardly surprising that the majority should bend what they observed to fit prevailing medical theories, rather than the other way round. As the nineteenth century progressed and medical research slowly began to show signs of being productive, it became increasingly unlikely – if, indeed it ever had been likely – that medical theories would change in any way to accommodate the awkward behaviour of asylum inmates. Another reason why psychiatry must follow medicine was that the last decades of the nineteenth century, like the first, lacked anything resembling a scientific theory of behaviour. This is not to suggest that had such theories been available psychiatrists would have gladly used them; professional considerations must still be taken into account. Those psychiatrists who wished to be scientific, however, could see no way of doing so that did not involve imitating medicine. The alternative, as they saw it, was to return to abstract philosophy or, worse, to theology or mysticism.

This insistence on 'scientific' practice, and the conviction that it involved studying the brains of those who behaved strangely, was particularly strong in Germany where neurology and psychiatry were virtually indistinguishable. There were, however, limits to the extent to which medicine could be imitated. Virchow's theory that classification and diagnosis consisted in naming pathological organ changes obviously could not be taken up, as so many asylum inmates did not show them and any changes which could be found could not be systematically related to behaviour. Nevertheless, the search for disease entities must proceed. There were some attempts to characterise these in terms of 'psychological structures', but no agreement could be reached on what these might be and the theories were short lived. In the absence of well-demonstrated physical lesions, it became increasingly necessary to emphasise the importance of phenomena which presented themselves directly to the clinician. Fortunately, this emphasis had a long and respectable history in medicine, even if it was now being replaced by an emphasis on laboratory analysis. In line with this, in the last decades of the nineteenth century Kahlbaum reiterated Sydenham's view that progress would only be made by observing the onset, course and outcome of various groups of symptoms. It is interesting to note that it seems to have been taken for granted that these groups of symptoms would somehow present themselves to the physician in a readily recognisable form; his main task was to chart their course, to discover whether or not they constituted specific disease entities.

There can be little doubt that the growing body of evidence about the nature of infectious diseases, including syphilis, must have helped to convince psychiatrists that they were on the right track as far as methodology was concerned. For probably the first time in medical history there were strong indications that adopting a particular theoretical framework would lead to a successful outcome. Moreover, medicine's successes had begun with – indeed would never have been attainable without – careful observation of phenomena as they presented themselves to the clinician, *not* by speculation about unknown causes. Dementia paralytica appears to have been particularly common in northern Germany, and Kraepelin – who was greatly influenced by Kahlbaum – wrote extensively on the subject. The role of the discovery of the dementia paralytica/syphilis link may therefore have been to confirm and extend the belief in a particular way of working, rather than in a somatic theory of deviant behaviour, which was in any case already well established. And the length of time it had taken to discover the link may have given psychiatrists hope in the face of their poor empirical results.

These, then, are some of the 'conditions of possibility' (Foucault, 1976) of the concept of dementia praecox/schizophrenia: the conditions which made it seem reasonable for a neurologist/psychiatrist to 'discover' a specific mental disease which explained a wide range of bizarre behaviour. However, if we look at this quest to discover disease entities in its own terms – as part of a scientific, medical enterprise – then it is clear that it proceeded in apparent ignorance of or disregard for the considerable conceptual and methodological problems it presented. These will be discussed in detail in the next chapter, but one obvious problem was that of knowing which behaviours should be thought of as symptoms, given that no pathology could be demonstrated in many inmates and, in those in which it could, there were no clear links between it and behaviour. Instead, it was implicitly reasoned that people were confined to asylums because they suffered from mental diseases. Therefore, what the clinician observed in the asylum, and considered abnormal, must be the symptoms of mental disease. But the concepts of insanity and mental disease were lay and not scientific concepts and their referents were idiosyncratic, many and varied. It is also possible, as I mentioned earlier, that definitions of insanity had broadened in the latter part of the nineteenth century; it is certainly beyond dispute that the apparent number of cases of insanity increased considerably. Indeed, Zilboorg (1941) has suggested that detailed clinical observation had to be stressed to bring order to 'the welter of clinical material which accumulated with such suddenness' (447). It is not being suggested here that theoretical order could never have been brought to the apparent chaos of the inmates' behaviour. What is suggested is that mad-doctors had failed to confront the consequences of their history, the implications of their ignorance, and the conceptual and methodological difficulties of the task they had taken on. Nevertheless, it is against this difficult background that Kraepelin is credited with having 'delineated syndromes from the midst of chaos' (Kendell, 1975b: 62) and with having 'identified a syndrome' (Andreasen and Carpenter, 1993: 200–201). Given the enormity of the task, and the fact that these statements – together with the continued use of 'schizophrenia' – amount to a claim that the necessary (and just sufficient) conditions for inferring the concept have been fulfilled, it is important that Kraepelin's putative achievements be examined in detail.

# Chapter 3

# The necessary conditions for inferring schizophrenia

## The work of Kraepelin, Bleuler and Schneider

This chapter will examine in detail the writings of Emil Kraepelin, Eugen Bleuler and Kurt Schneider to assess the extent to which they provide evidence that the necessary condition for inferring dementia praecox or schizophrenia – i.e. the initial observation of a set of regularities – has been fulfilled. These writers have been chosen because Kraepelin's ideas are said to mark the beginnings of the modern construct of schizophrenia; because Bleuler and Schneider were influenced by him, though in different ways; and because all three profoundly influenced future generations of psychiatrists. Bleuler's influence has been stronger in the United States, while Schneider and Kraepelin have proved more influential in Europe. The three also represent a chronological sequence which illustrates not only the development of the concept of schizophrenia but also many of the problems associated with it. Others, notably Adolf Meyer, were involved in the development of the construct but their work will not be examined here because their ideas post-dated those of Kraepelin and Bleuler, their influence has been less and the criticisms which could be made of them are similar to those which will be made of Kraepelin *et al.*

It must be emphasised that the issue being addressed here is not whether Kraepelin and his successors observed bizarre behaviours in asylum inmates; it is beyond doubt that the inmates behaved in ways which were both uncommon and incomprehensible to observers. Neither is it questioned that many of the inmates were distressed by their experiences. What *is* being examined is whether Kraepelin *et al.* were justified in claiming to have observed regularities amongst this mass of deviant behaviours which would justify inferring the concepts of dementia praecox and schizophrenia.

The writings of Kraepelin, Bleuler and Schneider will not be assessed in terms of whether they discovered discrete disease entities. As I noted in Chapter 1, although this was Kraepelin's goal it is widely acknowledged that he never achieved it. It is also not necessary for dementia praecox/schizophrenia to represent a discrete disease entity in order for it to be valid. The idea of a disease entity represented a theoretical or philosophical ideal or fantasy, rather than a scientific requirement. What *is* required, however, is that the concepts

of dementia praecox/schizophrenia should have been derived from the observation of a pattern of regularities; the work of Kraepelin, Bleuler and Schneider
will therefore be assessed in terms of the extent to which they support the
observation of a pattern of phenomena which would justify the label 'syndrome'. This criterion has been chosen for two reasons. First, as I noted in
Chapter 1, modern writers are apparently agreed in claiming that schizophrenia is inferred from such a pattern (what is actually and misleadingly claimed
is that schizophrenia is a syndrome). Second, this pattern is the minimum
which allows the conclusion that a postulated cluster is not either the chance
co-occurrence of unrelated phenomena or illusory (see, e.g., Chapman and
Chapman's 1967 demonstration of the perception of co-occurrences in random
data). It is not possible to apply a less stringent criterion to the work of those
said to have 'discovered schizophrenia' and maintain any semblance of support
for its claims to scientific status. Finally, it is important to emphasise that the
discussion here is about the initial introduction of the concepts of dementia
praecox and schizophrenia and *not* about the diagnosis of schizophrenia. The
modern focus on diagnosis and diagnostic criteria has succeeded in obscuring
the fact that the process of diagnosis is dependent on, and is meaningless
without, prior evidence that the introduction of the concept of schizophrenia
was justified in the first place.

## The work of Emil Kraepelin

The term 'dementia praecox', which Kraepelin was to bring to such prominence, had been introduced (as *démence précoce*) by Morel in 1852 – but with
referents different from those suggested by Kraepelin in 1896. Kraepelin himself had used the term in 1893 with referents somewhat similar to Morel's but
different from those he was later to employ. Kraepelin's 1896 writings are the
starting point of this evaluation because it is these which are most frequently
said to mark the beginnings of the modern concept of schizophrenia. Kraepelin
developed his ideas in a series of texts published between 1896 (5th edition)
and 1913 (8th edition). Material from the latter was published separately in
1919. I will discuss writings from the 1896, 1899 and 1913/19 texts in order
to describe both the introduction and development of Kraepelin's 'modern'
concept of dementia praecox. Two aspects of his work will be examined in
detail. First, the evidence he presented in support of his claim that a particular cluster of phenomena could be the source of the concept of dementia
praecox; second, the way in which his population and the setting in which he
worked might have influenced his theorising.

### Some general considerations

One problem which is immediately encountered in any attempt to describe the
evidence Kraepelin presented in support of his concept is that he more than

once changed his mind about the putative regularities which allowed dementia praecox to be inferred. In 1896, for example, he described what he claimed was a meaningful cluster of behaviours from which he inferred dementia praecox. He also described a second cluster from which he inferred catatonia and a third from which he inferred dementia paranoides. Kraepelin suggested that the second cluster probably had the same antecedents as the first, although he offered no direct evidence for this; he therefore suggested that both clusters should be the source of dementia praecox. The cluster from which dementia paranoides was inferred was thought to have different antecedents, although again no direct evidence was offered; Kraepelin therefore suggested that this cluster should continue to be the source of a construct different from dementia praecox (Kraepelin of course did not use this language but talked misleadingly of separate illnesses). By 1899, in the 6th edition of his text, Kraepelin had apparently reversed this decision. He now postulated a new set of putative regularities said to justify inferring dementia praecox and which included some of the behaviours from which he had previously inferred dementia paranoides.

Between the 6th and 8th editions of his text, Kraepelin further increased the number of behaviours said to be symptoms of dementia praecox. The scale of the increase can be gauged from the fact that in 1896 a discussion of the constructs of dementia praecox and catatonia took up about thirty-seven pages. In the 6th edition, 'dementia praecox' occupied seventy-seven pages; by the 8th edition, the discussion had grown to 356 pages. This increase was almost wholly accounted for by the proliferation of behaviours said to be symptoms of dementia praecox. As the number of behaviours said to fall within the scope of the concept increased, so too did the number of sub-groups (i.e. regularities within the larger pattern) which Kraepelin claimed to have observed. In the 6th edition he suggested three major sub-groups: putative regularities from which he inferred dementia praecox, hebephrenic type; dementia praecox, catatonic type; and dementia praecox, paranoid type. Within each of these, Kraepelin made further sub-divisions but without inferring new constructs. In his 1913 text, he claimed to have observed eleven major sub-groups within the larger dementia praecox cluster.

These changes in what Kraepelin claimed to have observed parallel apparent changes in the criteria he used to attribute meaningfulness to any postulated cluster. Both changes reflect the conceptual and methodological problems he encountered, but did not always recognise, in trying to make sense of the multitude of bizarre behaviours displayed by asylum inmates. Because of these apparent changes in criteria, Kraepelin's earlier and later writings will be discussed separately.

## Kraepelin's early writings: 1896 and 1899

In 1896, Kraepelin adopted the criterion of similarities in onset, course and outcome to assign meaningfulness to any postulated cluster of bizarre behaviours whose antecedents were unknown. He was thus claiming that if he could identify a group whose behaviour changed in a similar way at one point (onset), showed further similarity in development over a period of time (course) and reached a similar end point (outcome), he would be entitled to postulate a common, as yet unobserved, event or process to account for this supposed pattern and to infer a new hypothetical construct – in this case dementia praecox.

Some of the problems of this argument have already been mentioned but are sufficiently important to be repeated here. First, although the terms 'onset', 'course' and 'outcome' are often used as if they referred to simple, discrete events, in practice they are usually summary terms for a set of extremely complex and continuous processes, particularly when they are applied to behaviour. Thus, what is actually recorded under these headings may be quite arbitrary and will differ across researchers. Second, the complexities of describing 'onset', 'course' and 'outcome' are compounded by the difficulties in specifying *important* similarities among the range of phenomena observed. An investigator using this criterion to assign meaningfulness and faced with a heterogeneous population showing a wide range of similarities and differences in behaviour (as was the case with Kraepelin's population) has no easy way of knowing which similarities are important, i.e. which groupings are likely to result in the observation of 'new' phenomena. If this criterion of similarities in onset, course and outcome is applied to a heterogeneous population, the likely result is unstable and ever-changing groupings as different investigators, or the same investigator at different times, apply varying rules for assessing importance. Thus, the mere description of a set of similarities within a population, and of differences between it and other populations, is not enough to attribute meaningfulness to the 'pattern' of similarities described. It is for this reason that evidence is demanded that these are a function of another independently and reliably measurable event – in medical parlance, a sign. A third problem of this criterion is that the inclusion of 'outcome' requires that no statement be made about the population of interest until all members have reached a point where no further change is possible. Even if this were achieved – say the population was studied until every member was dead – it would still not be possible to identify any new exemplars of a postulated pattern until they too had reached an agreed end-point. Thus, diagnosis would be delayed and research progress minimal. Taken together, these problems account for the unpopularity of this criterion in medicine.

Kraepelin is unlikely to have been wholly unaware of these problems; it is more likely that he employed the criterion as a last resort, having been unable to establish order from the apparent chaos of the inmates' behaviour using more useful and conventional criteria. He certainly did not adopt similarities in onset, course and outcome as a general criterion for classification. It might be argued, however, that Kraepelin's employment of a problematic criterion does not invalidate his work; that if he did describe a pattern of similarities in onset, course and outcome it would at least be a starting point for a search for an independently measurable event associated with this supposed cluster. As this analysis will show, however, there is no evidence from Kraepelin's early writings that he even reached this starting point.

## Similarities in onset, course and outcome?

At first glance, it might appear that Kraepelin did indeed make use of his stated criterion to identify a pattern of behaviour from which he inferred dementia praecox. He suggested, for example, that the phenomena from which he inferred catatonia probably shared an antecedent with those from which he inferred dementia praecox because 'both in their development and in their origins and prognosis we find an extensive correspondence between the two forms of illness' (1896: 461). He also suggested that the events from which he inferred dementia paranoides were different from these because '[n]ot only does [dementia paranoides] develop on average at a rather higher age, it has a course and an outcome which is considerably different' (1896: 469). Indeed, the name Kraepelin chose for his construct – early dementia – reflects his belief that he was using this particular criterion: dementia refers to the alleged outcome and praecox to the time of onset. A closer examination of Kraepelin's work, however, gives a much less orderly impression of his methods and conclusions.

If medical researchers are engaged in a search for regularities in a heterogeneous population we would expect them to present data showing that some members of this population share features which are either not present in other groups or, if present, appear to have different antecedents (e.g. congenital vs. acquired immune deficiency). Data should also be presented in support of any claim that the first group is homogeneous in some important respect, that the features they share do not co-occur by chance. Having presented these data, the researchers would *conclude* by inferring a new hypothetical construct. Although Kraepelin saw himself as a scientific medical researcher, his presentation of the concept of dementia praecox in 1896 was quite different from that outlined here. Instead of *concluding* by inferring his concept, having presented evidence in support, Kraepelin *began* with the concept and proceeded to describe what he called cases of dementia praecox. He did not report the number of these who conformed to the descriptions he presented. These data, however, are crucial to claims that important shared features have been identified. Rather, Kraepelin's descriptions are in the form: 'one often notices'; 'it is occasionally observed'; 'in some cases', etc. Thus, for much of the time, Kraepelin wrote as if someone else had already introduced the concept of dementia praecox and presented valid evidence in support of it, so that he – Kraepelin – had been able to diagnose dementia praecox (i.e. identify new exemplars of an already recognised pattern) in his asylum inmates and was now merely recording his impressions of the group. He wrote, that is, as if data supporting the introduction of his concept had already been presented when in fact they had not.

If Kraepelin failed to follow the required first step to inferring new concepts in medicine, the question remains as to the evidence he did present in support of his contention that he had identified a group of asylum inmates who had in common that their behaviour developed and changed in similar ways and reached a similar end-point. The only source of evidence is Kraepelin's subjective and unquantified accounts of alleged cases of dementia praecox, with all the conceptual confusion such accounts imply. In this analysis, these will be examined under the headings of onset, course and outcome, although Kraepelin did not use these headings himself in spite of the importance he is supposed to have placed on them. Readers of his work can only extract information which appears to be relevant from the global accounts he provided.

### Initial changes in behaviour (onset)

Kraepelin appears to have paid scant attention to two fundamental problems of discussing 'onset' in this context. There is, first, that of knowing which behaviour changes were important within his framework (i.e. indicative of some unobserved but assumed biological change), and, second, that of the reliability of information collected retrospectively. The problems of retrospective data collection are well known – events may be distorted in memory by the passing of time, by attempts to understand the present, by leading questions from an interviewer, and so on. Kraepelin, however, does not say from what source or how he obtained his accounts of alleged behaviour changes, how long after the event or what efforts were made to verify the information. These problems are highlighted by Kraepelin's claims that:

> The whole upheaval can take place so imperceptibly and with such indefinite indications that those around imagine that they are confronted simply with the outcome of an unhappy development, perhaps even of some character fault.
>
> (1896: 426)

> In more than half the cases, the upheaval occurs so imperceptibly and with such indefinite indications that its actual beginning cannot be determined in retrospect.
>
> (1899: 149)

It is difficult to understand how Kraepelin could have made use of his stated criteria of similarities in onset, course and outcome when he believed that onset could not be observed in more than half of those to whom he applied the term 'dementia praecox'.

The issue remains of the extent of within-group similarity and between-group differences in what were claimed to be important initial changes. It is an issue which is impossible to resolve from the information provided by Kraepelin. Not only are his accounts of the postulated changes so vague that the observations which led to them are obscured, there is no indication of the number of people to whom each applied. Clearly, they did not apply to everyone labelled as suffering from dementia praecox, otherwise it would have been unnecessary for Kraepelin to have qualified his accounts thus:

> Somewhat less often the beginning of the illness is signalled by a markedly unhappy mood.
>
> (1899: 150)

> One often notices, particularly at the beginning, hypochondriacal complaints, self-recriminations, fears for the future . . .
>
> (1896: 427)

> One is often struck at this stage by a bluntness of feeling and indifference . . .
> (1896: 431)

It appears that quite different, indeed sometimes opposite, behaviour could signal the onset of dementia praecox:

> In the patient's behaviour, either a marked inertia and lassitude or typically childish characteristics make themselves apparent.
>
> (1896: 428)

> The psychosis begins as a rule with indications of a light or severe psychological depression . . . In a second group of cases one sees the illness set in with the sudden onset of a state of excitation with little prior warning.
>
> (1896: 442–443)

But Kraepelin also appeared to use the age at which some change was said to have occurred, rather than any specific changes, as one criterion for inferring dementia praecox. He suggested, for example, that: 'I think it is useful to divide dementia paranoides from the first named illnesses. Not only does it develop on average at a rather higher age' (1896: 469). The use of age of onset, of course, begs the question of how Kraepelin could possibly know that some alleged change was a function of whatever processes were said to underlie the illness of dementia praecox; in other words, of how he could claim that it marked the onset of dementia praecox as well as the question of why age was considered to be a useful criterion. It is difficult to avoid the conclusion that the population from whose behaviour Kraepelin inferred dementia praecox had in common only that their behaviour had changed in *some* disturbing way and to an extent sufficient for their relatives or the authorities to report them to the medical profession. Even those said to have 'collapsed imperceptibly' must have changed perceptibly at some point in order to be brought to Kraepelin's notice. But Kraepelin's account of the changes is so vague and the changes themselves apparently so varied that little else can be said about the extent of similarity within the group, far less about the extent of difference between it and groups to which the term 'dementia praecox' was not applied.

It might be objected that for any diagnostic category in medicine, similar variability would be observed: that for a group given label X, some would report initial changes A, B and C and others D, E and F. And while this is certainly true, the crucial point is that such an observation makes no sense without the previous observation of a pattern of regularities which would have justified inferring the hypothetical construct which is now the diagnostic label. It is this first step which is missing in Kraepelin's work.

## Changes in behaviour over time (course)

Kraepelin introduced his 1896 concept because he claimed to have observed a group of people whose behaviour initially changed, developed and 'ended' in similar ways. It is therefore somewhat surprising to find reference to large amounts of within-group variability in the way in which the behaviour of the group was said to change over time:

> The course of this process of illness can take the most varied forms.
>
> (1896: 426)

> The further course of the illness in these cases is a varied one insofar as the imbecility sometimes develops more rapidly, sometimes more slowly and can in fact stop progressing at very different stages.
>
> (1896: 429)

Kraepelin thus appears to be claiming that the course of the illness in different people was simultaneously very similar and very different.

I mentioned earlier that in 1896 Kraepelin suggested that the constructs of dementia praecox and catatonia were probably synonymous and gave as one of the reasons that the behaviour of those to whom the two constructs were applied changed in similar ways over time. It is therefore, again, surprising to find him describing the putative courses of these two 'illnesses' in quite different ways:

> The course of dementia praecox is in general one of regular progression. Only very seldom does one see an extensive remission of the signs of illness . . .
>
> (1896: 436)

An unusually important phenomenon of the course of catatonia is the remissions which occur.

(1896: 455)

Just as Kraepelin had attempted to 'join' the constructs of dementia praecox and catatonia in 1896, he wished to keep separate the construct of dementia paranoides, arguing that 'it has a course and an outcome which is considerably different' (1896: 469). It is not unreasonable, then, to expect that the later 'joining' of 'dementia praecox' to some of the behaviours which had been the source of dementia paranoides, should, within Kraepelin's framework, have been accompanied by an explanation of why what had been, in 1896, 'a considerably different course' was now, in 1899, apparently a similar one. Not only was such an explanation not forthcoming, Kraepelin appeared to be unaware that it was called for. In 1896 he apparently used extensive and persistent visual and auditory hallucinations and delusions as one source of dementia paranoides; less extensive and transient displays of these phenomena were one source of dementia praecox. In 1899, Kraepelin did not offer evidence that the extent and persistence of these phenomena were actually the same in both groups; nor did he indicate that a common antecedent had been found to justify disregarding differences in behaviour. Rather, he apparently abandoned 'extent and persistence of hallucinations and delusions', just as arbitrarily as he had chosen it, as a criterion for differences in course. Alternatively (and it is difficult to know from Kraepelin's writings which was the case) he may have abandoned 'course' altogether as part of the criterion for assigning meaningfulness, and merged the constructs on the basis of alleged similarities in outcome. This still, however, leaves the problem of how a 'considerably different outcome' had now become a similar one.

Kraepelin's own admission of a large amount of within-group variability and his apparently arbitrary choice of criteria for similarity, cast serious doubt on his claim to have identified a group who showed important similarities in behaviour change over time. The group to whom the term 'dementia praecox' was applied presumably did show some similarities in their behaviour but, as with Kraepelin's discussion of 'onset', it is impossible to know from his account either their extent or their significance.

### 'End-point' behaviour (outcome)

In trying to identify regularities in the behaviour of asylum inmates, Kraepelin appeared to place more emphasis on 'outcome' than on 'onset' and 'course', although there is no obvious justification within his framework for doing so; certainly, Kraepelin never offered one. An early attempt to clarify the concept of dementia praecox illustrates this emphasis on an alleged end-point:

> Dementia praecox is the name we give to the development of a simple more or less severe state of psychological weakness with manifestations of an acute or sub-acute disturbance of mind.
>
> (1896: 426)

This statement also, however, illustrates one of the major problems in Kraepelin's discussion of 'outcome', as indeed of 'onset' and 'course' – his failure to specify the referents of the term, although he did provide descriptions of some of the behaviour from which he inferred 'simple more or less high grade state of psychological weakness'. The descriptions, however, are highly varied and no indication is given of the number of inmates to whom they applied. For the most part, however, the reader is left not with descriptions but with only vague statements about psychological weakness with no indication of the observations which were the source of this term or its (apparent) synonyms:

> although patients are more placid, it is only to reveal ever more clearly the indications of a fairly high grade psychological weakness.
>
> (1896: 433)

> The common outcome of all severer forms of dementia praecox is idiocy.
>
> (1896: 436)

> The end state [of one type of paranoid form of dementia praecox] is feeble minded confusion.
>
> (1899: 188)

> Most frequently, however, the illness seems to lead to an insane confusion.
>
> (1899: 200)

Kraepelin's failure to specify behaviours which were the source of the concepts of feeblemindedness, idiocy, etc., or of the gradations of which he wrote, makes it impossible to know the extent of similarity amongst those to whom 'dementia praecox' was applied or of difference between them and other inmates. This problem is compounded by Kraepelin's indirect admission that the same behaviour might lead him to infer feeblemindedness in one inmate and not in another, depending on past behaviour:

> so that often enough we must remain in doubt as to the meaning of a particular final condition, should we be without the preceding history.
>
> (1905: 205)

Not only did Kraepelin apparently use past behaviour to decide whether feeblemindedness should be inferred from present behaviour, he also used present behaviour to reconstruct the past when no information was available:

Still, even now, in a considerable number of cases, the careful observation of clinical symptoms makes it possible for us to trace out at least a rough outline of what has gone before from the final stages of the malady.

(1905: 205)

But Kraepelin's claim that this was possible is difficult to understand in the light of his statement that:

Unfortunately, I have not yet been able to discover particular indicators for drawing conclusions about the likely outcome of the illness in individual cases.

(1899: 180)

Kraepelin confirmed his pessimism in 1920 when he again claimed that it was impossible to predict prognosis in spite of careful observation (Astrup and Noreik, 1966).

Kraepelin therefore fell into the trap of interpreting the present to fit constructions of the past and of reconstructing an unknown past to fit present observations and diagnosis. In other words, his assessments of onset, course and outcome were not independent. The tendency to indulge in these dubious practices is yet another reason for the disfavour with which 'similarities in onset, course and outcome' is viewed as a criterion for assigning meaningfulness to a postulated cluster.

A further problem in Kraepelin's discussion of outcome is that if he had been following his own rules, then no judgements should have been made about inmates until they had reached a point where no further change was possible, if indeed such a point could be identified before death. But Kraepelin provided no information about the point(s) at which he made decisions about 'outcome', although photographs suggest that the label 'dementia praecox' was applied to some inmates while they were relatively young. The important point, however, is that there is no reason to believe that the alleged end-point behaviour from which Kraepelin inferred idiocy, feeblemindedness, etc. did not change at some future point. Kraepelin in fact failed to provide any evidence that he had identified a group of people who displayed similar 'end-point' behaviours.

I suggested earlier that the mere description of a set of similarities in behaviour change at one point, in changes over time and in end-point behaviour, does not in itself justify inferring a new hypothetical construct but that it might serve as a starting point in a search for a meaningful cluster. It appears, however, that Kraepelin came nowhere near even this starting point; rather, he fell victim to the problems known to attend the use of this criterion for grouping a heterogeneous population.

### Kraepelin's later writings: 1913/1919

A recurring problem in Kraepelin's early writings is that of knowing what he actually *did* – what data he collected and how. The problem is partly a result of his question-begging approach, where he often wrote as if he had already established the validity of 'dementia praecox', and of his use of popular lay terms of the day such as 'weak-minded' or 'degeneration', whose referents were never specified. But in these early writings, although he often confused the processes of concept development and diagnosis, Kraepelin did remind himself intermittently that he was required to demonstrate that certain phenomena 'went together' – that they co-occurred above chance level – in order to justify his construct of dementia praecox. Although he chose a highly problematic criterion and failed to provide evidence that a group of people conformed to it, at least his goal (to demonstrate co-occurrence) was appropriate. In his later writings, Kraepelin's goals are obscure. Wender (1963) claims that Kraepelin had now adopted a new criterion – that of identifying 'common characteristics of the disorder' – for assigning meaningfulness to a postulated cluster. It is, however, very difficult to know from Kraepelin's writings if this was his intention; he appears largely to have lost sight of the importance of demonstrating that certain phenomena 'went together', possibly because he mistakenly thought that the demonstration had already been made.

What *is* clear is that in 1913 Kraepelin placed much less emphasis on putative similarities in type and timing of initial behaviour changes, in changes over time and in end-point behaviours, and instead introduced the new topic of 'disorders which characterise the malady'. This change of emphasis is signalled by his introductory statement:

> Dementia praecox consists of a series of states the common characteristic of which is a peculiar destruction of the internal connections of the psychic personality.
>
> (1919: 3)

The new emphasis on a 'common characteristic' was probably at least in part the result of criticism of his earlier emphasis on 'similarities in onset, course and outcome'. Unfortunately, criticism was not based mainly on the deficiencies of this criterion; rather, it was based on the claim that it was possible to find cases of dementia praecox whose behaviour had changed in some disturbing way relatively late in life and whose end-point behaviour, or, more accurately, behaviour at the last point at which observations were made, apparently differed little from what the medical profession designated as normal (see, e.g., Bleuler, [1911] 1950). Kraepelin appeared partly to accept these criticisms:

> It has since been found that the assumptions upon which the name chosen rested are at least doubtful . . . the possibility cannot in the present state

of our knowledge be disputed that a certain number of cases of dementia praecox attain to complete and permanent recovery and also the relations to the period of youth do not appear to be without exception.

(1919: 4)

Highlighting the apparent inappropriateness of the term 'dementia praecox', Serbski (cited in Zilboorg, 1941), commented on Kraepelin's statement that about 13 per cent of his cases apparently recovered, and inquired whether these were to be thought of as deterioration without deterioration, as dementia without dementia. Rowe (1906) pointed to the lack of reliability in the measurement of 'outcome', to the fact that the term 'deterioration' was used very loosely, and to its questionable use as a diagnostic criterion.

Kraepelin's critics are interesting, however, not so much for the problems they saw as for those they missed: the fallacy of their arguments was apparently overlooked. If Kraepelin's justification for originally inferring dementia praecox was the claim that he had identified a group that showed similarities in type and timing of initial behaviour changes, change over time and end-point behaviour, then it was logically impossible to have 'some cases of dementia praecox' whose behaviour changed relatively late in life and then reverted to 'normal'. Such a claim was incompatible with the use of Kraepelin's concept *unless* evidence was presented that a new and different set of regularities had been observed which would justify inferring dementia praecox without recourse to 'onset, course and outcome'. This evidence was never presented. Rather, by the early 1900s, 'dementia praecox' seemed to have taken on a life of its own, quite detached from any examination of its origins. Critics spoke as if a new 'disease' had been 'discovered' which had, perhaps, been inappropriately named, about whose symptoms there might be disagreement, but which could easily be recognised in 'unequivocal cases':

A clinical picture is necessary to a concept of disease, and the predominant symptoms are what in the majority of cases will give us the classification. I would throw out the weak, meaningless, ill-defined symptoms which serve only to confuse and lessen the wealth of more reliable data; and the stilted verbosity and generalisation should be replaced by constant and well-cut symptoms true to the disease. These not being present, I should hesitate before stamping it dementia praecox.

(Rowe, 1906: 393; see also Bleuler, [1911] 1950)

It was against this background of ill-informed discussion, characterised by reification and question-begging, that Kraepelin published what was to be his last major set of writings on the construct of dementia praecox. Before these are examined, it is important to note the methods by which Kraepelin reached the conclusion that 'there are apparently two principal groups of disorders which characterise the malady'. He appears in doing so to have committed the same fallacy as his critics: in claiming that 'the possibility cannot in the present state of our knowledge be disputed that a certain number of cases attain to complete and permanent recovery' and that 'the relations to the period of youth do not appear to be without exception', Kraepelin was admitting that the group of people from whose behaviour he had originally inferred dementia praecox, did *not* show the kind of similarities in 'onset, course and outcome' he had first claimed. Given that he had used this criterion to assign meaningfulness to a putative cluster and, therefore, to justify the introduction of his 1896 construct, it follows that, within his own framework, he was no longer justified in using it; nor could he arbitrarily alter its correspondence rules. Instead, he must restart his search for regularities amongst the heterogeneous group of asylum inmates whose behaviour did not conform to any known pattern. Not only is there no evidence that Kraepelin did restart his search, he appeared, like his critics, to have been unaware of the problem. His writings, however, are in a form from which it is extremely difficult to deduce what he actually did; not only did he fail to describe how he sought 'disorders which characterise the malady' (he claimed only to have found them), he failed also to describe what he meant by 'characterise the malady'. It is possible that he meant 'criteria I use to infer dementia praecox', but, if so, these should have been derived only after abandoning the construct, and should have been accompanied by evidence that they were a set of regularities which would justify reintroducing the concept. Alternatively, Kraepelin may have meant 'disorders shared by every inmate called a case of dementia praecox'. The problem here, of course, is that in order to seek such 'disorders', 'dementia praecox' must first, by some independent and valid criteria, be identified. Kraepelin was no doubt helped in this task by his belief that he too could recognise unequivocal cases when he saw them:

> In the first rank of course the delimitation of dementia praecox comes into consideration. We shall see later that on this point, in spite of the ease with which the great majority of cases can be recognised, there is still great uncertainty.
>
> (1919: 186)

Unfortunately, Kraepelin did not even describe the criteria by which he recognised this great majority, far less provide evidence of their validity. Instead, he continued to beg the question of the validity of 'dementia praecox'. His failure to deal with these fundamental problems makes it extremely unlikely that his later writings will allow the conclusion that he was justified in introducing and later using the construct. Nevertheless, they will be examined here in order to emphasise the weakness of the foundations on which his considerable influence rests and because the analysis is relevant to the work of Bleuler, which will be discussed in the next section.

*'. . . two principal groups of disorders . . .'*

On the one hand we observe a *weakening of those emotional activities which form the mainsprings of volition.*

The second group of disorders, which gives dementia praecox its peculiar stamp . . . consists in the *loss of the inner unity* of the activities of the intellect, emotion and volition in themselves and among one another.

(1919: 74–75; emphasis in original)

Unfortunately, Kraepelin did not describe the observations on which these inferences were based. What he did instead was to list literally hundreds of what were claimed to be 'psychic symptoms of dementia praecox', grouped according to unstated but apparently multiple criteria. The headings included: 'Influence on thought'; 'Hallucinations of sight, smell and taste'; 'Morbid tactile sensations and common sensations'; 'Sexual sensations'; 'Orientation'; 'Consciousness'; 'Retention'; 'Association experiments' and 'Evasion', with some headings claimed to be disorders of others. It is difficult to understand the rules by which Kraepelin generated these headings and listed behaviour under them, particularly as apparently identical phenomena appear to be listed under several different symptom headings.

Under many of the headings, Kraepelin discusses behaviours or 'states' which he claims are connected in some way with disorders of volition, to which he apparently attached much importance. It is, however, impossible to deduce which behaviours Kraepelin used to infer the putative disorders or the nature of the connection between the behaviours and the 'disorders of volition'. Some behaviours and 'states' are presented as alleged *results* of a disorder of volition; others are apparently cited as *causes* of disorders of volition; still others are used to infer this concept. There is no indication of how these choices of behaviour were made and, for the most part, Kraepelin writes of the putative association between various behaviours and 'disorders of volition' in such a way that it is extremely difficult to know what he is trying to convey.

*'. . . which characterise the malady.'*

I noted earlier that it is difficult to interpret what meaning Kraepelin attached to 'characterise the malady'. His writings not only fail to clarify this problem, they obscure it. One interpretation of the phrase is that Kraepelin was claiming to have identified behaviour shared by all those to whom he had already applied the label 'dementia praecox', but not by other inmates. On Kraepelin's own admission, however, this does not appear to have been the case:

We may well suppose that also the development of such stereotypes, which give such a peculiar appearance to the terminal states of the disease *and likewise to many forms of idiocy*, is specially favoured by the failure of healthy volitional impulses.

(1919: 45; emphasis added)

More specifically, a group of inmates from whose behaviour Kraepelin inferred paraphrenia appeared also to display behaviour which Kraepelin had previously connected with 'disorders of volition':

At the same time there are also abnormalities in the disposition, but till the latest stages [of paraphrenia] not that dullness and indifference which so frequently form the first symptoms of dementia praecox.

(1919: 283)

It may be, then, that Kraepelin was suggesting that those he called dementia praecox had in common that they displayed whatever behaviours were the source of disorders of volition with greater intensity or frequency than did other inmates. As Kraepelin failed to identify the behaviour in question, far less the intensity and frequency in all inmates, it is impossible to know whether this was the case. The details are hardly relevant, however, unless accompanied by evidence that grouping inmates according to such variations is useful, i.e. leads to the prediction of previously unobserved events. An alternative interpretation of 'characterise the malady' is that Kraepelin was proposing that the two 'principal disorders' could be used as diagnostic criteria. Setting aside for the moment the necessity for a prior demonstration that the principal disorders referred to a pattern of behaviour, it is clear from Kraepelin's discussion of 'diagnosis' that, whatever his intentions, he did not consistently use these criteria to diagnose dementia praecox.

The meaning which Kraepelin attached to 'characterise the malady' remains obscure. What is clear, however, is that in his later writings as much as in his earlier work, he failed to provide evidence that he was justified in inferring and using the construct of dementia praecox. His failure is well illustrated by his discussion of diagnosis. If Kraepelin had identified a pattern which justified inferring a new hypothetical construct, the chapter entitled 'Diagnosis' would have contained a clear description of this pattern, accompanied, perhaps, by discussion of how to avoid confusing it with other overlapping patterns (e.g. the pattern from which lung cancer is diagnosed may be confused with the pattern from which tuberculosis of the lungs is diagnosed unless certain discriminating observations are made). Kraepelin did indeed include a discussion of possible confusion between the alleged symptoms of dementia praecox and alleged symptoms of other 'disorders'. But quite apart from the fundamental problem of justifying any choice of behaviour as symptomatic of dementia praecox or any other 'condition', Kraepelin gave the asylum doctors the futile if not impossible task of distinguishing the unstated referents of various popular lay terms:

From genuine impulsive negativism there must be distinguished the surly, stubborn self-will of the paralytic and the senile dement, the playful reserve of the hysteric, the pertly repellent conduct of the manic and from the senseless perversities in action and behaviour, as they occur in dementia praecox, the conceited affectation of the hysteric, as also the wantonly funny solemnity of the manic patient.

(1919: 258)

Kraepelin in fact appeared to use different criteria for diagnosing dementia praecox in different inmates, while claiming that he was actually using the 'whole clinical picture'. This claim might have been quite reasonable if the 'clinical picture' corresponded to a previously observed pattern, but it clearly did not. On the contrary, it is interesting to note that when he talked of the 'whole clinical picture', Kraepelin appeared to fall back on his old, problematic criterion of similarities in onset, course and outcome:

But what hardly ever is produced in quite the same way by morbid processes of different kinds is . . . *the total clinical picture*, including development, course and issue.

(1919: 261; emphasis in original)

The states in dementia praecox which are accompanied by confused excitement and numerous hallucinations, have often been called amentia and traced to exhausting causes. Experience has shown me that cases of that kind cannot be separated from the remaining forms of dementia praecox according to the origin, course and issue.

(1919: 275)

But that the judgement of 'issue' still lay in the eye of the beholder is illustrated by Kraepelin's justification for separating out a group of inmates to whom he applied the term 'paraphrenia systematica', but in whom other doctors diagnosed dementia praecox because, they claimed, the outcome of the two groups was indistinguishable. While agreeing that the outcome of 'dementia praecox, paranoid form' and of 'paraphrenia systematica' might *look* the same, Kraepelin nevertheless claimed that:

it is obvious that in the terminal states [of those I call dementia praecox, paranoid form], we have to do with morbid processes which have run their course and ended in recovery with defect, and just on that account these cases have not progressed to the more severe forms of dementia such as form the issue of other paranoid cases of dementia praecox. We may well imagine, and may occasionally even really experience it, that a fresh outbreak of the disease may yet transform the

hallucinatory or paranoid weak-mindedness into a drivelling, silly, neg-
ativistic or dull dementia.

(1919: 299)

It is perhaps not surprising to find Kraepelin noting that agreement
amongst observers about putative outcome, and many other aspects of the
inmates' behaviour, was virtually non-existent. Indeed, he goes even further to
note the obvious fact, applicable to himself, that:

> In this uncertainty about the delimitation the statements of different
> observers can in the first place not be compared at all, not even the diag-
> noses of the same investigator at different periods of time separated by a
> number of years.

(1919: 186)

Unfortunately, having noted this lack of reliability, Kraepelin proceeded as if he
had noted exactly the opposite. Kraepelin did, of course, have the option of
searching for regularities which would justify inferring a new construct by the
accepted medical method of identifying a pattern of signs and symptoms. He
certainly tried to find biological events, including changes in brain structure,
which reliably co-occurred with whatever behaviours he thought of as symptoms
of dementia praecox. By his own admission, however, the attempt failed and it
is interesting to note, in spite of his claim to be a medical scientist, Kraepelin's
repeated appeals to his own authority, rather than to empirical evidence, in support of his claim to have identified a pattern which justified his concept:

> we shall no longer need to refute in any detail the objection formerly
> brought from different sides against the establishment of [dementia prae-
> cox] that it was a case of unjustified grouping of uncured psychosis of very
> different kinds . . . Clinical experience has demonstrated innumerable
> times that it is possible from the conception of the pathology of demen-
> tia praecox to tell with great probability the further course and issue of a
> case belonging to the group.

(1919: 252)

> We have therefore even yet to rely purely on the valuation of clinical
> experience . . .

(1919: 255)

> Although I must doubt that all of the disease pictures of Kahlbaum actu-
> ally belong together, I nevertheless feel that my extensive experience
> justifies the recognition of the great majority of these cases as examples of
> a single characteristic illness form.

(1899: 160)

## The context of Kraepelin's work

Kraepelin arrived at the study of deviant behaviour after most of the events described in Chapter 2 had taken place. He was therefore the product of an environment which accepted unquestioningly the appropriateness of the methods and theories of medicine to the study of disturbing behaviour, but which had never seriously considered the problems this might present. While Kraepelin has been mildly criticised by modern writers for his insistence on a disease entity model, it may be argued that this aspect of his belief system, by acting as an obvious target for attack, has tended to obscure the problems of the wider framework within which he worked, as well as the fact that he failed to provide any evidence in support of his concept, (see, e.g., Wing, 1988). Kraepelin in fact appears to have been unaware of, or to have chosen to ignore, even the most basic principles of empirical enquiry – the need to present systematically gathered data, rather than to rely on personal experience and beliefs; the importance of clear description so that others can try to replicate the observations; the importance of reliability of observations and the dangers of question-begging. He appears also to have been unaware of the problem of how he could possibly know, in the absence of independent evidence, which of the many disturbing behaviours shown by asylum inmates were products of an unspecified brain disease. Given that the social context in which Kraepelin worked was one of relative *naïveté* in conceptual and methodological matters, perhaps these deficiencies are not surprising. What is surprising is that Kraepelin's work is given serious consideration by his successors – Strauss and Carpenter (1981) even claimed it to be the cornerstone of scientific psychiatry – and is subjected only to mild criticism by modern writers.

One further aspect of Kraepelin's working environment and population deserves detailed comment, but as the discussion applies equally to the work of Bleuler it will be postponed until the end of the next section.

## The work of Eugen Bleuler

Bleuler's major text – *Dementia Praecox or the Group of Schizophrenias* – was published in 1911. Gottesman and Shields (1982) noted that 'Bleuler had no major disagreements from Kraepelin's views on schizophrenia' (39). This was unfortunate, for it meant that Bleuler took for granted that Kraepelin had described a pattern which justified introducing the new concept of dementia praecox. Bleuler compounded the error by adopting his own set of criteria for inferring the concept as well as suggesting the new word schizophrenia, although he continued to use the term 'dementia praecox'. Wing (1978a) claims that Bleuler's 'schizophrenia covered all Kraepelin's sub-classes with the addition of paraphrenia' (2). But the lack of specificity of Kraepelin's descriptions, the confusion of his account of diagnosis and the lack of specificity in

Bleuler's account make it impossible to know whether the two were using the construct(s) as Wing claims. Because Bleuler, like Kraepelin, took for granted the validity of 'dementia praecox', his work was at best misconceived and at worst futile. In addition, most of the criticisms which were made of Kraepelin's writings apply also to Bleuler's. His work will therefore be reviewed less extensively than was Kraepelin's.

### The word 'schizophrenia'

Bleuler put forward three reasons for introducing the word 'schizophrenia'. He claimed, first, that the term 'dementia praecox' (which he called the name of the disease) 'only designates the disease, not the diseased' ([1911] 1950: 7). Why he thought it appropriate to coin a term denoting the person is not clear, and Bleuler offered no explanation. Wing (1978b) claimed that the availability of an adjectival form of the word made it more convenient, but for what or whom he does not explain. Bleuler's second reason reflected his belief that certain behaviours were 'characteristic of the illness': 'in every case we are confronted with a more or less clear-cut splitting of the psychic functions' ([1911] 1950: 11). The problems of the first part of this belief will be discussed below; it is worth noting, however, that Bleuler used the term 'splitting of the psychic functions' so loosely that it is impossible to know what range of behaviour was its source. Bleuler's third and, he suggested, most important reason for 'coining a new name' was that although he believed that the *construct* of dementia praecox was properly applied to people whose behaviour changed (in some unspecified way) relatively late in life and who did not merit the term 'demented', the *words* were inappropriate. The problems of holding this belief and retaining the construct, albeit retitled, were discussed in the previous section.

Bleuler created two dichotomies, in writing at least, within whatever behaviours were the source of his concept of schizophrenia. He called these fundamental and accessory symptoms and primary and secondary symptoms. Although the two are sometimes, apparently, taken as synonymous, (see, e.g., Gottesman and Shields, 1982), Bleuler's writings give no indication that he meant this to be the case; on the contrary, he appears to have attached quite different meanings to 'primary' and 'fundamental' and to 'secondary' and 'accessory'. In addition, some behaviours called fundamental symptoms appear later as secondary, while behaviours called accessory symptoms were later labelled primary. The number of dichotomies Bleuler created and the names he attached to them, however, are of much less importance than are the justifications he advanced for creating them. Because Bleuler did apparently create two dichotomies, they will be discussed separately.

## The fundamental/accessory dichotomy

Bleuler claimed that:

> Certain symptoms of schizophrenia are present in every case and at every period . . . Besides these specific, permanent or fundamental symptoms, we can find a host of other, more accessory manifestations . . . As far as we know, the fundamental symptoms are characteristic of schizophrenia.
>
> ([1911] 1950: 13)

Bleuler's claim to have identified behaviour 'permanently displayed in every case of schizophrenia' raises problems similar to those discussed in relation to Kraepelin's discussion of 'disorders which characterise the malady': Bleuler's claim demands that an independent and valid criterion be used to infer schizophrenia in the first place, before any statements can be made about 'behaviour displayed in every case'. Alternatively, if Bleuler was claiming to have observed a group, all of whom displayed behaviour not observed in other inmates, and that he introduced *his* schizophrenia on the basis of these, he was not justified in doing so unless he also provided evidence that the behaviours formed a meaningful cluster. A third interpretation, that these behaviours were Bleuler's diagnostic criteria, makes the statement self-evident, as every 'case' would have to display these to qualify as a 'case'.

Bleuler failed to meet either of the requirements demanded by the first two interpretations; indeed, he seemed to be unaware of the problem. He also made no attempt to provide evidence to support his assertion that all those whom he called schizophrenic, by whatever criteria, showed the same behaviour permanently. Bleuler dealt with this detail simply by claiming that 'it was proven that there exist certain constant symptoms' ([1911] 1950: 284). Bleuler appeared to contradict even his own use of 'fundamental symptoms' by claiming that 'at . . . times [the accessory symptoms] alone may permanently determine the clinical picture' ([1911] 1950: 13). This claim is apparently incompatible with his earlier claim that whatever behaviours he called fundamental symptoms were permanent and were present 'at every period of the illness', although it must be admitted that Bleuler's meaning here is obscure.

Bleuler claimed that certain behaviours were displayed only at some times by some of those he called schizophrenic; these were also, he claimed, shown by other inmates. The scope of the term 'accessory symptoms', which he applied to these behaviours, was sufficiently wide for Bleuler to group them into twenty-eight categories. The question arises of why Bleuler believed he was entitled to call the hundreds of behaviours in these categories symptoms of schizophrenia. This is not to suggest that his designation of some forms of behaviour as fundamental symptoms raises no problems; far from it, but Bleuler at least advanced criteria, however inadequate and unfulfilled, which he believed himself to be using. No criteria were put forward for the choice of behaviour as accessory symptoms. Nor did Bleuler describe any consistent relationship between fundamental and accessory symptoms, making it difficult to avoid the conclusion that the choice was arbitrary.

Although Bleuler did not spell out any clear relationship between fundamental and accessory symptoms, he appeared at times to imply that the latter were a result of the former. If Bleuler had observed a syndrome pattern, then such a claim might have been reasonable if 'fundamental symptoms' merited the term signs and if plausible theoretical links existed between his signs and symptoms. Not only did Bleuler fail to describe any of this, he apparently suggested a variety of directional links between fundamental and accessory symptoms. For example, fundamental symptoms were said to cause other fundamental symptoms and accessory symptoms were said to cause fundamental symptoms.

### Primary and secondary symptoms

Bleuler's second dichotomy was, he claimed, one which separated 'the symptoms stemming directly from the disease process itself' from 'those . . . which only begin to operate when the sick psyche reacts to some internal or external processes' ([1911] 1950: 348). Bleuler also claimed that '[t]he primary symptoms are the necessary partial phenomena of the disease' (349), thus seeming to imply that whenever events designated as the disease process occurred, then primary symptoms must follow. Yet Bleuler also stated that '[t]o start with [the disease] remains latent until an acute pathological thrust produces prominent symptoms, or until a psychic shock intensifies the secondary symptoms' ([1911] 1950: 463). He therefore implied that primary symptoms could not always be observed, which raises the interesting question of how Bleuler could infer them. He did not deal with this important problem, but it appears that his reasoning could be tautological. The secondary symptoms of hallucinations and delusions, for example, indicated to Bleuler the presence of a primary symptom, the predisposition to hallucinations, which was, in turn, claimed to be a necessary condition for the development of hallucinations ([1911] 1950: 349).

### The choice of primary and secondary symptoms

Bleuler stated that '*We do not know what the schizophrenic disease process actually is*' ([1911] 1950: 466; emphasis in original). Yet he still felt able to provide a list of 'symptoms stemming directly from the disease process'. It is difficult to understand how Bleuler was able to recognise the consequences of a totally unknown antecedent; inevitably, then, his criteria for applying the term 'primary symptom' varied from symptom to symptom.

The 'disturbance of association', for example, was regarded as primary 'insofar as it involves a diminution or levelling of the number of affinities', and because some 'confusional states usually occur without psychic occasion' and are 'sometimes . . . accompanied by a syndrome which we ordinarily associate with signs of infection or autointoxication' ([1911] 1950: 350). Certain pupillary disturbances were regarded as primary symptoms for no stated reason, but the conclusion was said to be 'assisted' by the claim that when such disturbances were observed, the 'cases . . . show a poorer termination than those with other kinds of pupillary disturbances' ([1911] 1950: 352). Bleuler at least made some attempt to justify these choices; with other types of behaviour said to be primary symptoms, no justification was given. Bleuler claimed, for example, that:

> most of the manic episodes appear to belong to the disease process itself.
>
> ([1911] 1950: 351)

> We can assume that the tendency towards stereotypy originates directly from the disease process.
>
> ([1911] 1950: 351)

> A part of these edemas appear to be directly conditioned by the disease process.
>
> ([1911] 1950: 352)

Bleuler's choice of behaviours as secondary symptoms appears to be based on the belief that they were 'subject to psychic influences'. Quite apart from the problem of how this decision was made and of the justification for calling some of the many inmate behaviours which must have varied with the environment, symptoms of schizophrenia, there are some interesting inconsistencies in Bleuler's writing. He claimed, for example, that the disturbances of affect were secondary because 'real destruction of affectivity cannot be proved, even in the most severe cases . . . some affects may be present and others not' ([1911] 1950: 353). But Bleuler also claimed that '[e]ven in the most severe cases the majority of the associations take the usual pathways' ([1911] 1950: 355), which can reasonably be interpreted, using Bleuler's language, to mean that 'real destruction of associational activity cannot be proved, even in the most severe cases'. Whatever Bleuler thought of as the associational disturbances, however, were 'conceived of as being primary' ([1911] 1950: 355).

As with 'primary symptoms', Bleuler designated various unspecified behaviours as secondary symptoms on the basis only of his authority:

> negativism is certainly a complex secondary phenomenon.
>
> ([1911] 1950: 354)

> it should need no proof that the disturbance of the complex functions of intelligence . . . the impaired synthesis of the total personality, the disordered strivings and efforts of the patients . . . the altered relations to

reality . . . are comprehensible only in connection with the already mentioned secondary symptoms; therefore they themselves are secondary
manifestations for the most part.

([1911] 1950: 354)

These problems highlight yet again the important general issue of how the
'symptoms of schizophrenia' were chosen. It must be borne in mind that
Bleuler, like Kraepelin, assumed that the brains of those called schizophrenic
had changed in some uniform way in structure or function. Whatever behaviour was said to be symptomatic of schizophrenia was assumed to be a direct or
indirect consequence of these changes. Bleuler, however, never demonstrated
that either of these assumptions was justified; indeed, he did not even systematically investigate them. Nevertheless, he believed that he could diagnose
schizophrenia and correctly designate some forms of behaviour as symptoms of
schizophrenia. Bleuler's account of diagnosis shows that, like Kraepelin, he
used many different criteria. These included unspecified styles of writing or
playing the piano; a 'will o' the wisp' gait; pupillary disturbances; the overall
impression (unspecified) received from an inmate and the inmate's remaining
'quantitatively and qualitatively rigid with regard to the same feelings, even
though he responds to ideas of varying values' ([1911] 1950: 300). If Bleuler's
criteria appear non-specific, this may be because '[j]ust how prominent the various symptoms have to be in order to permit a diagnosis of schizophrenia can
hardly be described' ([1911] 1950: 298). In addition to these diagnostic criteria, Bleuler designated many other behaviours as symptoms of schizophrenia.
*Which* behaviours were rarely specified, perhaps because, according to Bleuler,
speaking of his criteria for inferring affective disturbance 'it is easier to sense
these phenomena than to describe them' ([1911] 1950: 42).

One criterion which Bleuler did appear to use in designating behaviours as
symptoms was his belief about how normal people reacted to events:

> Even when the affects change, they usually do so more slowly than in the
> healthy . . . During an interview, a female patient was repeatedly shown
> the picture of a child. It took one-quarter of an hour for the corresponding
> sorrowful affect to appear.
>
> ([1911] 1950: 45)

> All the nuances of sexual pleasure, embarrassment, pain or jealousy may
> emerge in all their vividness which we never find in the healthy when it
> is a question of recollecting the past.
>
> ([1911] 1950: 46)

> During celebrations one can observe how much longer it takes the schiz-
> ophrenic to get into the party mood than it does the healthy person.
>
> ([1911] 1950: 45)

With this criterion in mind, it is interesting to note Bleuler's general account of some of the phenomena from which he inferred schizophrenia simplex:

> On the higher levels of society, the most common type is the wife (in a very unhappy role, we can say), who is unbearable, constantly scolding, nagging, always making demands but never recognising duties. Her family never considers the possibility of illness, suffers for many years a veritable hell of annoyances, difficulties, unpleasantnesses from the 'mean' woman . . . the possibility of keeping the anomaly secret is facilitated by the fact that many of these patients still manage to conduct themselves in an entirely unobtrusive way. Frequently, one is veritably forced to keep the situation secret from the world at large because there are many people who readily step in and defend these women who themselves know how to play the role of injured and persecuted innocence.
>
> ([1911] 1950: 236)

## Kraepelin's and Bleuler's population

Several writers (e.g. Strauss and Carpenter, 1981; Cutting, 1985; Hare, 1986; Der *et al.*, 1990; Brewin *et al.*, 1997) have remarked on the fact that the kind of 'severe and long-standing cases' described by Kraepelin and Bleuler are no longer seen, that certain symptoms of schizophrenia, particularly catatonia, are now rare or that the incidence of 'schizophrenia' appears to have sharply declined. These persistent observations suggest that there is some notable difference between Kraepelin's and Bleuler's population and that called schizophrenic today. There are indeed striking differences between the two populations. It is possible to say this because, although both Kraepelin and Bleuler consistently failed to specify the range of phenomena which was the source of their concepts, they did provide many specific descriptions of the behaviour of inmates said to be cases of dementia praecox or schizophrenia. Those few attempts to clarify the differences between early and modern populations always assume that Kraepelin and/or Bleuler 'discovered' or 'described' schizophrenia and that 'it' has somehow changed in presentation. Strauss and Carpenter, for example, imply that the difference might have arisen because 'schizophrenia' has inexplicably become less severe or is halted by modern drugs, but they provide no evidence that this is the case. But given the fact that neither Kraepelin nor Bleuler provided any evidence to justify their concepts, such question-begging explanations will not do. Instead, any explanation of the population differences must start from the premise that whatever Kraepelin and Bleuler did, it did not involve 'discovering' or 'describing' 'schizophrenia'. A more plausible explanation of the difference is that Kraepelin and Bleuler were dealing with a quite different population from that called schizophrenic today, and one to which the term would not now be applied.

I mentioned earlier that in Europe close links existed at this time between neurology and psychiatry and that, in Germany at least, the two professions were virtually one, in contrast with the modern position of two quite separate groups. The close links between psychiatry and neurology were in part the result of ignorance about both brain and behaviour; the separation of the groups increased as neurologists' and not psychiatrists' knowledge increased. Inevitably, then, Kraepelin and Bleuler would have seen people who would now fall within the orbit of neurology and not psychiatry. There is, in fact, a remarkable similarity between their descriptions of 'cases of dementia prae-cox/schizophrenia' and later descriptions of people said to be showing Parkinsonian sequelae to the (assumed) viral infection called encephalitis lethargica. These sequelae included dramatic and often bizarre cognitive, behavioural, affective and motor abnormalities. It is important to note that the pattern from which the concept of post-encephalitic Parkinsonism was inferred was first described in 1917 by Constantin von Economo – *after* Kraepelin and Bleuler had completed their major writings. Sacks (1971), however, has pointed out that various singular phenomena which were part of this pattern had been described often in the past, but without anyone 'seeing' the overall pattern, and that each generation apparently 'forgot' the observations of the previous one. Von Economo himself acknowledges that he was helped in 'seeing' the pattern by the sheer number of examples produced by the devastating European epidemic of encephalitis and its sequel between 1916–27, and by his mother's recollection of the Italian epidemic (the great *nona*) of the 1890s. Just how similar are the descriptions of Kraepelin, Bleuler and von Economo, and how different from modern descriptions of 'schizophrenia', can be seen from Table 3.1. In addition to the phenomena listed there, Kraepelin, Bleuler and von Economo also described marked peculiarities of gait (Bleuler considered that he could diagnose schizophrenia simply by watching inmates walking); excess production of saliva and urine; dramatic weight fluctuations; tremor; cyanosis of hands and feet; constraint of movement and the inability, in spite of effort, to complete 'willed' acts. All three also described delusions and hallucinations of many sensory modalities while both Kraepelin and von Economo provided details of the severe structural brain damage which was revealed microscopically at post-mortem. Both stressed the great damage to nerve tissue and the proliferation and 'infiltration' of abnormal glia cells. Given that Kraepelin and Bleuler are credited with having first described schizophrenia 'so thoroughly and sensitively' (Gottesman and Shields, 1982) it is remarkable that with the exception of delusions and hallucinations, not one of the phenomena described above, and in Table 3.1, appears in the index of a comprehensive academic text on 'schizophrenia' (Neale and Oltmanns, 1980). This striking discrepancy provides further support for the conclusion that Kraepelin and Bleuler derived their concepts from a population which has little in common with today's 'schizophrenics'.

*Table 3.1*  Descriptions of dementia praecox, schizophrenia and encephalitis
lethargica/post-encephalitic Parkinsonism

---

The spasmodic phenomena in the musculature of the face and speech which often
appear, are extremely peculiar.

(Kraepelin, 1919: 83)

Fibrillary contractions are particularly noticeable in the facial muscles and 'sheet lightning'
has long been known as a sign of a chronically developing [schizophrenic] illness.

(Bleuler, [1911] 1950: 170)

As a rule, other spontaneous movements are associated with the choreic movements of
Encephalitis Lethargica, the myoclonus and fascicular twitches of the disease: an
important rhythmical and symmetrical flash-like short twitches of separate muscles or
groups of muscles.

(von Economo, 1931: 39)

Dufour has described disorders of equilibrium, adiadochokinesia and tremor which he
regards as the expression of a 'cerebellar' form of dementia praecox.

(Kraepelin, 1919: 79)

Constraint is also noticeable in the *gait* of the patients. Often indeed it is quite
impossible to succeed in experiments with walking. The patients simply let themselves
fall down stiffly, as soon as one tries to place them on their feet.

(Kraepelin, 1919: 148; emphasis in original)

In some cases the ataxia attains such a degree that the instability of gait, the deviation
towards one side, the tendency to fall backwards on standing, the tremor, the giddiness
and the nystagmus can only be ascribed to an involvement of the cerebellum in the
inflammatory process.

(von Economo, 1931: 32)

[Ermes] found that a fall of the leg held horizontally only began after 205 seconds [in
cases of dementia praecox], while in healthy persons it made its appearance on an
average after 38 seconds, at latest after 80 seconds. There followed then [in dementia
praecox] either a repeated jerky falling off with tremor or a gradual sinking.

(Kraepelin, 1919: 79)

if . . . one lifts up the forearm of a patient [suffering from the amyostatic-akinetic form of
encephalitis lethargica] the arm remains raised for quite a time after having been
released, and is only gradually brought back in jerks and with tremors.

(von Economo, 1931: 44)

During acute thrusts [of schizophrenia], though rarely in the chronic conditions, we
often encounter somnolence. Patients are asleep all night and most of the day. Indeed,
they often fall asleep at their work. Frequently, this somnolence is the only sign of a new
thrust of the malady.

(Bleuler, [1911] 1950: 169)

In the now increasing somnolence [of the acute phase of the somnolent ophthalmoplegic
form of encephalitis lethargica] one often observes that the patients, left to themselves,
fall asleep in the act of sitting or standing or even while walking . . . [somnolence] is
repeatedly found in quite slight cases as the only well marked symptom.

(von Economo, 1931: 27)

*Table 3.1* continued

Hoche also mentions the markedly increased secretion of the sebaceous *glands* [in schizophrenic patients].

(Bleuler, [1911] 1950: 167; emphasis in original)

A hypersecretion of the sebaceous glands (probably centrally caused) causes the peculiar shining of the faces of these patients.

(von Economo, 1931: 46)

The tendency to edema [*sic*] is usually ascribed to poor circulation, but it may have other causes . . . in a physically strong female patient with a beginning mild schizophrenia, edemas were noted in the thigh area . . . At times more severe edemas may make movement painful.

(Bleuler, [1911] 1950: 173)

oedema of hands and feet . . . are . . . more frequent in the amyostatic than in the other forms of encephalitis lethargica.

(von Economo, 1931: 46)

In the most varied [schizophrenic] conditions, [the pupils] are often found to be unequal without having lost their ability to react . . . this pupillary inequality is rarely persistent; it often varies within a few hours, becoming equal or reversed.

(Bleuler, [1911] 1950: 173)

[The] behaviour of the pupils is of great significance. They are frequently in the earlier stages [of dementia praecox] and in conditions of excitement conspicuously wide . . . here and there one observes a distinct difference in the pupils. The light reaction of the pupils often appears sluggish or slight.

(Kraepelin, 1919: 77)

pupillary disturbances are very common. In patients [with the hyperkinetic form of encephalitis lethargica] one generally finds unequal and myopic pupils with a diminished and sluggish reaction but sometimes also one-sided or double or complete absence of reaction or an absence of light reaction only. These pupillary disturbances often vary considerably [in the same patient].

(von Economo, 1931: 38)

A differential diagnosis between [encephalitis lethargica and chorea] must necessarily be very difficult except where there exist for our guidance pupillary disturbances or other objective signs of encephalitis lethargica.

(von Economo, 1931: 39)

Contemporary neurologists, of course, noticed that von Economo's descriptions of 'encephalitis lethargica' and the sequelae, were very similar to what they had been used to calling dementia praecox or schizophrenia. Von Economo claimed that some people said to be suffering from schizophrenia were in fact cases of encephalitis lethargica, while Hendrick (1928) pointed to cases, supposedly of dementia praecox, where the diagnosis of encephalitis lethargica was confirmed at post-mortem. The problem was, however, that the validity of 'dementia praecox/schizophrenia' was taken for granted, so that it was assumed that Kraepelin and Bleuler had described a different disorder from von Economo but that it could be very difficult indeed to tell the difference between them. The criteria suggested for making this differentiation were, inevitably, vague, subjective and inconsistent:

> the [encephalitis lethargica] patient . . . can be shown much more easily than the schizophrenic to be highly sensitive and his withdrawal from contact with others is a motivated defence rather than a product of preoccupation and dulling of external interests . . .
>
> (Hendrick, 1928: 1007)

> Stransky in 1903 established the fundamental thesis that in the schizophrenic diseases an intra-psychic ataxia (that is a dissociation of the 'noö- and thymo-psyche') exists as a basic symptom. In this division he meant 'noö-psyche' to be the representative of the purely intellectual functions, while the 'thymo-psyche' embraced the urges, emotions and volition . . . In encephalitis lethargica, though no genuine dissociation as in dementia praecox occurs, an isolated disturbance of the thymo-psyche takes place, leaving the noö-psyche intact . . .
>
> (von Economo, 1931: 163)

By contrast, McCowan and Cook (1928) claimed that close observation would show 'some degree of mental degeneration in nearly every case [of post-encephalitic Parkinsonism]' (1316). They also claimed that 'The main criteria [for differentiating dementia praecox from post-encephalitic Parkinsonism] lie in the constant absence of inaccessibility and indifference in the typical emotional reactions of the encephalitic' (1318). But several of the cases they described and to whom they had given a definite diagnosis of post-encephalitic Parkinsonism, were said to show such indifference. This was then described as 'schizophrenic indifference', so great as to 'mask successfully the customary interest of the encephalitic in his illness' (1318).

The confusion was compounded not only by taking for granted the validity of dementia praecox, but also by the fact that the diagnosis of encephalitis lethargica was not straightforward. As von Economo pointed out, the initial infection was sometimes mild and sometimes severe and the sequelae could appear immediately or after many trouble-free years. In addition, what von Economo described as 'a remarkably constant' picture of brain damage was obviously not visible until post-mortem, while many other physiological functions were apparently within normal limits. It is likely, then, that in trying to tell the difference between 'schizophrenia' and 'encephalitis lethargica', the psychiatrists and neurologists were actually distinguishing amongst exemplars of 'encephalitis lethargica'. We must be very careful, however, of concluding that Kraepelin's and Bleuler's 'schizophrenics' were simply all

examples of post-encephalitic Parkinsonism. There is no reliable way of check-
ing the diagnostic status of Kraepelin's and Bleuler's populations and,
certainly, it might be objected that before the great epidemic the prevalence of
encephalitis lethargica/post-encephalitic Parkinsonism in Europe would be
insufficient to account for the large numbers said to be suffering from dementia praecox or schizophrenia. Sacks (1971), however, has claimed that the
prevalence of Parkinsonian sequelae of encephalitic infection prior to the great
epidemic may have been underestimated; he argues that variously named
European epidemics from the sixteenth to the nineteenth centuries may well
have been forms of post-encephalitic Parkinsonism. It is also interesting to
note here William Perfect's suspicion, recorded in 1787, that one contributor
to the increasing prevalence of insanity was 'the epidemic catarrh, more generally known by the name of the *Influenza* which raged with such violence . . .
in the year 1782' (Hare, 1983: 449; emphasis in original). It could be speculated that if these epidemics increased in extent or frequency in the nineteenth
century, possibly as a result of urban development, or if more people survived
the initial infection only to experience the sequelae, then this – and not an
increase in 'schizophrenia', as Hare claims – might in part account for the
rising numbers of cases of insanity. But to return to Kraepelin and Bleuler:
there are at least good circumstantial grounds for supposing that Kraepelin
and Bleuler were for the most part dealing with the consequences of some
forms of encephalitic infection and that a sizeable number of their patients
would later have been diagnosed as cases of post-encephalitic Parkinsonism. It
is notable, too, that papers which appeared at the time on 'organic aspects of
schizophrenia' (e.g. Hoskins, 1933; Hoskins and Sleeper, 1933), described
phenomena – pupillary disorders, polyuria; cyanosis – certainly not claimed
today to be part of 'schizophrenia' (see APA, 1980, 1987, 1994). And it was
exactly these symptoms, amongst others such as chronic constipation and
greasy skin, which were said to be shared by patients with schizophrenia and
encephalitis lethargica (Farran-Ridge, 1926).

   What appears to have happened since is that as post-encephalitic
Parkinsonism and other severe infectious diseases with their neurological
sequelae became rarer, and as neurology and psychiatry separated into two distinct specialisms, then the referents of 'schizophrenia' gradually changed until
the term came to be applied to a population who bore only a slight and possibly superficial resemblance to Kraepelin's and Bleuler's. This gradual
transformation of the concept, while at the same time retaining the idea that
Kraepelin and Bleuler discovered or first described schizophrenia, has probably proceeded without critical comment for several reasons. First, the habit of
taking for granted the validity of 'schizophrenia' has now, as much as in the
1920s, encouraged the idea that the concept, although problematic, could
eventually be sorted out and has discouraged any fundamental reassessment; its
gradual transformation might therefore have been mistaken for progress
because the nature of the transformation – from a neurological, physical and

behavioural concept to an entirely behavioural/experiential one – and its implications, were never made explicit. The transformation may have been aided,
secondly, by the fact that changes in the social and 'moral' behaviour of those
said to be suffering from encephalitis lethargica were emphasised by some
writers. A gradual shift in emphasis to types of disturbing *behaviour* as diagnostic criteria for schizophrenia might not, therefore, have been very obvious,
particularly as the same profession claimed jurisdiction over both disturbing
behaviour and disturbing neurology. Thus, the events described in the previous chapter, and particularly those at the end of the nineteenth century, were
especially important in allowing the transformation to a behavioural concept,
and in allowing the retention of somatic explanations. The idea that Kraepelin,
Bleuler and modern psychiatrists are studying the same phenomena may,
finally, have been encouraged by an emphasis on the similarities in Kraepelin's,
Bleuler's and modern descriptions of 'schizophrenia', and by a lack of discussion of the differences.

Those who use the modern construct of schizophrenia might object that any
similarity between Kraepelin's and Bleuler's populations and that of von
Economo is irrelevant, for two reasons. First, because Kraepelin's and Bleuler's
inclusion of these people was as a simple case of misdiagnosis and, second, that
the validity of the modern construct of schizophrenia does not depend on
Kraepelin and Bleuler but is justified by later research. Both of these arguments are questionable. To talk of *misdiagnosis* requires accurate *diagnosis*,
which in turn requires researchers' prior observation of a pattern of signs and
symptoms. It is precisely this prior observation which Kraepelin and Bleuler
were supposed to make but did not, and which therefore renders nonsensical
any arguments about misdiagnosis, or diagnosis, of schizophrenia or dementia
praecox. If Kraepelin and Bleuler did use phenomena from which we would
now infer post-encephalitic Parkinsonism, as part of a putative pattern said to
justify the introduction of dementia praecox, then, if these are removed, it *must*
be demonstrated that the remaining phenomena form a pattern which justifies
inferring a new construct. This rule is central to the construction of scientific
theories (Cronbach and Meehl, 1955). It is clear from Kraepelin's and Bleuler's
writings that neither the separation nor the demonstration was even
attempted, far less achieved. The second possible objection to the relevance of
any similarity between von Economo's and Kraepelin's and Bleuler's populations – that the modern concept of schizophrenia is not dependent on the
latter's work but has been validated by later research – is, of course, one of the
major issues being addressed in this book, but it is worth noting here that it
is difficult to reconcile with the attention paid by modern writers to the work
of Kraepelin and Bleuler and with persistent attempts to present the modern
concept of schizophrenia as 'originating' in this work (I will return to this issue
in Chapter 7).

We could reasonably argue, of course, that the question of Kraepelin's and
Bleuler's populations is irrelevant because their writings provide no evidence

that they were justified in inferring any hypothetical construct. The issue is raised here because it may help explain some of the undoubted differences between Kraepelin's and Bleuler's population and that called schizophrenic today, and help account for some of the problems encountered by the modern concept.

Before the work of Kurt Schneider is reviewed, it would be useful to jump forward for a moment, because the suggestions made here about the origins of 'schizophrenia' might encourage the conclusion that later suggestions of it being an infectious disease have some validity (see, e.g., Crow, 1984; Hare, 1983, 1986). There are, however, good reasons for assuming that this is not so. The first is that the suggestions take no account of the lack of evidence to justify the introduction of 'dementia praecox' and 'schizophrenia': they are based, as were the writings of neurologists at the time, on the assumption that Kraepelin's and Bleuler's concepts were valid. The same confusion is evident in Crow's (1984) and Tyrrell et al.'s (1979) suggestion that schizophrenic symptoms are found in a variety of disorders, including infectious encephalitis. It might as well be claimed that humoral disorders are infectious diseases, or that symptoms of humoral disorders are found in a variety of other disorders. The second reason for doubting the validity of these claims is that the results of research relating to them are both inconsistent and extremely difficult to interpret (Crow, 1984; King and Cooper, 1989; Kirch, 1993). What might reasonably be suggested, however, is that some instances of bizarre behaviour which are at present construed as symptomatic of schizophrenia may have a viral or other infection as one antecedent. This is quite different from arguing that some types of schizophrenia may be viral in origin. Again, to use the previous analogy, that is like arguing that some types of humoral disorder may have been viral in origin. Looked at in one way, of course, they probably were, but we no longer consider it a useful kind of statement to make.

## The work of Kurt Schneider

Schneider's ideas have exerted a considerable influence on modern psychiatry, including on the development of DSM-IV's diagnostic criteria for schizophrenia, and on the diagnostic criteria for research which accompany the 10th edition of the International Classification of Mental and Behavioural Disorders (WHO, 1993). Schneider's 1959 writings will be examined here as they are a comprehensive and representative expression of his views (see also 1974).

Three aspects of Schneider's writings are noteworthy. First, he too begged the question of the validity of 'schizophrenia'. He took for granted that there existed a disease called schizophrenia but failed to provide any evidence in support of this notion. This is unfortunate – not only because none of his predecessors had provided the necessary evidence but also because Schneider added to the confusion by adopting yet another set of correspondence rules for inferring schizophrenia; more correctly, he adopted several sets because, like

Kraepelin and Bleuler, he used different criteria to diagnose schizophrenia in different people. Second, Schneider was closer to Kraepelin than to Bleuler in his orientation in that he tended to eschew theory and claimed to prefer pragmatic description. It is perhaps not surprising that many of his conclusions conflict with Bleuler's. Third, unlike Kraepelin and Bleuler, Schneider made virtually no mention of inmates' neurological or physical state but concentrated on behaviour; but he was still unable to ignore the fact that no reliable organic antecedents of whatever behaviour was the source of his concept of schizophrenia had been identified.

Schneider saw his major task as that of setting out criteria whereby schizophrenia might be recognised. He was therefore particularly interested in diagnosis or, more accurately, the identification of new exemplars of a previously observed pattern. Given that neither Schneider nor any of his predecessors presented evidence that such a pattern had been observed, it was inevitable that any attempt to pursue the task of diagnosis – which depended on such evidence – would end in confusion.

### Schneider's concept of illness

Schneider stated that:

> Illness is always a bodily matter . . . if [some organic disease process] is absent, description of psychic or indeed social peculiarities as if they were illnesses involves the use of unscientific metaphor . . . our criterion for psychiatric illness becomes reduced to the simple establishment of morbid organic change . . . our concept of psychiatric illness is based entirely on morbid bodily change.
>
> (1959: 7)

> In medicine, we take [symptom] to mean the sign of an illness, an understandable indication of an illness.
>
> (1959: 130)

Setting aside Schneider's confusion of the two very different terms 'sign' and 'symptom', he was apparently claiming that phenomena designated as symptoms are those which indicate that some morbid bodily change has occurred. Schneider also admitted, however, that morbid bodily change could not reliably be demonstrated in those whom he wished to call schizophrenic. The logical conclusion to have drawn, therefore, was that the terms 'illness' and 'symptom' were inappropriately being applied to 'social peculiarities'. But Schneider could hardly abandon these terms and still claim expertise over these behaviours. He therefore retained them by *assuming* an as yet unobserved morbid bodily change and by altering the meaning he had previously applied to 'symptom':

It would be wiser . . . [in the case of psychosis with no demonstrable somatic base] to understand by 'symptom' some generally characteristic, constant feature of a purely psychopathological nature that can be structured into an existing state with a subsequent course. In this case, the medical connotation of 'symptom' is abandoned . . . Thought withdrawal is at bottom not a symptom of the purely psychopathologically conceived state of schizophrenia, but is frequently found and therefore a prominent feature of it.

(1959: 131)

Schneider offered no justification for this question-begging argument nor for having altered what he claimed was the medical meaning of 'symptom' other than that 'It seems well worth preserving this particular meaning of "symptom"' (1959: 131–132).

Schneider thus appeared to designate as symptoms of schizophrenia any phenomena claimed to be frequently found and therefore a prominent feature of schizophrenia. This reasoning is of course similar to Kraepelin's and Bleuler's when they spoke of 'characteristic' or 'fundamental' symptoms, and the same problems attend it: Schneider's statement demands the use of valid criteria for inferring schizophrenia in the first place and ones which are independent of whatever behaviours are said to be found in association with 'it'. Because no such criteria were available, and Schneider certainly did not suggest any, his rule for calling certain behaviours 'symptoms of schizophrenia' must have been other than he claimed. It is, however, extremely difficult to deduce from his writings what it might have been.

### First- and second-rank symptoms

Schneider divided whatever phenomena he had chosen as symptoms of schizophrenia into first rank and second rank. The former included audible thoughts, the experience of influences playing on the body and delusional perceptions; the latter consisted of '[a]ll the other modes of experience that attend schizophrenia' (1959: 134). Schneider's criteria for calling some phenomena first-rank symptoms are unclear. At one point, he seemed to suggest that they are behaviours which appear only in schizophrenia and not in cyclothymia (1959: 135), and that some of them are highly specific for schizophrenia (1959: 120). These arguments, however, can be criticised on the same grounds as was Schneider's definition of symptoms of schizophrenia – that an independent criterion is needed for diagnosing schizophrenia before we can meaningfully talk of behaviour which only appears in schizophrenia. Alternatively, these statements may be interpreted to mean that 'first-rank symptoms' form a pattern which would justify inferring a hypothetical construct. Schneider, however, did not even attempt to present evidence that this was the case. He did, however, appear to make use of another criterion for choosing first-rank symptoms, which was the reliability with which it was claimed they could be observed. But no data were actually provided on reliability, and in any case it would have been irrelevant without evidence that the behaviours formed a pattern.

Schneider claimed that his first-rank symptoms had 'special value in diagnosis' (1959: 133) and were (for various individual 'symptoms') 'of extreme importance in the diagnosis of schizophrenia' (1959: 97); 'a particularly important sign for the diagnosis of schizophrenia' (1959: 99); 'of exceptional diagnostic importance' (1959: 104). It might be supposed that if Schneider had followed his own reasoning he would infer schizophrenia only if these behaviours were observed, although such an inference would not, of course, be justified. But this was not the case. Clinicians were apparently 'often forced to base their diagnosis on the symptoms of second rank importance, occasionally and exceptionally on mere disorders of expression alone, provided these are relatively florid and numerous' (1959: 135). Why these clinicians should be forced to make a diagnosis, rather than admit ignorance, is not explained. It is rather like claiming that a clinician was forced to make a diagnosis of diabetes mellitus in the absence of an abnormal response to glucose intake or of sugar in the urine, or forced to make a diagnosis of cancer in the absence of cells of a certain type, simply because someone reported tiredness or nausea. The analogy is not exact, however, because Schneider had never identified events of the status of glucose tolerance, etc., so that even in the presence of 'first-rank symptoms' he would still not be entitled to make a diagnosis.

The problem is compounded by Schneider's apparent confusion over the status of his first-rank symptoms. He claimed, for example:

> Delusional perception . . . is always a schizophrenic symptom, if not always an indication of what we clinically are used to calling a schizophrenia.
>
> (1959: 104–105)

and

> Where there is delusional perception we are always dealing with schizophrenic psychosis . . .
>
> (1959: 106)

Further evidence of Schneider's limited understanding of the close relationship in medicine amongst the activities of concept formation, theory construction and diagnosis is provided by his claim that:

> [The value of first-rank symptoms] is . . . only related to diagnosis; they have no particular contribution to make to the theory of schizophrenia . . .
>
> (1959: 133)

## An overview of the work of Kraepelin, Bleuler and Schneider

I suggested earlier that Kraepelin and Bleuler described a population quite different from that which would be diagnosed as schizophrenic today. There are indications that Schneider was already working with a rather different population from his predecessors, although the paucity of his descriptions makes it difficult to know if this was the case. Schneider, for example, placed much less emphasis on problems of voluntary movement and on various physical features (indeed, he scarcely mentioned them). He claimed also that insight into the illness was rare, where Bleuler had claimed it to be typical. (By 'insight' they apparently meant simply that the person agreed that their behaviour was strange or alien to them; von Economo and Kraepelin also provided many very similar descriptions of patients' attempts to account for their, to them, bewildering behaviour.) Schneider also mentioned a group of what he called elderly cranks who showed unspecified eccentric movement and speech; he claimed that these people were quite dissimilar to those to whom the term 'catatonic' was now applied, but unfortunately he did not say in what ways.

But the nature of the population studied by Kraepelin, Bleuler and Schneider is less important than the fact that none of them presented evidence of having observed a set of regularities which would justify inferring a new hypothetical construct, even without attendant assumptions about brain disease. Certainly, none of them identified a syndrome, although their frequent misuse of the term 'sign' might convey the erroneous impression that they, or someone, had done so. But what is perhaps most remarkable about their work is that, in spite of aligning themselves to a scientific framework, not one of them presented a single piece of data relevant to their assumption that they were justified in introducing and using the concepts of dementia praecox and schizophrenia. They presented instead their own beliefs, backed up by authority.

Nevertheless, in spite of the lack of evidence that the necessary conditions for inferring schizophrenia had been fulfilled, the concept continued – and continues – to be used. This raises the important questions of what correspondence rules are now used to infer the concept and where have they come from? As correspondence rules can be seen, at their most basic level, as a statement of 'necessary conditions which have been fulfilled', the question is obviously an interesting and extremely important one. The next two chapters will therefore examine what are conventionally known as diagnostic criteria for schizophrenia but which I will also call here official correspondence rules for inferring schizophrenia.

# Chapter 4

# The official correspondence rules for inferring schizophrenia

## I The development of diagnostic criteria

Official guidelines as to what should be observed for schizophrenia to be inferred have been set out in a series of publications by the World Health Organization (WHO) and the American Psychiatric Association (APA). WHO guidelines for inferring schizophrenia are included in the medical manual, *The International Statistical Classification of Diseases and Related Health Problems*, previously *The International Classification of Diseases, Injuries and Causes of Death*. Their inclusion there implies that the concept of schizophrenia is similar to concepts used in medicine and that the activity of psychiatric diagnosis is similar to that of medical diagnosis. The guidelines for inferring schizophrenia are therefore best examined, and the problems surrounding them best understood, in the context of a general discussion of medical diagnosis. The first part of this chapter will therefore be concerned with describing the activity of medical diagnosis and its theoretical background, as well as with some of the most frequent misconceptions to be found in the literature on psychiatric diagnosis. The second part will describe and evaluate the early development of 'official' diagnostic criteria for inferring schizophrenia.

## The nature of diagnosis

The word 'diagnosis' is derived from Greek and means to distinguish, to discern through perception. It is unfortunate that the term has come to be closely associated in the public mind with 'finding out what is wrong with someone' or with their functioning, and, indeed, has even been used in this way by some professionals (e.g. Silberman, 1971; Clare, 1976; Wakefield, 1999a, 1999b). Just as misleadingly, Kendell (1975b) has described 'diagnosis', in its active sense, as 'the process by which a particular disease is attributed to a particular patient' and, as a noun, as 'the decision reached, the actual illness attributed to that individual' (23). These definitions are unfortunate not only because Kendell's reifies concepts inferred from various biological and behavioural phenomena, and misleadingly calls them diseases and illnesses, but also because they obscure the complexity and variety of activity subsumed under the term 'diagnosis'. They also obscure its relationship to the activities of non-medical scientists. Given that users of the concept of schizophrenia claim scientific status for it, i.e. claim that their activities in relation to it are similar to the activities of other scientists in relation to their concepts, it is particularly important that these two aspects of diagnosis are not obscured if we are to evaluate claims made about 'schizophrenia'.

Put at its simplest, diagnosis is a matching task. Medical practitioners faced with people displaying various physical phenomena ask themselves to which if any pattern or set of regularities *already observed by researchers* these phenomena correspond. Obviously, in order to answer that question, the clinician must collect a considerable amount of information about the phenomena displayed by the patient, few of which may be visible at first examination. Clinicians will, however, look only at those aspects of the person's functioning they think likely to yield useful information. They will, in other words, ask themselves which already observed patterns include the immediately available information (e.g. headache, blurred vision, nausea, etc.). As I pointed out in Chapter 1, the same 'symptoms' form part of a number of different patterns which may only be differentiated by the presence or absence of events not immediately observable by the clinician (e.g. a malignant brain tumour). But the clinician may not be sufficiently knowledgeable about what researchers have observed and/or be unskilled at eliciting information about symptoms and so make investigations which lead nowhere. Those who earn a reputation as good diagnosticians tend to be distinguished by their extensive knowledge of patterns suggested by researchers, by their skill in eliciting information about symptoms and by their unwillingness to reach hasty conclusions as to which set of regularities is matched by the phenomena displayed by their patients. It may happen, of course, that an experienced clinician does not know of any already observed pattern which matches a patient's signs and symptoms. This may mean that the signs and symptoms are unrelated or that they represent a 'new' pattern – one which has not been previously observed.

Clinicians, however, do not communicate their conclusions in this kind of language. They do not say that Mr X displays a set of physical phenomena which match those observed by Dr Y in a group of research participants. Instead, they use one or two words, usually with the verb 'to have' – Mr X has multiple sclerosis/throat cancer/osteoarthritis, and so on. There are two main reasons for this. The first is that when researchers, both medical and non-medical, observe what is considered to be a set of regularities, their habit is to infer constructs from them in the way described in Chapter 1 and it is the construct name which often becomes the diagnostic label. The second reason for adopting this style of communication is quite different. It seems to stem from our persistent and problematic habit of talking about concepts inferred from biological or behavioural phenomena as if the concepts denoted real entities which were located somewhere within the person (Mr X *has* tuberculosis). To be accurate in communication, diagnosticians would have to report that, 'The phenomena observed in Mr X seem to match those already observed by Dr Y in research participants and from which Dr Y inferred the construct Z. I am therefore inferring the construct Z from the phenomena I have observed in Mr X.' Not surprisingly, doctors rarely make such cumbersome, if accurate, speeches.

Part of the complexity of medical diagnosis arises from the fact that the various sets of regularities suggested by researchers, and which form the basis of the matching task, are of very different types. Engle and Davis (1963) have outlined five different forms of regularity, which vary in terms of their specificity, the amount of variability shown from person to person and the extent to which the antecedents are known. Those clusters known as syndromes, and which were described in detail in Chapter 1, have been placed at the bottom of the list. This is because their antecedents are generally unknown and there is considerable variability amongst those who share some of the features which make up the clusters. Engle and Davis describe diagnoses based on these different sorts of pattern – that is, claims to have observed a new exemplar of the pattern – as being of 'decreasing orders of certainty' from the first to the fifth type of pattern. By this is meant simply that as the patterns suggested by researchers become less distinct and the variability amongst those who share some of the features increases, then the less 'certain' can a diagnostician be that the phenomena displayed by a particular patient correspond to one of them. The patterns from which, for example, frostbite and to a lesser extent cholera are inferred, are more specific and show less variability from person to person than do the patterns from which multiple sclerosis or rheumatoid arthritis are inferred. It follows that concepts derived from these different types of pattern will have more or less well-developed theoretical networks. Some are hypothetical constructs with well-developed networks; others, such as essential hypertension or dermatitis, are little more than summary descriptions with no theoretical network to speak of. It is the richness of the theoretical networks of concepts that determines the amount of information clinicians can give patients about 'their illnesses'. If concepts invoked at diagnosis have previously enabled predictions to antecedent events or processes, then patients will be told about 'causes'; if the progress of the pattern over time and the variables which influence it are known, then information about 'prognosis' can be offered. And, if it is known what can reliably be done to alter the pattern in a desired direction, then 'effective treatment' may be given.

Kendell (1975b) rightly describes the concepts which researchers infer from these different types of pattern (and which he misleadingly calls diseases; see also Kendell 1991) as having variable conceptual bases. For example, the correspondence rules for some of the constructs are based on morbid anatomy, for some on histopathology, and for others on the presence of a particular antecedent (e.g. a bacterial or viral agent). Kendell has therefore suggested that 'our present [medical] classification is rather like an old mansion which has been refurnished many times but always without clearing out the old furniture first, so that amongst the new inflatable plastic settees and glass coffee tables are still scattered a few old Tudor stools, Jacobean dressers and Regency commodes and a great deal of Victoriana' (20). Kendell appears, however, to be unnecessarily disparaging of medicine here. The range of patterns on which diagnosis is based will *always* be a mixture because they represent all that is hypothesised in medicine at any time. Because knowledge is always imperfect and some areas are always better described than others, the result will inevitably be this kind of hierarchy. As research proceeds, some concepts (e.g. Down's syndrome) move 'up' as their theoretical networks expand; others (e.g. wasting diseases, general paralysis) are abandoned as it is realised that they referred to several different patterns. Still others (e.g. tuberculosis) 'expand' as a common antecedent is found for what were once thought to be different patterns. And new concepts will be added as new patterns are described. There is no reason to suppose that this process of grouping and regrouping phenomena, of enriching, abandoning and adding concepts will not continue indefinitely. The result will only be a hierarchy whose contents change, so that two centuries from now it may look, to use Kendell's analogy, like a mixture of Art Deco, High Tech and whatever style is in vogue at the time. The twenty-third century's medical constructs will no doubt have as varied conceptual bases as have ours.

## International classification systems in medicine

When clinicians officially record the results of their assessments of patients, including their diagnoses, they do so in accordance with the 10th edition of the *International Classification of Diseases and Related Health Problems* (ICD) (WHO, 1992–4). The starting point of attempts to devise international classifications is usually taken to be 1853, when the International Statistical Congress asked William Farr and Mark d'Espine to draw up a nomenclature of the causes of death, which could be used in all countries. It was hoped that this would bring some order to the then rather chaotic system of recording medical statistics. Some clinicians, for example, were in the habit of recording a proximal cause of death (e.g. renal failure), but not the events leading up to it (e.g. carcinoma of the liver). Others might record a major antecedent but not its sequelae. Similarly, only some might record that the patient had just given birth or was known to be a heavy drinker. To add to the confusion, different names might be given to one concept, so that it looked as if two patterns were being referred to instead of only one.

The term 'nomenclature' refers to a list of approved terms for recording observations. In this context, nomenclature is in fact mainly a list of concepts and summary descriptive labels, derived from patterns of varying complexity suggested by researchers. The lists devised by Farr and d'Espine were regularly revised. Such revisions are essential in order to incorporate new concepts suggested by researchers as well as modifications of existing concepts. In 1899, the International Statistical Congress approved a resolution recommending that revisions be made every ten years. The modern International Classifications are not simply of causes of death. Their title – the *International Classification of Diseases, Injuries and Causes of Death* (until the 9th edition; now *Diseases and Related Health Problems*) – reflects the fact that a much wider range of phenomena are incorporated, an expansion which began in 1949 with the 6th revision. But nor is the International Classification just a nomenclature or list of concepts. It attempts to group together patterns from which the concepts are derived and which are thought to have important features in common, like an admittedly primitive Periodic Table. What might be called higher-order concepts, whose names usually reflect the supposedly important shared features, are then inferred from these larger groupings (e.g. 'infectious diseases'). It is this attempt at grouping which earns the title 'classification system'.

I pointed out earlier that the concepts included in medical classification systems are derived from different types of patterns. Some include events thought to be antecedents of other phenomena in the cluster; in other patterns, the antecedents are unknown. In the first type, the antecedents are varied – genetic, traumatic, viral, bacterial, and so on. Some patterns are defined in terms of a type of bodily reaction or by site of visible damage. Because some patterns meet more than one criterion for grouping them, and because our ignorance of bodily 'dis-ease' is so great, any attempt to group patterns according to what are thought to be important shared features will inevitably be both a compromise and temporary. The groupings and headings, or 'higher-order constructs' adopted by the 10th revision conference include Diseases of the Respiratory System; Diseases of the Nervous System; Endocrine, Nutritional and Metabolic Diseases and Symptoms, Signs and Abnormal Clinical and Laboratory Findings not Classified Elsewhere. Each heading is allocated a range of letter/digit combinations (e.g. infectious and parasitic diseases are coded A00–B99); the number of three-character categories (in this case 200) represents the number of concepts or terms which have been included under the main heading (i.e. the number of clusters which have been grouped together to form the larger group). This number represents a best guess as to how many, given the present state of medical knowledge, are necessary and may be the subject of heated debate within the revision committees. The clusters may be sub-divided again according to various criteria, by the use of a fourth digit (e.g. by body site or aetiological agent). The International Classification was thus envisaged by Farr and remains today a best estimate of the state of medical knowledge, with implications beyond the mere listing of approved medical terms. Researchers of course are not bound by this classification; indeed, as the system reflects a mixture of well-agreed empirical data, best guesses and ignorance, it is their task to provide data which will alter it. It is to this system that diagnosticians refer when they record their assessments of new patients or complete death certificates or other official forms. The system, however, tells them only in what terms and in what order to record their observations; it does not tell

them how to make a diagnosis. It does not, in other words, set out the correspondence rules for the concepts it lists. It does not do this because its
devisers are presumably aware that these are set out in numerous specialist
texts; it is to these that clinicians can refer to familiarise themselves with patterns suggested by researchers, with concepts derived from them, with their
theoretical networks and with the empirical data offered in support. Indeed,
ICD-10 describes itself as 'a system of categories to which morbid entities are
assigned *according to established criteria*' which is used to 'translate diagnoses of
diseases and other health problems from words into an alphanumeric code
which permits easy storage, retrieval and analysis of the data' (WHO, 1993:
2; my emphasis). In other words, it is rightly assumed that correspondence
rules already exist for the concepts included in the classification system. The
assumption is entirely reasonable, given that the very existence of the concepts implies the existence of patterns, of sets of observations, from which the
concepts were initially inferred. As we shall see, it was precisely the lack of
such patterns which caused so much trouble for psychiatric classification
systems.

## The ICD and 'abnormal' behaviour

Since 1949, the ICD has included a section (Chapter V) whose subject matter
is not unwanted physical phenomena but unwanted or disturbing behaviour.
Some of the events which led to medical men claiming expertise in deviant
behaviour were described in Chapter 2. It was emphasised there that in order
to claim equality with their colleagues in physical medicine, alienists had to
behave as far as possible in similar ways. It is therefore not surprising that as
well as calling the odd behaviour of asylum inmates 'symptoms of illness', and
searching for a particular type of pattern amongst these 'symptoms', alienists
also sought to develop international classification systems of their subject
matter. Having done so, they tried, like their physician colleagues, to use
them as a basis for diagnosis. Before their development is described, however,
some common misconceptions about diagnosis in psychiatry, and in some
cases about diagnosis in general, will be discussed.

## Diagnosis: some misunderstandings

### The subject matter of diagnostic systems

Many of those who apply the diagnostic terms of psychiatry and medicine
seem to believe that their subject matter is 'diseases', 'illnesses' or 'disorders'
(e.g. Stengel, 1959; Engle and Davis, 1963; Silberman, 1971; Kendell,
1975b; Klein, 1978; Spitzer and Endicott, 1978; WHO, 1992; APA, 1994).
These claims are suspect because they smuggle into existence the problematic
terms 'disease' and 'illness' and give the false impression that there exist 'out

there' readily recognisable phenomena called diseases which naturally form the subject matter of psychiatry. In doing so they obscure the fact that the terms 'disease' and 'illness' are popular or lay constructions whose referents change in idiosyncratic ways with time and place. This leads to reification and to the erroneous belief that researchers and diagnosticians 'name diseases' which are somehow possessed by people. WHO (1974) for example, claimed that 'the classification of diseases cannot begin without a list of agreed names of diseases in which each name stands for only one disease' (11), while DSM-IV talks of 'dysfunction[s] *in* the individual' and states that '[a] common misconception is that a classification of mental disorders classifies people, when actually what are being classified are disorders that people have' (APA, 1994: xxi–xxii; my emphasis).

Problems with the ideas of disease and disorder will be discussed in more detail in Chapter 7; for the moment, it is important to emphasise that it is no more possible accurately to define the 'natural' subject matter of medicine or psychiatry than that of, say, chemistry or geography. All that can be said is that people who call themselves psychiatrists or geographers or whatever tend by convention or even by public demand, to study certain phenomena. For medicine, these are usually physical events or processes which are distressing to and unwanted by the sufferer or others. For psychiatry, the phenomena of interest are experiences and behaviours which unwanted by the person themselves or by others and which are often assumed to be outside the person's control. The fact that some of these phenomena have in our culture been popularly construed as 'illnesses' or 'diseases', and have had various popular assumptions made about them, is no more relevant to their scientific study than is the fact that some of the phenomena now studied by astronomers or physicists were once popularly construed as 'magical' or 'miraculous'. What psychiatrists and medical researchers therefore try to classify are putative patterns of unwanted physical and behavioural phenomena. The arbitrariness with which particular phenomena are deemed to be part of or not part of the subject matter of psychiatry, and therefore deemed to form illnesses or disorders, can be seen in the way in which 'homosexuality' was removed by committee vote from the subject matter. This behaviour pattern therefore ceased, from one moment to the next, 'to be a disease'.

Because what are seen as unwanted and uncontrollable behaviours and experiences vary with time and place, so too does psychiatry's subject matter. The variation is more noticeable in psychiatry because what are construed as unwanted behaviours are generally more variable than are unwanted physical phenomena, although there is considerable variation even in these. It follows that any attempt to define the subject matter of medicine or psychiatry (which usually appears as attempts to define disease) can amount to nothing more than a description of how the term 'disease' is currently used. This point is emphasised by the views of Spitzer and Endicott in their discussion of the 3rd edition of the APA *Diagnostic and Statistical Manual of Mental Disorders*:

We believed that without some definition of mental disorder, there would be no guiding principles that would help determine which conditions should be included in the nomenclature, which excluded and how conditions should be defined. As we considered the many conditions traditionally included in the nomenclature, we realized that although the definition of mental disorder proposed at the time of the controversy regarding homosexuality was suitable for almost all of them, a broader definition seemed necessary.

(1978: 18)

Unfortunately, Spitzer and Endicott did not say for what or whom a broader definition seemed necessary, and it is notable that the devisers of the DSM are now castigated for adopting an overly broad definition (Wakefield, 1997a; Kutchins and Kirk, 1997). It is clear, however, that all anyone seeking to define 'mental disorder' can do – and, indeed, all that they actually do – is to attempt to find common features amongst behaviours said *by tradition* to form the subject matter of psychiatry, or behaviours they would like to form the subject matter of psychiatry, and call this a definition of mental disorder. Such an exercise would be of interest mainly to etymologists were it not for the fact that definitions constructed in this way are then illogically used to 'prove' that certain behaviours 'are manifestations of mental illness' and that they should therefore fall under the jurisdiction of psychiatrists.

The ideas that the subject matter of medicine and psychiatry is diseases or illnesses which exist 'out there', and that practitioners find diseases in people, are extremely tenacious. This is perhaps best illustrated by the fact that even those writers who are clearly well aware of the popular roots of terms like 'disease' and of the dangers of reification, persist in talking as if they had never made these points. Klein (1978), for example, after thoughtfully discussing the social conventions surrounding the terms 'disease' and 'illness', proceeded to put forward his own definition, as if it were somehow independent of these, as if it enabled him properly to call some behaviours manifestations of mental disorder or mental illness. Kendell (1975b, 1991), although clearly aware of the problem of reification, talks of 'diseases as concepts'. The confusion here is that it is not diseases that are concepts but that Kendell and others talk of *concepts* which claim scientific status as if their referents and theoretical networks were synonymous with those of the popular term 'disease'. In other words, they misleadingly call concepts, diseases.

### Syndrome as a cluster of symptoms

I pointed out in Chapter 1 that the term 'syndrome' refers to a type of pattern made up of events known as signs and symptoms, where the signs are antecedents of the symptoms and where the antecedents of the cluster are unknown. It is the presence of the signs in the cluster which suggests that it is not the chance co-occurrence of unrelated phenomena and which enables clinicians, however tentatively, to claim to have observed a new exemplar of a cluster. It follows that the term 'cluster of symptoms' means something quite different from that of a 'cluster of signs and symptoms'. There are, however, many examples in the psychiatric literature of the term 'syndrome' being used to mean a cluster of symptoms, as if this usage were synonymous with a cluster of signs and symptoms. Kendell (1975b), for example, appears to use the word syndrome to mean both a constellation of symptoms and a constellation of symptoms and signs. He also (1991) claims that a syndrome denotes 'a cluster of symptoms with a characteristic temporal evolution' (63); Spitzer and Endicott (1978) claimed that '[a] syndrome is a collection of symptoms (or signs) that co-vary' (29), while Miller and Flack (1991), in discussing 'the syndrome of schizophrenia', ask whether there is a universal 'group of symptoms' (146).

Spitzer and Endicott's definition seems to treat symptoms and signs as interchangeable, and there are many references in the literature to 'symptoms or signs' as if it did not really matter which was which. This confusion is echoed in the WHO (1994) listing of diagnostic criteria for research on 'schizophrenia' which calls its criteria a listing of 'syndromes, symptoms and signs' but without specifying which is which or how any of the criteria come to merit these labels. Similarly, Keith and Matthews (1991) provide a list of behaviours and complaints which are called 'symptoms' in the table heading but 'signs' in the following text. The problem with these loose usages of 'sign' and 'syndrome' is not that they violate some absolute or correct definitions of the terms, but that they obscure what is required in order to claim that the concept of schizophrenia refers to a meaningful pattern (i.e. that it has some claim to validity). I noted in Chapter 1 that before a hypothetical construct can be inferred from a putative cluster, there must exist some evidence that the cluster is meaningful, that it is not the chance co-occurrence of unrelated events or even illusory. I also noted that we may 'find' clusters in random data or mistake chance co-occurrence for meaningful covariation, and that the kinds of events called symptoms – subjective, overdetermined, widely distributed – were particularly likely to cluster or seem to cluster in ways which might or might not be meaningful. The inclusion of an event which can be reliably observed, and which is thought to be an antecedent of the symptoms, is therefore not an optional extra; it is crucial in helping to identify valid rather than illusory patterns. The use of the word 'syndrome' to refer to suggested clusters both with and without signs may therefore create the spurious impression that one is as likely to be meaningful as is the other. Similarly, using 'sign' and 'symptom' as if they were interchangeable, or without specifying which phenomena each term is being applied to, creates the impression that it does not really matter how we use these terms, when in fact it is crucial. These issues are not simply semantic niceties; the misuse of the terms 'syndrome' and 'sign' can create a spurious impression of validity for 'schizophrenia', an issue I shall return to in Chapter 7.

## The validation of psychiatric diagnoses

There are a number of references in the psychiatric literature to the idea that diagnoses should be valid or can be validated (e.g. Robins and Guze, 1970; Kendell, 1975b; Neale and Oltmanns, 1980; Andreasen and Flaum, 1991; Klosterkötter et al., 1995; Mason et al., 1997). But because diagnosis is a matching task, the result can only be described as more or less accurate, in the sense that what is claimed to be a new exemplar of a previously observed pattern is more or less similar to it. The term 'validity' is, of course, applicable to the construct originally inferred when the pattern was first described; obviously, if the construct was not derived from a meaningful cluster there can be no matching and no diagnosis. Thus, to make a diagnosis is to claim, implicitly, that the validity of the concept invoked has already been established. The confusion in the literature seems to arise from a failure to make the crucial distinction between the original research which seeks to identify new patterns and infer new constructs, and the later activity of identifying new exemplars of these patterns (i.e. diagnosis). As we saw in Chapter 3, this confusion was frequent in Kraepelin's, Bleuler's and Schneider's writings and is widespread in the psychiatric and psychological literature; part of its importance lies in the fact that to talk of 'validating diagnoses' can create the impression that repeatedly adjusting diagnostic criteria and then 'trying them out' is an appropriate route to progress, whereas it simply obscures the fundamental question of whether the concept invoked at diagnosis should have been introduced in the first place.

## The confusion of reliability and validity

The issue of reliability has been prominent in the psychiatric literature for at least the last forty years. This is perhaps not surprising given that concepts which claim scientific status should be derived from observations about which there is a high level of agreement. Early studies of diagnostic reliability, however, suggested that agreement amongst psychiatrists as to whether a particular concept should be inferred from someone's behaviour could be unsatisfactorily low (e.g. Beck, 1962; Beck et al., 1962; Ward et al., 1962; Spitzer and Fleiss, 1974; Kendell, 1975b). Perhaps because of this, when high levels of agreement have been achieved, they have often been overvalued. This issue of reliability, and the value which is placed on it, has now become so prominent in psychiatry that it deserves detailed discussion, not least for the ways it helps misrepresent the problems surrounding 'schizophrenia'; I will return to this issue in Chapter 7, but note here an important way in which agreement amongst clinicians about diagnoses of schizophrenia is often misrepresented as if it indicated validity. This is achieved through language such as 'core symptoms', 'characteristic symptoms', 'pathognomic symptoms' or 'salient features' to indicate behaviour which seems to be observed more often in those called schizophrenic than in people with other diagnoses, or to indicate behaviour which many clinicians seem to agree should be used in diagnosing schizophrenia. All that is happening here, of course, is that researchers are 'discovering' what definitions clinicians use, or what instructions they follow, in applying 'schizophrenia' or other diagnostic labels, and then talking as if this told us something fundamental about 'schizophrenia' rather than something about clinicians. It is like our agreeing to call 'tall' only people over 6 feet and then 'discovering' that being over 6 feet is characteristic of, or a core or salient feature of, 'tallness'. Similarly, clinicians agreeing on a diagnosis may indicate nothing more than their similar training or that they have been convinced by the same authorities; it certainly tells us nothing about the validity of any concept invoked at diagnosis.

### Categories versus dimensions

As Hempel (1961) has pointed out, the development of classification systems may be thought of as a special case of scientific concept formation. Unfortunately, these systems are often described in a language which obscures this important similarity and the impression is often given that classification systems consist of a set of entities which 'possess' certain definite characteristics: the idea that medical classification systems name single diseases is an example of this fallacy. As I noted earlier, classification systems are in fact attempts to group what are assumed to be meaningful patterns, on the assumption that some patterns are similar in important ways. But the patterns which form these groupings are often not discrete in that it may be difficult to observe a clear division between their presence and absence. The question then arises as to whether the same concept should be inferred from the 'semi-pattern' as from the 'full pattern'. An answer can only be derived empirically by asking in what way it would alter the construct's predictive power. It is this problem which is sometimes, rather misleadingly, referred to as that of borderline cases versus clear cases or typical cases. It is more usefully described by asking whether the correspondence rules should be stated in a dimensional (quantitative, quasi-linear) fashion and if so at what point it apparently ceases to be useful to infer the construct. Even when there is general agreement about this, there may still be gradations within the patterns. In medicine, these are usually called more or less severe cases. Some of the patterns which form the basis of medical classifications are thought to represent the co-occurrence of dimensional attributes, others categorical. In fact it is rarely possible to claim that a pattern either does or does not 'exist'. A pattern which appears to be either present or absent may only seem so because measurement is unsophisticated and subtle gradations in the attribute in question cannot yet be detected. The claim can perhaps most confidently be made for those few patterns whose antecedents include a known single dominant gene or a specific traumatic event, such as a snake bite or a gunshot wound.

Although it appears regularly in the literature of 'schizophrenia', and has apparently been used in an attempt to defend the concept (see Wing, 1988) or as a possible solution to its difficulties (Kendell, 1991; and see Chapter 8 of this book), the issue of categories versus dimensions is not especially relevant to schizophrenia, for two reasons. First, to ask whether a postulated pattern represents the co-occurrence of graded characteristics or is qualitatively distinct is to assume that a pattern has been observed in the first place. Discussion about whether schizophrenia should be a categorical or a dimensional concept therefore begs the more important question of whether the concept is justified at all. Second, it might be argued that the discussion is of limited relevance in the more general sense that constructs are inferred to aid the observation of 'new' events. This can be achieved by grouping either graded *or* either/or characteristics, although the theoretical networks derived from the former may be more complex. Perhaps the best reason to be aware of the issue is that ordinary language encourages us to believe that we are dealing with distinct and specific 'things'.

## The development of International and United States classification systems for 'abnormal' behaviour

Some of the many attempts by medical men to describe patterns of disturbing behaviour were briefly described in Chapter 2. These were distinguished mainly by their vagueness and multiplicity; by the last decades of the nineteenth century it was obvious, even to the most uncritical observer, that the result was chaos. In 1885, the Congress of Mental Medicine appointed a Commission to consider existing classifications and to derive one system 'which the various associations of alienists could unite in adopting' (Kendell, 1975b: 87). It is unfortunate that the Commission's brief was not more modest and realistic: that they should consider *why* classification systems were so numerous, why no two of them were in agreement, why the concepts were not tied to specified phenomena and whether it was possible at that time to derive *any* system based on more than the opinion of authority. Unfortunately, these issues were never given serious consideration; the Commission duly devised a system which can at best be described as arbitrary but which was officially adopted by the now renamed International Congress of Mental Science in 1889. The system consisted of eleven concept names and included those 'upon which the majority [of the Commission's members] were unanimous' while omitting those 'upon which opinion was divided'. The Commission claimed to have attempted, in spite of these disagreements, to include 'the principal forms of madness' (Kendell, 1975b: 88). The list included Moral and Impulsive Insanity, Insane Neurosis and Progressive Systematic Insanity.

There is no indication that the choice of concepts was based on anything other than the opinions of the commissioners; certainly no reference was made to where the empirical evidence which would have justified inferring them was to be found. Not surprisingly, the system was not much used. Indeed, in the absence of clear statements in the psychiatric literature of the concepts' correspondence rules and evidence of their validity, most of it *could* not be used for any constructive purpose, apart from to discover which terms were fashionable amongst some medical men of the day. This official attempt to classify disturbing behaviour was paralleled and followed by numerous others, equally devoid of an empirical base; none of them enjoyed extensive usage.

Kendell has suggested some reasons why these systems were not accepted by asylum doctors. The Commissioners, he suggests, were:

> forced to chose between several existing classifications, each acceptable only to its own authors; they were handicapped by ignorance of the aetiology of the conditions they were trying to classify; they were unable to agree amongst themselves whether classifications should be on the basis of symptomatology, psychology, aetiology or outcome or a combination of all four; and they were dealing with professional colleagues who were often as disinclined to have a uniform nomenclature imposed on them as they would have been to have uniform methods of treatment imposed on them.
>
> (1975b: 89)

These supposed reasons for the system's failure deserve comment, if only because they illustrate some of the ways in which psychiatric classification and diagnosis are misrepresented.

In the first place, neither the Commissioners nor the organisations they represented were *forced* – except by their own dictates – to choose between existing rival systems. They could have admitted the truth: that they were not in possession of the empirical data which would allow them to infer most of the concepts in their classification systems. Second, by claiming that the Commissioners were 'handicapped by ignorance of the aetiology of the conditions they were trying to classify', Kendell implies that patterns of deviant behaviour which would justify inferring hypothetical constructs ('conditions') had already been observed and that the problem lay in ignorance of the antecedents of these patterns. This was not so. It is worth remembering that these concepts were suggested before Kraepelin's 'dementia praecox'. Unfortunately, his habit of introducing concepts – of claiming to have observed patterns in the behaviour of asylum inmates – but without providing evidence in support, had a long history amongst asylum doctors, and the devisers of the early classification systems did not depart from this tradition. They were, in fact, hampered by nothing more – or less – than their ignorance of what might be the regularities in asylum inmates' behaviour *and* by their disregard of their ignorance. Kendell's accurate comment that the

Commissioners' colleagues were 'disinclined to have a uniform nomenclature imposed on them' reflects a remarkable state of affairs on which Kendell does not comment. Asylum doctors, or at least those desirous of professional advancement, repeatedly claimed to be scientific. They should, then, have recognised that this claim was incompatible with 'to each his own nomenclature' and have declared themselves powerless *without* agreement on concepts and their correspondence rules. This is not to suggest that they should have accepted the Commissioners' opinions but that they should at least have recognised the implications of their disagreements.

The next few decades saw no important developments in attempts to produce international classifications of deviant behaviour. Although Kraepelin's 'dementia praecox' and Bleuler's 'schizophrenia' were used by asylum doctors, their lack of an empirical base rendered them useless, except in so far as they gave an impression of progress where none existed.

### The beginnings of the modern International Classifications

In 1948, a major administrative change took place with the setting up of the World Health Organization. The old medical *International List of Causes of Death* was revised and renamed *The International Statistical Classification of Diseases, Injuries and Causes of Death*. This 6th edition contained, for the first time, a section listing concepts mainly derived from behaviour, so-called mental, psychoneurotic and personality disorders. The concept of schizophrenia appeared in this section as 'Schizophrenic disorders (dementia praecox)'. This was followed by a number of concepts, such as paranoid, paraphrenic and primary schizophrenia, said to represent sub-divisions of the major concept (the term 'concept' or 'construct' was never actually used). WHO obviously assumed that reliable correspondence rules were available for these and the many other concepts listed in Section V and took their validity for granted. The classification was therefore of very limited usefulness and inevitably was widely ignored. Those who did use the terms it contained presumably used their personal criteria for inferring them. This WHO attempt at the classification of deviant behaviour was ignored by United States psychiatrists (who had nevertheless co-operated in drafting it) to the extent of devising their own system: the 1st edition of the *Diagnostic and Statistical Manual of Mental Disorders* was published by the APA in 1952. The concept of schizophrenic reactions was used in place of schizophrenic disorders, and again the main concept was sub-divided.

Kendell (1975b) has claimed that the US classification was 'in many ways superior to its contemporaries elsewhere' (92). Given the purpose of the classification, the only relevant way in which it could have been superior would have been in listing concepts derived from reliably observed patterns and grouped according to shared features of demonstrated importance. There is no indication that this was the case. Rather, the 'superiority' apparently lay in the fact that the classification was 'widely available in a carefully prepared book-let' and that 'adequate publicity was given to its existence and to the need for all American psychiatrists to bring their own diagnostic predilections into line with its requirements' (92). Kendell has claimed that the new classification was also superior in that it provided 'working definitions or thumbnail descriptions of the syndromes concerned' (92). As with his comments on the earlier classifications, Kendell is again taking for granted that the concepts listed in DSM-I had been derived from previously observed patterns. The 'working definition' of 'schizophrenic reaction' was:

> This term is synonymous with the previously used term dementia praecox. It represents a group of psychotic reactions characterised by fundamental disturbance in reality relationships and concept formations, with affective, behavioural and intellectual disturbance in varying degrees and mixtures. The disorders are marked by a strong tendency to retreat from reality, by emotional disharmony, unpredictable disturbances in stream of thought, regressive behaviour, and in some, by a tendency to 'deterioration'. The predominant symptomatology will be the determining factor in classify-ing such patients into types.
>
> (1975b: 26)

Each 'sub-concept' was followed by a similar type of description, emphasising some aspect of the main description.

This kind of thumbnail sketch (though usually much less vague) is often used in medicine in answer to the question, for example, 'What is Aids?' The answers, which vary from writer to writer, are usually a mixture of imprecisely stated correspondence rules and parts of the construct's theoretical network. The accounts are not intended for diagnosticians but are often used to reduce a complex theoretical network to manageable proportions for non-specialists. Such accounts are often found in, for example, medical dictionaries or in books or magazines for the general public. But this kind of imprecise and incomplete account can only be given because a more complex set of correspondence rules and empirical data are available for the concept – the thumbnail description is merely a distillation of them. But neither reliable correspondence rules nor, therefore, a theoretical network existed for 'schizophrenic reaction'; the impres-sion of superiority produced by the working definitions was entirely spurious. The inevitable state of affairs prevailed after the introduction of DSM-I: many ignored it and those who tried to use it had to employ their own idiosyncratic correspondence rules.

### Attempts at solutions

In 1959, Erwin Stengel published a lengthy and influential report under the auspices of the WHO. He detailed the extent of rejection of Section V of the

6th (and similar 7th) edition of the International Classification. More important, he suggested possible reasons and remedies. Stengel described only some of the large number of classifications recommended for use by Psychiatric Associations in different countries and discussed some of those devised by particular individuals. He noted two features of these systems. First, they were based on what Stengel called symptomatology or syndromal classification; some classifications were based on assumed aetiology of putative clusters (usually simply organic or non-organic) and some on assumed psychological features. Second, Stengel noted that the concepts contained in these systems had not been defined; that is, there were no clearly stated rules for inferring them. Stengel's proposed solution to this problem was remarkable, as too was the fact that it had taken the best part of a century for the problem to be officially noted. In reaching his solution, Stengel was strongly influenced by a conference paper delivered by the philosopher of science, Hempel. Hempel had pointed out that the development of nomenclature and of classification systems was a special case of scientific concept formation and that the activities should therefore follow similar rules. He emphasised one of the fundamental tenets of scientific practice: that concepts must be tied to observable events. Where these consisted of a series of well-described operations, they might be called the operational definition of the construct. Hempel suggested, however, that 'mere observations' could and should count as operations. Hempel may have created some semantic confusion by suggesting this usage of operational definition, but the important point remains that he was simply emphasising that concepts must be tied to, and inferred from, an agreed set of observable events. Hempel then pointed out that psychiatric concepts were not tied to observables in this way; that is, there were no clear rules for inferring them.

Unfortunately, Stengel concluded from this that the answer lay in developing operational definitions for existing psychiatric concepts. It must be emphasised that Hempel had not suggested this solution but merely described the problem. Stengel's conclusion is false because, in scientific activity, the observations or 'operations' come *first* and the concepts *second as a consequence of them*. Concepts developed in this way come, as it were, ready equipped with correspondence rules; to suggest that it is reasonable to try to find these for existing concepts is nonsensical, a back-to-front view of research. This is of course not the case outside of scientific practice. In politics, law and religion, for example, authorities frequently suggest or impose new criteria for inferring what are acknowledged as non-scientific concepts, such as fair wage, criminal act, sin, basic necessities, and so on. These rules are developed according to a quite different set of procedures from those used by scientists. The rules vary, for example, with political or religious creed, with cultural beliefs or with economic factors. Concepts derived in this way are often then used for administrative purposes; they are certainly not expected to have predictive power.

In proposing that psychiatrists work in a direction opposite to that of scientists and try to find correspondence rules for their concepts, Stengel overlooked the resulting problem of how it could possibly be known which concepts justified the search, and what criteria were to be used in choosing them. Concepts are included in classification systems because they are assumed to be valid. But validity cannot be demonstrated without correspondence rules. Thus, to choose to include a construct in a classification system which claims scientific status is to imply that it is already tied to an agreed set of observables. Not surprisingly, Stengel's suggestions did not immediately result in the publication of a classification system complete with operational definitions. The Manual of the 8th edition of the International Classification was published without them. In 1968, a glossary of thumbnail sketches for each of the constructs in ICD-8 was published by the British General Register Office; in 1974 WHO published its own glossary. I noted earlier that these sketches presuppose that a concept is both tied to observables and has a theoretical network, and are neither intended for nor usable as diagnostic criteria. The compilers of the sketches were apparently unaware of this: Wing (1970) pointed out that the glossaries were produced in response to Stengel's call for operational definitions. The APA agreed, albeit reluctantly, to tailor the 2nd edition of their Diagnostic and Statistical Manual to the nomenclature of ICD-8 (APA, 1968). Like the HMSO and WHO glossaries, DSM-II presented thumbnail sketches for its constructs. 'Schizophrenia' (the DSM-I term schizophrenic reactions had been abandoned) now had three different sketches.

Unfortunately, it was still thought that the resulting confusion and rejection of the International and United States Classifications could be overcome by printing 'proper' operational definitions of, or correspondence rules for, schizophrenia and other concepts. Kendell (1972) for example, declared this the 'remedy for diagnostic confusion'. He reiterated Stengel's arguments and claimed that 'there is no alternative to defining schizophrenia in terms of its clinical features' (386). Kendell did not specify what he meant by 'clinical features', although he appeared to be using the term to mean certain types of abnormal behaviour. These must, therefore, be the behaviours from which schizophrenia is inferred. Kendell thus appeared to be arguing that there is no alternative to defining schizophrenia other than in terms of the behaviours from which schizophrenia is inferred. His argument in fact reduces to the circular statement that the devisers of the International Classifications must develop an operational definition (or correspondence rules) for schizophrenia in terms of its operational definition (or correspondence rules). In other words, Kendell, like Stengel, was instructing them to begin their task by assuming that they had already successfully completed it. This kind of tautological and question-begging argument is a predictable result of the suggestion that psychiatrists work backwards from concept to correspondence rules and of a failure to appreciate the problems which will inevitably result.

Neither Stengel nor Kendell was able to suggest how the devisers of the International Classification might find this operational definition or set of correspondence rules for schizophrenia, and the 9th edition (WHO, 1978) did not contain one. The Manual, however, did depart from tradition by including the thumbnail sketches which had previously been published separately. As before, the glossary was prepared for Section V only. Kramer *et al.* (1979) called this integral glossary a major innovation. It was certainly an innovation; it also highlighted the potentially embarrassing fact that the subject matter of Section V and the concepts based on it were claimed to be both the same as and different from those in the other, medical, sections. The devisers of Section V sought to explain this paradox:

> This section of the classification differs from the others in that it includes a glossary, prepared after consultation with experts from different countries, defining the contents of the rubrics. The difference is considered to be justified because of the special problems posed for psychiatrists by the relative lack of independent laboratory information on which to base their diagnoses. The diagnosis of many important mental disorders still relies largely upon descriptions of abnormal experience and behaviour and, without some guidance in the form of a glossary that can serve as a common frame of reference, psychiatric communications easily become unsatisfactory at clinical and statistical levels. Many well-known terms have different meaning in current use, and it is important for the user to use the glossary descriptions and not merely category titles when searching for the best fit for the condition he is trying to code.
>
> (Kramer *et al.*, 1979: 247)

At first glance, these arguments may have an air of reasonableness, but it is fallacious. The 'special problems' referred to are not, as is claimed, a lack of *laboratory* information (criteria) on which to base diagnoses, but a lack of *any* independent, agreed criteria. It was precisely this lack which led to the inappropriate call for operational definitions. It is not a necessary condition of medical classification systems that the patterns included in them include events observed in a laboratory. It happens, however, that 'laboratory information' often refers to phenomena which can be reliably observed and which reliably co-occur with symptoms. Without information of this type, whether observed in or out of a laboratory, there can be no claim to have observed a pattern and therefore no concept and no diagnosis. The devisers of ICD-9 thus overlooked the same problem as had their predecessors: how could a concept such as schizophrenia, lacking an agreed and valid set of correspondence rules and, thus, a theoretical network, come to have a thumbnail sketch based on these? The development of ICD-9 was, in fact, preceded by a series of international seminars attended by 'experts' (Kramer *et al.*, 1979); the results of the seminar concerned with 'schizophrenia' were published in 1965 (WHO,

1965). Participants took part in 'diagnostic exercises' in which they inferred concepts from written descriptions of people and from video recordings of interviews. The results were then scrutinised for areas of agreement in the use of the concepts. This kind of opinion survey could equally be used to discover how people use popular terms like 'moral' or 'ambitious' and so on, but it implies nothing about validity. How the results of this seminar were translated into the sketch of 'schizophrenic psychosis' is unclear. It is difficult to avoid the conclusion that the development of this sketch, and those which preceded it, represents simply an amalgam of the personal beliefs of prominent users of the concept of schizophrenia; that is, it is a social and professional stereotype.

## The development of DSM-III

ICD-9 was criticised for failing, yet again, to provide clear operational definitions of the concepts it contained; the sketches were rightly seen as unusable as diagnostic criteria. They were seen as such, however, not because of the way in which they had been developed but because they were not specific enough. It is difficult to overestimate the potential of this lack of specific criteria to cause real difficulties for the psychiatric profession. These debates on diagnostic criteria were taking place at a time when critics, particularly Thomas Szasz and Ronald Laing, were raising vociferous objections not only to aspects of psychiatric practice but also to its fundamental concept of mental illness. Yet here was a profession which could not even defend itself by describing the criteria used to identify the illnesses it claimed to diagnose and treat. The situation threatened to be not only a professional but a public embarrassment, or worse. The devisers of the 3rd edition of the *Diagnostic and Statistical Manual of Mental Disorders* (APA, 1980) were therefore determined to provide clear definitions or rules for inferring its major concepts and the manual therefore represents a landmark in psychiatric classification. It does so not only because it included specific diagnostic criteria but because, it was claimed, the committee which devised it made a conscious effort to use available 'scientific information in the development and evaluation of proposed nosological changes' (Kendler, 1990: 969). It was also claimed that on the publication day of DSM-III, 'the ascendance of scientific psychiatry became official' (Maxmen, 1985: 35). It was at this point, then, that references to 'science' became central in the presentation of psychiatric diagnosis. But I have argued here that the strategy used by the devisers of DSM-III and its successors – that is, to search for correspondence rules for an existing concept – is likely to be incompatible with claims for scientific status. The methods used for the search, and the claims made about the results, therefore deserve detailed consideration.

# Chapter 5

# The official correspondence rules for inferring schizophrenia

## 2 DSM-III, IIIR and IV

This chapter is concerned with the 'official' rules for inferring schizophrenia, as set out in the 3rd and 4th editions of the DSM. Although it is DSM-IV which is currently in use, I shall also examine DSM-III in some detail.[1] There are several reasons for this. First, as I noted at the end of the previous chapter, DSM-III was the landmark edition of the DSM, the first to include correspondence rules (diagnostic criteria) for its concepts. Subsequent editions have not made fundamental changes to the actual criteria for inferring 'schizophrenia', although the justifications given for producing particular criteria have changed. It is therefore important to examine DSM-III to evaluate the process by which the initial criteria were produced. Second, although the process of producing diagnostic criteria is presented as one of continual progress, in practice it is one of trying to repair the shortcomings of previous versions of the DSM while avoiding a fundamental examination of the validity of its diagnostic concepts. It is therefore difficult to appreciate the approach to producing schizophrenia's correspondence rules which was taken in DSM-IV, the reasons why it was taken and the problems encountered, without knowing something about the approach adopted in DSM-III and *its* problems. Finally, it is not unlikely that the approach or justificatory framework adopted by DSM-III will resurface at some future time when its problems have been obscured or forgotten, so that it might be as well to keep them in mind.

## DSM-III

The correspondence rules which DSM-III suggested as the source of schizophrenia are listed in Table 5.1. I emphasised in Chapter 1 that diagnostic criteria represent a statement of a pattern observed by researchers and from which they inferred the concept now to be invoked in diagnosis; that is, to be invoked in the process of recognising new exemplars of this previously

---

1 A text revision of DSM-IV was published in 2000, but the diagnostic criteria were not changed.

*Table 5.1*  DSM-III criteria for inferring schizophrenic disorder

A   At least one of the following during a phase of the illness:

   1  bizarre delusions (content is patently absurd and has no possible basis in fact),
      such as delusions of being controlled, thought broadcasting, thought insertion,
      or thought withdrawal;
   2  somatic, grandiose, religious, nihilistic, or other delusions without persecutory
      or jealous content;
   3  delusions with persecutory or jealous content if accompanied by
      hallucinations of any type;
   4  auditory hallucinations in which either a voice keeps up a running
      commentary on the individual's behaviour or thoughts, or two or more voices
      converse with each other;
   5  auditory hallucinations on several occasions with content of more than one
      or two words, having no apparent relation to depression or elation;
   6  incoherence, marked loosening of associations, markedly illogical thinking, or
      marked poverty of content of speech if associated with at least one of the
      following:

      (a)  blunted, flat, or inappropriate affect;
      (b)  delusions or hallucinations;
      (c)  catatonic or other grossly disorganised behaviour.

B   Deterioration from a previous level of functioning in such areas as work, social
    relations, and self-care.

C   Duration: continuous sign of the illness for at least six months at some time
    during the person's life, with some signs of the illness at present. The six-
    month period must include an active phase during which there were
    symptoms from A, with or without prodromal or residual phase, as defined
    below:

    *Prodromal phase:* A clear deterioration in functioning before the active phase
    of the illness not due to a disturbance in mood or to a Substance Use
    Disorder and involving at least two of the symptoms noted below.

    *Residual phase:* Persistence, following the active phase of the illness, of at least
    two of the symptoms noted below, not due to a disturbance in mood or to a
    Substance Use Disorder.

    *Prodromal or residual symptoms*
   1  social isolation or withdrawal;
   2  marked impairment in role functioning as wage-earner, student, or
      homemaker;
   3  markedly peculiar behaviour (e.g. collecting garbage, talking to self in public, or
      hoarding food);
   4  marked impairment in personal hygiene and grooming;
   5  blunted, flat, or inappropriate affect;
   6  digressive, vague, over elaborate, circumstantial, or metaphorical speech;
   7  odd or bizarre ideation, or magical thinking, e.g. superstitiousness,
      clairvoyance, telepathy, 'sixth sense', 'others can feel my feelings', over-valued
      ideas, ideas of reference;
   8  unusual perceptual experiences, e.g. recurrent illusions, sensing the presence
      of a force or person not actually present.

---

*Table 5.1*   continued

---

*Examples:* Six months of prodromal symptoms with one week of symptoms from A; no prodromal symptoms with six months of symptoms from A; no prodromal symptoms with two weeks of symptoms from A and six months of residual symptoms; six months of symptoms from A, apparently followed by several years of complete remission, with one week of symptoms in A in current episode.

D   The full depressive or manic syndrome (criteria A and B of major depressive or manic episode), if present, developed after any psychotic symptoms, or was brief in duration relative to the duration of the psychotic symptoms in A.

E   Onset of prodromal or active phase of the illness before age 45.

F   Not due to any organic mental disorder or mental retardation.

---

Source: Reprinted with permission from the *Diagnostic and Statistical Manual of Mental Disorders*, 3rd edn. Copyright 1980 American Psychiatric Association.

---

observed pattern. In suggesting these particular diagnostic criteria, DSM-III was therefore implicitly claiming that they represented a pattern of regularities, a group of phenomena which co-occurred above chance, which had previously been observed by researchers and which justified inferring the concept of schizophrenia. In support of this implicit claim, it was stated that:

> This manual utilises clinical criteria that include both a minimum duration and characteristic symptom picture to identify a group of conditions that has validity in terms of differential response to somatic therapy; presence of a familial pattern; and a tendency towards onset in early adult life, recurrence and deterioration in social and occupational functioning.
>
> (APA, 1980: 181)

This claim can be reworded to state that when individuals display particular behaviours in combination for a certain length of time, this is reliably associated with:

1   a different response to drugs (different, presumably, from instances where the same behaviours are displayed for a shorter period);
2   the presence of the same pattern in their family;
3   people of certain ages;
4   the recurrence of the same set of behaviours;
5   deterioration in social and occupational functioning.

It is this claim to predictive power which apparently justified the assumption that DSM-III's correspondence rules for inferring schizophrenia referred to a pattern and therefore that the diagnostic concept of schizophrenia had validity or some claim to scientific status. The arguments for and against the use of each of these standards for judging whether a pattern has been identified or whether an inferred concept is valid, are to some extent similar. But because they are complex and not identical, they are best discussed separately. It is important to emphasise that DSM-III was, in fact, making two claims about each of these five standards. First, that its correspondence rules for schizophrenia were reliably associated with them (i.e. that researchers had previously observed these associations), and, second, that the standards – age of onset, outcome, etc. – are appropriate for imputing meaningfulness to a proposed cluster (i.e. for claiming to have observed a pattern). These two claims will be considered separately for each standard.

## The diagnostic criteria for inferring schizophrenia are said to have validity in terms of:

### (1) . . . a differential response to somatic therapy

Unfortunately, it is not clear what specific claim was being made here, far less what evidence was offered in support. A paper describing the development of the criteria for inferring schizophrenia (Spitzer *et al.*, 1978a) was given in support of, apparently, all the alleged validating standards; no specific reference was given for the claim to a differential response to somatic therapy. Spitzer *et al.* claimed that DSM-III's diagnostic criteria were developed in order to relate diagnosis more closely to, amongst other things, treatment. They claimed to have done this, however, only whenever possible. The possibilities for relating the criteria to 'treatment response' were apparently limited: reference was later made to a 'vast literature' said to indicate that those called schizophrenic and who have a 'poor prognosis' differ from a 'good prognosis' group on a number of dimensions, including '*perhaps* treatment response' (491; emphasis added). From this 'vast literature', four papers were quoted. Two of these described the same study, written up by different members of the research team for different journals, and none of the four discussed response to somatic intervention. The devisers of DSM-III perhaps inferred response to somatic treatment from 'poor prognosis'; it appears that the diagnostic criteria were intended to identify a group who showed a 'poor prognosis' or tendency towards recurrence. The merits of this claim will be discussed later, but it is obvious that if certain phenomena persist or recur – that is, 'have a poor prognosis' – they have not been significantly altered by any intervention. Thus, DSM-III was apparently claiming two validating standards for the price of one. Certainly, no direct evidence was offered about the response to somatic intervention of people who show the phenomena listed in the diagnostic criteria.

But this hardly matters beside the fact that 'response to treatment' is almost always an inappropriate standard for claiming that a proposed cluster is meaningful. It is so because, as has so often been observed in medical practice, the same intervention is often appropriate for what are known to be different patterns as, for example, in the instance cited by Kendell (1975b) of aspirin being appropriate for rheumatism and toothache. And if response to intervention is often uninformative, then the *lack* of it, as apparently used by DSM-III, is even more so because the number of phenomena which do not change in response to a particular intervention is usually much greater than the number which do. Taking this argument to its conclusion, it might as well be claimed that the phenomena referred to by, say, multiple sclerosis, flat feet and brain tumours form a pattern because none of them is changed by treatment with antibiotics. Given these problems, it is extremely unlikely that *lack* of response to somatic intervention, which was apparently implied by DSM-III, can help to identify a pattern.

### (2) . . . the presence of a familial pattern

As with 'response to treatment' it is difficult to know exactly what was being claimed here. DSM-III, like its predecessors, included a long statement purporting to be what is known about schizophrenia. This sketch is organised under a number of headings, one of which is familial pattern. It was claimed that 'All investigators have found a higher prevalence of the disorder among family members' (186). This claim is a curious one. No explanation is given of how it could be possible to have studied 'the disorder', and to have charted its progress in families, in the absence of a reliable set of rules for inferring schizophrenia. The authors of DSM-III thus placed themselves in the paradoxical position (apparently advised by Stengel and Kendell) of devising criteria for inferring schizophrenia using research which assumed that the task had already been completed. The research to which DSM-III presumably refers will be discussed in detail in the next chapter, but some aspects of it need to be mentioned here.

First, because there were no agreed referents for schizophrenia, researchers have inevitably studied a variety of behaviours. Indeed, in many of the family studies it is impossible to know what was being studied because the specific criteria used to infer schizophrenia were not stated. Family members may well have resembled each other, but in what way is difficult to say. But even the conclusion that families resembled each other in some unspecified way is questionable – first, because researchers have not always reported the reliability of their inferences to schizophrenia, and when they have done (e.g. Gottesman and Shields, 1972) they have at times been dismayingly low; second, because researchers have rarely employed truly blind observation of participants and their family members. Taken together, these problems make the data from family studies virtually uninterpretable. Although it is presumably this research to which DSM-III was referring, it must be emphasised again that, in talking of a family pattern for the disorder, the authors of DSM-III are implying that *their* correspondence rules for schizophrenia have been found to run in families. Thus, the only admissible research for their purposes would be that which used the DSM-III criteria. There is no indication that any such research was carried out prior to the publication of DSM-III, far less that it supported its conclusions.

But even if it had been demonstrated that DSM-III's diagnostic criteria 'ran in families', this would not support the claim that the criteria denoted a meaningful pattern. It is easy to show that this is the case by taking any physical features or behaviour where family resemblance might be expected. Take, for example, large eyes, small nose and large mouth. If researchers could reliably identify people who showed all three features, then it is likely that the prevalence of *the cluster of three* would be higher in their family members than in the general population. It could not, however (and no doubt would not), be concluded that these three features formed a pattern which justified inferring a new construct. Rather, it would be correctly pointed out that each feature *independently* may show family resemblance and that their co-occurrence might therefore be by chance. Of course, people who have these features might be called attractive and mate with other 'attractive' people who are also more likely to show them. Their families might therefore show a considerably higher prevalence of the cluster of features than would the general population, but this would still not justify the conclusion that the three features formed a pattern. The same reasoning could be used for any arbitrarily chosen group of behaviours – for example, playing a musical instrument, smoking and attending church regularly. The mode of transmission from generation to generation might be different from that for physical features, but the argument remains the same.

The authors of DSM-III have therefore reached two false conclusions: one, that family studies show familial resemblance in a specified cluster of behaviours and, two, that even if this had been shown, it would justify imputing meaningfulness to this cluster. In referring to these family studies, DSM-III appeared to be confusing the original observation of a pattern with later attempts to elaborate the theoretical network of a concept derived from it. The presence or absence of family resemblance in an *already observed pattern* might help clarify the nature of its antecedents; they cannot themselves reliably indicate that a proposed cluster does form a pattern.

### (3) . . . a tendency towards onset in early adult life

In its sketch, DSM-III merely claimed that 'Onset is usually during adolescence or early adulthood' (184). This statement, of course, raises the same problems as does the use of 'family resemblance' – onset of what? The claim implied the existence of data which demonstrated that DSM-III's criteria first show themselves, as a cluster, during adolescence or early adulthood. The difficulties of using 'age of onset' as a standard for imputing meaningfulness to a proposed cluster were discussed in relation to Kraepelin's work in Chapter 3, but no mention was made of these problems in DSM-III; indeed, no justification at all was given in DSM-III for the claim that age of onset is usually during adolescence or early adulthood. Spitzer *et al.*, however, did attempt to provide one:

> [E]xperience in the DSM-III field trials forced us to re-consider the question of the appropriateness of a diagnosis of schizophrenia in an individual whose first episode of illness is diagnosed as Involutional Paraphrenia.
>
> (1978a: 492)

The language of this statement makes it difficult to know what was being claimed. Presumably the claim was that people who show a particular set of behaviours before age forty-five are different *in some important way* from those who show the same or similar behaviours at age forty-six or later. They presumably differ, that is, in some way which, if the groups were separated on the basis of it, would aid the prediction of previously unobserved events, different for the two groups. This interpretation is supported by Spitzer *et al.*'s conclusion that 'since it is likely that such conditions are fundamentally different from schizophrenia of early onset, we believe it advisable to limit the diagnosis of schizophrenia to individuals whose first episode of illness occurred before the age of 45' (1978a: 492). Unfortunately, Spitzer *et al.* provided no evidence that this was the case; indeed, they did not even say what this alleged fundamental difference might be. Rather, they resorted to their personal opinions and to unspecified experiences. That such a difference has never been reliably observed is attested to by the fact that no reference was made to it in the diagnostic criteria: the problematic 'age of onset' is used instead.

### (4) . . . a tendency to recurrence

Spitzer *et al.* (1978a) noted that in selecting criteria for inferring schizophrenia, one of their goals was to '[limit] the concept [of schizophrenia] so that it is not applied to individuals likely to return to an adequate premorbid level of adjustment' (490). (This did not, apparently, mean that those called schizophrenic using DSM-III's criteria would inevitably run a 'deteriorating course'.) DSM-III's claim that its criteria for 'schizophrenia' were reliably associated with particular events at follow-up (prognosis, outcome), appeared to be central to the assumption that they identified a group who shared *important* features and that they therefore allowed the inference to a hypothetical construct. As with the other standards for imputing meaningfulness, two separate issues need to be considered. The first is whether DSM-III's correspondence rules *were* reliably associated with whatever was meant here by a tendency to recurrence or poor prognosis; the second is whether, even if they were, this amounted to a demonstration of a pattern of events and therefore justified inferring a hypothetical construct.

*Do the correspondence rules indicate a 'poor prognosis'?*

Support for the assumption that the diagnostic criteria were reliably associated with 'poor prognosis' appeared to be drawn from three sources. The first was a study (Kendell *et al.*, 1979) purporting to show that a set of criteria very similar to those of DSM-III were 'the most predictive of incomplete symptomatic recovery and poor social outcome' (Spitzer *et al.*, 1978a: 490). The second source was research relating the initial persistence of 'abnormal' behaviour (i.e. the length of time the behaviour had been present before it was brought to the attention of a psychiatrist) and behaviour at follow-up. The third source was research purporting to investigate the relationship between 'prognosis' and the presence or absence of 'affective disorder' in those diagnosed as schizophrenic.

DSM-III's authors assumed that this research had identified a pattern of behaviours which were reliably associated with their own persistence or recurrence and with other negative phenomena such as unemployment or poor social relationships. Thus, the correspondence rules were based on those said to have 'most predictive power' in Kendell *et al.*'s study; they stipulated that certain deviant behaviours should have been 'continuously present' for six months and, finally, required 'absence of major affective disorder' before schizophrenia was inferred. Taken together, these phenomena were said to be associated with a 'poor prognosis'. The three sources of support for this assumption will be considered separately.

## KENDELL *ET AL.*'S STUDY

Between 1959, when Stengel first called for operational definitions of psychiatric concepts, and 1980, when the first 'official' set was published in DSM-III, a number of users of 'schizophrenia' published their own preferred sets of correspondence rules (e.g. Astrachan *et al.*, 1972; Feighner *et al.*, 1972; Carpenter *et al.*, 1973a; Spitzer *et al.*, 1978b). No two of these sets were the same and, as Fenton *et al.* (1981) have pointed out, all were to some extent arbitrary and none had demonstrated validity. Nevertheless, attempts were made to assess their relative merits, and the Kendell *et al.* study is an example of one such comparison.

Using their own preferred criteria, Kendell *et al.* inferred functional psychosis from the behaviour of 134 residents of a London hospital. Six to eight years later, 118 of these people were followed up and interviewed. On the basis of interview data and hospital notes, each of the 118 were rated on five variables: social isolation, persistent delusions or hallucinations, defect state, employment status and proportion of follow-up period spent in hospital. Scores on a sixth variable, called incomplete recovery from index episode, were derived from 'all the information available'. This score was called a global outcome rating. (Little information was provided about the specific phenomena used to infer these variables and to derive scores; no information was provided on the reliability of the ratings.) Shortly after these follow-up assessments had been made, the original interview data on the participants were examined to discover to what extent each person matched the (different) correspondence rules for schizophrenia suggested by Schneider (1959), Langfeldt (1960), Astrachan *et al.* (1972), Carpenter *et al.* (1973a) and Spitzer *et al.* (1978b). Seventy-five participants met none of these criteria; the remainder met between one and all of them (there is considerable overlap amongst the criteria). Kendell *et al.* then conducted a large number of paired comparisons to discover to what extent the application of each set of rules would separate subjects on each of the six outcome variables. Thus, all those who matched, say, Schneider's criteria were compared, as a group, with the group made up of all remaining participants, on every outcome variable. The same procedure was followed for each set of diagnostic criteria. Kendell *et al.* were thus able to construct, for each outcome variable, a kind of league table of the diagnostic criteria in terms of their ability to separate the groups on each outcome variable. For example, 45 per cent of those who matched Langfeldt's criteria were said to show incomplete recovery from index episode, versus 13 per cent of those not fulfilling the criteria. For Schneider's criteria, the figures were 31 per cent versus 17 per cent. Langfeldt's criteria were therefore placed higher on the 'league table', for this variable, than were Schneider's. For those outcome variables rated on a continuous scale, group mean ratings were compared.

It is from this data that Spitzer *et al.* (1978a) concluded that one of the sets of criteria used, the Research Diagnostic Criteria (RDC) (Spitzer *et al.*, 1978b), was the 'most predictive of both incomplete symptomatic recovery and poor social outcome'. For this reason, the RDC formed the basis of the DSM-III criteria. This conclusion is unwarranted because the data provided do not allow any comparisons *within each league table*; that is, they do not indicate whether any set(s) of diagnostic criteria were significantly better than any other at predicting outcome variables. Spitzer *et al.* appear to have drawn the false conclusion that a set of criteria which assigns 43 per cent of those who match it to 'persistent delusions or hallucinations', versus 8 per cent of those who do not, is 'more predictive' of this variable than a set of figures of, say, 36 per cent versus 8 per cent. The conclusion is false because no data are provided on the significance of the difference between the first and second sets of figures.

But even if Kendell *et al.*'s data *had* allowed statements about the 'most predictive set of diagnostic criteria', the implicit claim that the RDC are reliably associated with 'poor prognosis' is still problematic. It is so, first, because the RDC achieved the largest separation of groups on only two of the six outcome variables; on the remaining four, it achieved third, third, fourth and second places on the 'league table'. (It must be emphasised that all definitions of 'poor prognosis' are to some extent arbitrary; there is no question of Kendell *et al.*'s six variables necessarily being a 'better' definition than Spitzer *et al.*'s choice of two of these. The point is made merely to highlight the apparent arbitrariness of Spitzer *et al.*'s choice of the RDC as the basis of

DSM-III's criteria for inferring schizophrenia.) The implicit claim that the RDC are predictive of 'poor prognosis' is problematic, second, because on every outcome variable a large number of participants who fulfilled the RDC nevertheless did not conform to the criteria for poor prognosis. On the two variables for which Spitzer *et al.* claim the RDC was 'most predictive', 57 per cent and 35 per cent of subjects *failed* to show a 'poor prognosis'; that is, their delusions or hallucinations did not persist and their 'social outcome' was rated as good. On the remaining variables where either/or classifications were used, the figures were 57 per cent and 76 per cent. Thus, whatever definition of 'poor prognosis' is used, the RDC can hardly be claimed to identify a group which is homogeneous in terms of it. Spitzer *et al.* in fact claimed that they 'later concluded' that the RDC combined 'good' and 'poor' prognosis schizophrenia (491). They did not quote Kendell *et al.*'s study as having indicated this; they did not say what the source of their conclusion was. They did, however, claim that '[t]here is a vast literature indicating that [good and poor prognosis schizophrenics] differ markedly not only in prognosis, but also in family history, phenomenology, mode of onset, and, perhaps, treatment response' (491). The argument being pursued by Spitzer *et al.* is not clear; apparently, it is assumed that these alleged correlates of 'good and poor prognosis schizophrenia' justify the claim that the groups differ in important ways and so should be separated *and* that each group represents a pattern, thus justifying two hypothetical constructs – in this case 'schizophrenia' and 'schizophreniform disorder'.

Whether 'prognosis' can be used as a criterion of important within-group similarity will be discussed later. The problem here is to clarify Spitzer *et al.*'s arguments as to why and how the RDC should be modified so that they identify a group homogeneous for/reliably associated with, 'poor prognosis'. The solution – within Spitzer *et al.*'s framework – appears simple: if members of a group share some 'abnormal' behaviours but differ in prognosis and also differ *markedly* in family history, mode of onset and phenomenology, then the good and poor prognosis members can be identified using family history, phenomenology, etc. Inexplicably, again within their framework, Spitzer *et al.* did not choose to discriminate between the two groups in this way (i.e. they did not use family history, etc.) in the rules for inferring schizophrenia. On the contrary, they claimed that '[a]t the present time there is no entirely satisfactory method of separating [good and poor prognosis schizophrenics] on the basis of cross-sectional evaluation' (491). But cross-sectional evaluation, as used by Spitzer *et al.*, apparently means phenomenology. They are thus arguing both that good and poor prognosis schizophrenics differ markedly on phenomenology *and* that they cannot be separated on the basis of it. Then, instead of using any of the variables which they claim markedly differentiate good and poor prognosis groups, Spitzer *et al.* suggested that DSM-III's criteria should include six months of symptoms because '[s]ome evidence suggests that requiring 6 months of symptoms is among the most powerful diagnostic indicators' (491). This evidence, then, is the second source quoted in support of the association between a 'poor prognosis' and DSM-III's correspondence rules.

## PROGNOSIS AND 'SIX MONTHS OF SYMPTOMS'

Three references were quoted in support of the inclusion of six months of symptoms in DSM-III's correspondence rules. The first was a follow-up study by Astrup and Noreik (1966), the second a brief report (Sartorius *et al.*, 1978) on *Schizophrenia: An International Follow-up Study* (WHO, 1979) and the third a study by Tsuang *et al.* (1976). The three will be considered separately.

Astrup and Noreik claimed to have studied 'the natural course of illness in an unselected sample' because of 'varying diagnostic practices and diagnostic uncertainty' (12). In fact, their sample was pre-selected in two ways – in consisting of 'mental hospital cases' and of people to whom the term 'functional psychosis' had been applied, but by unspecified criteria. Astrup and Noreik reported follow-up data on two such groups, one admitted between 1938 and 1950 and one between 1951 and 1957. All were followed up at least five years after their first admission. Using information from a variety of sources – interviews with patients, their relatives or public health officers, questionnaires completed by patients and hospital notes – the participants were placed in one of five 'outcome' groups called: (1) severe schizophrenic deterioration; (2) characteristics of slight deterioration; (3) schizophrenic personality changes; (4) no schizophrenic personality change, but have had psychotic relapses during the last five years or reduced social adaptation because of neurotic or psychopathic traits; (5) well for at least five years. (1, 2 and 3 were together called schizophrenic outcome, with 4 and 5 being called non-schizophrenic outcome.) As well as being rated on 'outcome', participants were also rated on a number of variables using information recorded at admission and called, for example, symptomatology, intelligence, age of onset, body type, pre-psychotic personality and marital status.

There are a number of serious methodological weaknesses in Astrup and Noreik's study. They did not, for example, report on the reliability of outcome ratings nor on how the different sources of information – and these were different for different participants – were combined to give the global rating. They did report the extent of agreement on ratings of admission information. For some variables (e.g. marital status) this was obviously high; for others it was unsatisfactorily low. For the variable of interest here – 'duration of symptoms prior to first assessment' – raters disagreed on 29 per cent of participants. Spitzer *et al.* (1978a) however, made no mention of these problems and have apparently taken Astrup and Noreik's data at face value. The discussion here will therefore also do so to examine the extent to which these data, whatever their merits, justify Spitzer *et al.*'s conclusion that '6 months of symptoms is among the most powerful prognostic indicators'.

*Table 5.2* Outcome by prior duration of illness

| Outcome | Duration before admission (years) | | | | | | |
|---|---|---|---|---|---|---|---|
| | <½ | ½–1 | 1–2 | 2–5 | 5–10 | >10 | Total |
| Recovered | 93 | 12 | 10 | 4 | 2 | 0 | 121 |
| Improved | 138 | 35 | 18 | 22 | 9 | 9 | 231 |
| Schizophrenic personality change | 34 | 10 | 16 | 28 | 11 | 1 | 100 |
| Slight schizophrenic deterioration | 24 | 21 | 37 | 57 | 22 | 16 | 177 |
| Severe schizophrenic deterioration | 9 | 10 | 14 | 23 | 13 | 8 | 77 |
| Total | 298 | 88 | 95 | 134 | 57 | 34 | 706 |

Source: Astrup and Noreik, *Functional Psychosis: Diagnostic and Prognostic Models*, 1966. Courtesy of Charles C. Thomas, Publisher, Ltd., Springfield, IL.

Astrup and Noreik examined the relationship between the ratings made from admission information and outcome ratings using univariate and then multivariate analyses. In the first stage they calculated, for each admission variable, the distribution of participants on the five-point 'outcome' scale. Table 5.2 shows this distribution for the variable 'prior duration of illness'. No significance levels were reported; apparently on the basis of visual inspection, Astrup and Noreik chose a number of admission variables said to be related to 'favourable or unfavourable outcome' and used these in their multivariate analyses. Two aspects of the analyses are relevant here. The first is the way in which the variable 'prior duration of illness' was quantified and the second its fate in the multivariate analyses.

As can be seen in Table 5.2, Astrup and Noreik divided 'prior duration of illness' into six categories: <½ year, ½–1 year, 1–2 years, 2–5 years, 5–10 years and >10 years. If Spitzer *et al.*'s conclusion were reasonable, it would be expected that the outcome distribution for the <½ year group would be strikingly different from that for *all* other categories *and* that these would not differ significantly from each other. This last point is crucial: if two different constructs are inferred from 'less than 6 months' symptoms' and 'more than 6 months' symptoms' (as is the case in DSM-III) because their prognosis is said to be significantly different, it follows, using DSM-III's reasoning, that if '½–1 year of symptoms' is associated with a significantly different outcome distribution from, say, '2–5 years of symptoms', then a third construct should be inferred from this 'cluster'. This is exactly what emerges from an analysis of Astrup and Noreik's data. The outcome distributions for the <½ year and ½–1 year groups are indeed significantly different ($\chi^2$ = 32.46, df 4 $p$ > 0.001) but those for the ½–1 year and the 2–5 year groups are even more dissimilar ($\chi^2$ = 144.4, df 4, $p$ > 0.001). It can also be seen from Table 5.2 that the majority of those rated 'prior duration of symptoms ½–1 year' were rated as having recovered or improved. These figures hardly allow the conclusion that '6 months of symptoms' is reliably associated with a tendency to recurrence or a poor prognosis. Astrup and Noreik in fact chose to include 'prior duration of illness' in their multivariate analyses not because of differences between the <½ year and ½–1 year groups but because of the contrast between the <½ year and 2–5 year groups. It must be emphasised that it is not therefore being suggested here that Spitzer *et al.* should have chosen '2 years or more of symptoms' as part of the rules for inferring schizophrenia; to have done so would have been to ignore both the complexities of Astrup and Noreik's multivariate analyses and, more important, the problematic status of 'prognosis' as a validating standard.

Having chosen admission variables said to be associated with favourable or unfavourable outcome, Astrup and Noreik performed a number of multivariate analyses using, as is customary, different combinations of variables and different methods of analysis. As might be expected, their analyses showed that the power of the variable 'prior duration of illness' to predict 'outcome' varied from significant to non-existent, depending on which variables were included in the analyses – a point Astrup and Noreik emphasised. In one analysis, the independent contribution of each of seven admission variables, including 'prior duration' ½–2 years and >2 years, to an 'unfavourable outcome' was reported. For participants admitted between 1938 and 1950, the relative contribution of the two duration variables was 12.7 per cent (½–2 years; sixth highest out of seven) and 27.9 per cent (>2 years; second highest out of seven). For those admitted between 1951 and 1957, the corresponding figures were 19.1 per cent (third out of seven) and 31.3 per cent (first out of seven). The analyses were carried out again but now included thirteen variables, all said to be associated with an unfavourable outcome. For the 1938–50 sample (results were not given for the other group), the figures for the same two duration variables were 10.5 per cent (fifth out of thirteen) and 29.9 per cent (first out of thirteen). Although Spitzer *et al.* did not indicate from which of Astrup and Noreik's many analyses they drew their conclusion, it was probably from these. In doing so, however, they apparently overlooked not only the fact that it was 'more than 2 years' prior duration' and not 'more than 6 months' which made the *relatively* large contribution to the variance of 'outcome'; they overlooked also the remainder of Astrup and Noreik's analyses *and* their conclusions.

In eight later analyses (four each for the two samples), Astrup and Noreik used different combinations of variables to produce listings of the best predictors of 'unfavourable outcome'. For each set of participants, 'prior duration more than 2 years' was included in two of three listings (listings were not given for the fourth analysis). As would be expected, its predictive power varied depending on which variables had been included in the regression equation. Astrup and Noreik concluded from these analyses that the best predictors of unfavourable outcome in their data were clinical variables (i.e. ratings of initial symptoms), not prior duration.

The role of 'prior duration' was further examined in another series of analyses. These used a maximum likelihood method (Maxwell, 1961) which predicted the outcome rating which was most frequent for each paired combination of five 'symptoms' said to be displayed at admission. Astrup and Noreik's conclusions from this series of analyses are worth quoting in detail:

[T]he inclusion of duration of illness enhances the predictability to some extent (5.3% in the 1951–57 sample, 2.1% in the 1938–50 sample) but the number of symptoms predicts nearly as well as non-linear combinations of the five clinical symptoms . . . Though the inclusion of duration in a non-linear formula increases predictability for each of the original samples, these gains are not retained in cross-validation. It appears that the additive prediction based on the number of symptoms (excluding duration) leads to predictions that are about as good and more stable than the non-linear equation with or without duration.

(1966: 125, 128)

Three main conclusions can be drawn from Astrup and Noreik's study (ignoring its methodological problems). First, that Spitzer *et al.*'s conclusion that '6 months of symptoms is among the most powerful prognostic indicators' is, to say the least, an oversimplification of Astrup and Noreik's data. Second, the predictive power of 'prior duration' varies, depending on which variables are included in the analyses, from significant to non-existent. When it does emerge, it is as 'more than 2 years' prior duration' and not as 'at least 6 months'. Third, those variables which most consistently emerged as predictors of 'unfavourable outcome' were 'clinical symptoms at admission'. Because Astrup and Noreik rated the continued presence of these 'symptoms' as an unfavourable outcome, their data apparently suggest that one of the best predictors of extent of 'abnormality' at point B was extent of 'abnormality' at point A.

The second source of support quoted for Spitzer *et al.*'s conclusion that '6 months of symptoms is among the best prognostic indicators' is a brief report (Sartorius *et al.*, 1978) on *Schizophrenia: An International Follow-up Study*, a study conducted under the auspices of the World Health Organisation (WHO, 1979). This research was similar to that of Astrup and Noreik in that it examined the relationship between admission variables and outcome variables in a group to whom the term 'functional psychosis' had been applied. It is difficult to understand how Spitzer *et al.* reached their conclusion from Sartorius *et al.*'s report; certainly, it was not drawn by the report's authors. Sartorius *et al.* in fact concluded that 'no single factor and no combination of a small number of factors appear to be strongly associated with the course and outcome of schizophrenia' (107), and that:

the three classes of predictor (i.e. admission) variables [1. *sociodemographic*: social isolation, social status and marital status. 2. *past history*: history of psychiatric treatment, poor psychosexual adjustment and unfavourable environment. 3. *factors relating to the initial psychotic episode*: length of episode before initial evaluation, insidious onset, presence of precipitating factors, presence of derealization, affective symptoms or flattening of affect] were found to be about equal in their predictive power.

(1978: 108)

It was also noted, however, that the 'length of the psychotic episode before the patient's entrance in the study' was amongst the best (albeit weak) predictors of every outcome measure in both 'developed' and 'developing' countries. It may be that it was this last point which encouraged Spitzer *et al.* to draw their conclusion about six months of symptoms. The actual data reported by WHO, rather than Sartorius *et al.*'s report, will therefore be reviewed briefly here to assess the validity of Spitzer *et al.*'s conclusion.

The 1979 WHO report forms part of a larger study, divided into three phases – preliminary, initial evaluation and follow-up. Participants were drawn from psychiatric centres in nine countries. Diagnostic terms were applied to them in the second phase of the study, using the guidelines for Section V of the ICD-8 and the Present State Examination (Wing *et al.*, 1974). Forty-seven independent (predictor) variables were chosen for investigation in the third, follow-up, phase. These were rated from information collected at initial evaluation. The forty-seven predictor variables were divided into the three classes mentioned earlier – sociodemographic, past history and factors relating to the initial psychotic episode. Initially, 1,202 participants were evaluated; 906 were included in the multivariate follow-up analyses. Of these, 609 received a diagnosis of schizophrenia.

Participants were assessed by interview at two-year follow-up using four assessment instruments: The Present State Examination (PSE) to assess 'symptoms', a Psychiatric History schedule, a Social Description schedule and a Diagnostic Assessment schedule. With the exception of the PSE, no data were reported on the reliability of these instruments. Follow-up information from the Psychiatric History and the Social Description schedules was converted, by a different set of raters, to five 'outcome' measures; ratings on these served as the dependent variables in the multivariate analyses. The five measures were called social functioning, length of episode of inclusion, percentage of time spent in psychotic episodes during follow-up period, pattern of course and overall outcome. The relationships between the forty-seven predictor variables and the five outcome categories were calculated mainly by multiple regression. In some analyses, the results for the whole sample were reported with 'country' included as a predictor variable. In other analyses, results were reported separately for 'developed' and 'developing' countries; in yet others, they were reported separately for each country. The results can be summarised briefly. First, the proportion of variance accounted for by the five best predictors of any of the 'outcome' measures in either type of country was always small, with a range of 8–22 per cent. Indeed, WHO emphasised the weak relationship between its predictor and outcome variables. Second, the best predictors were different for the different outcome measures and for different countries. Third, although 'prior duration' appeared frequently amongst the five best predictors, it did not appear for every outcome measure. Nor did it appear for every country as a predictor of 'overall outcome'.

There is little in these results to support Spitzer *et al.*'s and DSM-III's assumption that the inclusion of '6 months of symptoms' in the correspondence rules for schizophrenia will reliably identify a group homogeneous for 'poor prognosis/tendency to recurrence'. Its inclusion becomes even more puzzling when two additional factors are taken into account. First, the variable 'social isolation' also emerged frequently amongst the best predictors of 'outcome'; like 'prior duration', it emerged on every outcome measure in both groups of countries. It is difficult to understand why DSM-III's authors did not therefore follow their own reasoning and include this variable in the correspondence rules for schizophrenia. Second, in all of these analyses, the predictor variable 'prior duration' was *continuous* with a range from 'less than one week' to 'five years or more'. It is therefore impossible, as with Astrup and Noreik's data, to draw any conclusions about the predictive power of a specific 'prior duration' – in this case '6 months or more'. Indeed, WHO mentioned 'more than or less than 6 months prior duration of symptoms' only to point out that dividing participants in this way could *not* explain the fact that almost twice as many of those from the 'developed' as from the 'developing' countries were placed in the 'worst outcome' category.

A third source of support was quoted by Spitzer *et al.* for the inclusion of '6 months of symptoms' in the criteria for inferring schizophrenia. This is a study by Tsuang *et al.* (1976) which compared three groups who had been given different diagnostic labels, on five variables. The three groups were called: schizophrenia, atypical schizophrenia and primary affective disorder; the five variables were called family history of psychiatric illness, precipitating factors, outcome, age at admission and sex. None of these had been used as a criterion for assigning the diagnostic labels.

Tsuang *et al.* chose a sample which had originally, between 1935 and 1944, been given a diagnosis either of schizophrenia or primary affective disorder, using unspecified criteria. This population was then re-divided by the authors, using hospital records, into 'schizophrenia', 'atypical schizophrenia' and 'primary affective disorder (unipolar or bipolar)', using the criteria based on those of Feighner *et al.* (1972). Spitzer *et al.* appear to have drawn their conclusion that '6 months of symptoms is among the most powerful prognostic indicators' from the fact that on follow-up, 44 per cent of the 'atypical schizophrenia' group were rated as recovered compared with only 8 per cent of the 'schizophrenia' group. An examination of Tsuang *et al.*'s criteria, however, shows that this conclusion is, once again, questionable. The 'atypical' group could differ from the 'schizophrenia' group in many ways apart from '6 months of symptoms'. They could, for example, have differed on social variables such as marital status (which appeared frequently in the WHO study discussed earlier, amongst the best predictors of 'outcome'). On the other hand, the two groups were not even required to differ on 'at least 6 months of symptoms', and data on participants' characteristics were not reported. It is thus impossible to deduce from Tsuang *et al.*'s data whether 'at least 6 months of symptoms' made *any* contribution to outcome ratings, far less how powerful its effect might have been. Certainly, the authors of this study drew no conclusions about '6 months of symptoms'.

None of the three studies quoted by Spitzer *et al.* justified the conclusion that including 'at least 6 months of symptoms' in the correspondence rules for schizophrenia would identify a group which was reliably associated with a 'poor prognosis/tendency to recurrence'. What may cautiously be concluded (bearing in mind the considerable methodological weaknesses of all three studies) is that, depending on the variables included in the analysis and on the culture in which participants live, there may be a relationship amongst the prior duration (unspecified) of some behaviours, their persistence, and other variables such as employment and social activities. How this conclusion might be interpreted will be discussed later.

### PROGNOSIS AND AFFECTIVE DISORDER

The third source of support for the assumption that DSM-III's diagnostic criteria are reliably associated with a 'poor prognosis' appeared to be the claim that those who displayed *both*, whatever behaviours are called symptoms of schizophrenia *and* behaviours called symptoms of affective disorder, had a more 'favourable prognosis' than did those who displayed only the first set of behaviours. It is, in fact, extremely difficult to know what DSM-III's authors *were* claiming. Spitzer *et al.* (1978a) claimed that the controversy over the relationship between affective disorder and schizophrenia was part of the good versus poor prognosis controversy. Unfortunately, they did not say in what way the two controversies are related. They claimed also that good prognosis and poor prognosis groups of schizophrenics 'differ markedly . . . in family history, phenomenology, mode of onset and perhaps treatment response' (490); but, as I noted earlier, they did not say what these differences were.

DSM-III's reasoning was further obscured by the fact that the correspondence rules for schizophrenia did not stipulate an *absence* of whatever behaviour is used to infer affective disorder; they merely stated that such behaviours 'if present [should have] developed after any psychotic symptoms or [should have been] brief in duration relative to the duration of the psychotic symptoms' (190). There is certainly no piece of research quoted in DSM-III which compares the 'prognosis' of two or three groups – one which displayed behaviours A, B and C ('schizophrenia') and then behaviours D, E and F ('affective disorder') and one which displayed behaviours D, E and F and then A, B and C, or one which displayed both sets, in any order, but with D, E and F displayed for a shorter period. Yet it is difficult to see how DSM-III's authors could have reached their conclusions about this part of the correspondence rules without the benefit of such research.

Of the studies which were quoted, none even allowed the conclusion that simply the absence of whatever was meant by 'affective disorder' was reliably associated with a 'poor prognosis' or its presence with a 'good prognosis'. Vaillant (1964), for example, followed up a group of people who had been admitted to hospital between 1947 and 1950 and given, by unspecified criteria, a diagnosis of schizophrenia. These people were rated on a 'prognostic scale' of seven variables claimed by Vaillant to be highly correlated in the literature with remission in schizophrenia. These were called: acute onset, confusion, depressive heredity, non-schizoid pre-morbid adjustment, clear symptoms of an affective psychosis, precipitating factors and concern with death. Seventy-seven per cent of those said to have achieved full remission were rated as showing clear symptoms of an affective psychosis; but so too were 49 per cent of those said not to have achieved full remission. From a correlational analysis, Vaillant concluded that 'the diagnosis "schizoaffective" attained prognostic significance only when the six other criteria were also applied to those schizophrenics who showed any depressive features' (i.e. those rated as showing clear symptoms of an affective disorder) (514).

Stephens (1970) reported a follow-up study of 349 people previously given a diagnosis of schizophrenia, reactive psychosis or cycloid psychosis. Forty-three variables 'thought to have possible prognostic significance' were correlated with ratings of 'outcome' as recovered, improved or unimproved, in two samples followed up for less than or more than ten years. In the first sample, the correlation between 'depressive features' and 'outcome' was 0.25 ($p < 0.01$); in the second it was 0.19 ($p < 0.05$). These figures did not apparently reflect the independent relationship of 'depressive features' to 'outcome'; it is likely to be lower than that reported here if the prognostic variables are correlated with each other. And Vaillant noted that in his data 'every favourable prognostic factor is positively correlated with every other favourable factor' (1964: 514). As would be expected from these low correlations, positive ratings of 'depressive features' did not identify a group homogeneous for 'good' or 'poor prognosis'; 43 per cent of those rated unimproved were said to have shown depressive features.

Three studies not quoted in DSM-III likewise cast doubt on the validity of its (apparent) conclusion that the presence of whatever behaviour is used to infer affective disorder is associated with 'good prognosis' when it appears in conjunction with the 'symptoms of schizophrenia'. Carpenter et al. (1978), as part of the WHO International Pilot Study of Schizophrenia, found no relationship between those behaviours whose absence or 'secondary presence'

DSM-III apparently requires, and ratings of 'outcome'. Vaillant (1978) found no differences in admission ratings of 'affective symptoms' amongst those participants whose 'schizophrenic' behaviour had persisted or recurred and those who no longer displayed this behaviour. And Gift *et al.* (1980) found a complex series of relationships between 'affective symptoms' and 'outcome' which depended on the criteria used both for diagnosis and for ratings of 'outcome'. (DSM-III criteria were not used.) In particular, higher ratings of 'depression' at admission, in conjunction with a diagnosis of schizophrenia according to Schneider's (1959) or Carpenter *et al.*'s (1973a) criteria, were associated with *lower* ratings of 'quality of work' at follow-up. This result is the opposite of that implied by DSM-III's criteria.

The authors of DSM-III appeared to have accepted as methodologically sound those research studies quoted in support of their claim that DSM-III's concept of schizophrenia was valid in terms of a 'tendency to recurrence' or 'poor prognosis'. But, as the analysis here has shown, even when methodological problems are ignored, the available data were not consistent with DSM-III's claim. On the contrary, the data here suggest that the correspondence rules were likely to be reliably associated with considerable heterogeneity in 'prognosis', however this is defined.

### Can 'prognosis' define a meaningful pattern?

I emphasised earlier that, as with the other standards for imputing meaningfulness to a suggested cluster, two separate issues were raised by DSM-III's implication that their correspondence rules for schizophrenia were reliably associated with 'poor prognosis'. The first is the extent to which this was in fact the case; the second is whether *even if it were* it could be concluded that the correspondence rules represent a pattern of regularities or events which co-occur above chance. As we have seen, the correspondence rules do not seem to be reliably associated with any particular 'prognosis'. For the moment, however, I will put aside that conclusion and assume that they are.

It would be tempting to conclude that the diagnostic criteria therefore represent a pattern of regularities, especially in the face of assertions such as that of Gift *et al.* that 'prognosis has often been used as a validating criterion for identifying disease entities' (1980: 580). The conclusion would, however, be false – as indeed is Gift *et al.*'s claim. Many of the problems of using 'prognosis' or 'outcome' as a standard for assigning meaningfulness to a cluster have already been discussed in detail in Chapters 2 and 3; I will mention here only some additional points of particular relevance to DSM-III.

In the research quoted by DSM-III's authors, 'prognosis/outcome' was defined in a number of different ways. The various definitions had in common that they reduced to statements about the *persistence* of various odd behaviours and to statements about their personal and social correlates (employment, social relationships, self-care, etc.). But the fact that behaviours persist does not indicate that they co-occur above chance; the behaviours could develop and persist independently, under the control of quite different antecedents and maintaining factors. Nor would the greater persistence of behaviours which had already been displayed for at least six months indicate anything other than that past behaviour predicts future behaviour. The same effect would be expected for many behaviours which may co-occur – smoking, learning a new language, taking up a sport, etc.; we should hardly be surprised to find that a greater proportion of those who have persisted at these activities for six months or more are likely to continue with them than is the case for those who started yesterday. Certainly, no conclusions can be drawn about the relationship of the behaviours to each other nor assumptions made about common antecedents. It would also be unremarkable to find that behaviours which represent considerable deviation from social norms, as do the so-called symptoms of schizophrenia, are associated with other social and personal difficulties. But neither this association, which is common to much socially deviant behaviour, nor its persistence allows the conclusion that these 'symptoms' form a meaningful pattern. Because social and personal difficulties may increase as the number of deviant behaviours increases, the spurious impression may be given that the 'symptoms' cluster together simply because they become more noticeable in combination. To draw this conclusion, however, is rather like concluding that the phenomena from which, say, multiple sclerosis, Parkinson's disease and rheumatoid arthritis are inferred form a pattern because the presence of all three sets is more likely to be associated with social and personal difficulties than is the presence of only one. Similarly, the 'outcome' of 'multiple sclerosis' may in some cases be identical, in social and personal terms, to that of 'rheumatoid arthritis', while two cases of 'multiple sclerosis' might have quite different 'outcomes'. But if the social and personal correlates of 'symptoms of schizophrenia' are omitted from a definition of outcome, all that remains is the persistence of the 'symptoms', which, as I have already noted, cannot tell us whether the behaviours in question form a pattern.

### (5) . . . Deterioration in social and occupational functioning

The authors of DSM-III claimed that its concept of schizophrenia was valid, finally, in terms of a deterioration in social and occupational functioning. No attempt was made to provide evidence that this was the case. Instead, DSM-III simply stated that '[s]chizophrenia always involves deterioration from a previous level of functioning during some phase of the illness in such areas as work, social relations and self-care' (181). The implication here was that a pattern of phenomena, from which schizophrenia could be validly inferred, had been found invariably to be associated with whatever was meant by a deterioration in social and occupational functioning. But it is then difficult to

understand why this 'deterioration' should have been included in the correspondence rules for schizophrenia in DSM-III. If 'schizophrenia' is invariably
associated with 'deterioration', then it follows that, whenever schizophrenia is
diagnosed, 'deterioration' will invariably be found.

Spitzer *et al.* failed to clarify the problem. As before, they offered only their
opinion in relation to this validating criterion:

> Central to our concept of Schizophrenia is the notion that the disorder
> interferes with normal social and occupational functioning. Yet occasion-
> ally one encounters individuals with one or more of the characteristic
> schizophrenic symptoms, such as bizarre delusions of longstanding, with-
> out any apparent disruption of their functioning. We believe that in such
> problematic cases the diagnosis of Atypical Psychosis is preferable.
>
> (1978a: 493)

It must be said that this use of 'deterioration in social and occupational
functioning' as a standard for claiming that a cluster of phenomena associated with such deterioration forms a meaningful pattern is unique in the
history of medicine, and it is not difficult to see why. Negatively valued
changes in these areas, which is presumably what DSM-III meant by 'deterioration', are common to so many physical and behavioural problems, and
may be the product of so many idiosyncratic factors, such as the level of skill
needed for an occupation or the presence of a supportive partner, as to be
useless as indicators of whether any of these physical and behavioural problems co-occur above chance. Where 'deterioration in social or occupational
functioning' is found in association with a cluster of behaviour, it could be
a result of just one of the behaviours in the cluster or the result of the
simple accumulation of independent problems. To these difficulties with the
criterion has to be added that of reliably describing this 'deterioration', free
of value judgements as to how people *should* behave in their working and
social lives.

## DSM-III's correspondence rules for schizophrenia: an overview

Relatively little attention has been paid here to the considerable methodological problems of the research quoted in DSM-III in support of its criteria for
inferring schizophrenia. This is for two reasons. First, the authors of DSM-III
have ignored most of them and I have tried here simply to compare their conclusions with the available data, whatever its merits, in order to indicate that
even these do not allow the conclusions. Second, to have concentrated on
methodological issues might have created the false impression that DSM-III's
authors simply needed to find or commission 'better' research. This might have
distracted attention from the three major issues raised by the development of

diagnostic criteria for schizophrenia – the inappropriateness of the task, the question-begging approach used and the use of inappropriate standards to assign meaningfulness to a cluster of behaviour.

It is clear that DSM-III's authors tried to create an impression of similarity between their work and that of medical and other scientists. They suggested that certain phenomena co-occurred above chance because their co-occurrence is reliably associated with other events; in this case, family history, age of onset, tendency to recurrence, treatment response, deterioration in social and occupational functioning. In doing so, however, they ignored the fact that they have worked in a direction, from construct to correspondence rules, opposite to that of the researchers they have tried to imitate *and* that they have used inappropriate standards to impute meaningfulness. They also argued, in a circular fashion, that DSM-III's concept of schizophrenia was valid in terms of some of the phenomena from which it was inferred. In addition, with the exception of deterioration in social and occupational functioning, not one of the events said to be reliably associated with schizophrenia could be measured *independently of the cluster from which schizophrenia was inferred*. The use of each of these standards therefore implied that a valid set of correspondence rules already existed for the concept, otherwise it was nonsensical to talk of family history (of schizophrenia), age of onset (of schizophrenia), etc. But it is axiomatic that in any attempt to demonstrate that a set of phenomena co-occur above chance, the cluster, and the event(s) said to be reliably associated with it, must be capable of being measured independently. Medical researchers do, of course, investigate family resemblance, 'prognosis', etc., but do so *after* a pattern has been observed and in order to elaborate a construct's theoretical network. The question arises, of course, of why DSM-III's authors used inappropriate criteria to impute meaningfulness. The answer, presumably, is that had they adopted appropriate criteria they would have been forced to the conclusion that no set of regularities which would justify inferring schizophrenia had ever been observed.

### A syndrome?

I pointed out in Chapter 1 that the term 'schizophrenia' is said to refer to a syndrome. This term was also adopted by DSM-III, but it is clear that DSM-III's correspondence rules for schizophrenia do not refer to such a pattern. There is no event included in them which could claim the status of a sign. Alpert (1985) has suggested that diagnosticians should give more weight to those events which can be reliably observed in the cluster from which schizophrenia is inferred; these, he has suggested, should be called signs. It is, of course, true that in medicine signs are, by definition, events which can be reliably observed. Alpert, however, was also suggesting that whichever of DSM-III's criteria could be reliably observed should be called signs of schizophrenia. But this ignores the important fact that the second part of the requirements for a sign, used in this sense, is that it be reliably associated with whatever events are called symptoms in such a way as to support the assumptions that the whole cluster forms a pattern *and* that the sign is an antecedent of the symptoms. It is not sufficient to take, as Alpert has done, a suggested cluster like DSM-III's for which this demonstration has not been made and arbitrarily choose to label as signs whichever of its elements clinicians can be trained to reach agreement about. It might as well be suggested that diagnosticians should place more emphasis on someone's height or weight, both of which can be reliably measured, in making a diagnosis of schizophrenia. If the analogy seems absurd, it is only because of the strong a priori belief that certain phenomena, which do not happen to include height or weight, are symptoms of schizophrenia.

Finally, two more aspects of DSM-III should be mentioned here – its description of 'sub-types of schizophrenia' and its use of 'multi-axial classification'. These are apparently seen as attempts to improve the classification system and to describe those to whom it is applied in more useful ways. But both of these 'improvements' are dependent on the assumption that the 'overall' correspondence rules for schizophrenia refer to a meaningful pattern. Thus, the grouping of this supposed pattern into subtypes is an attempt to specify patterns within the larger pattern, while multi-axial classification groups people simultaneously on several axes, the major one of which, in DSM-III, is the diagnosis. If, as seems to be the case, no larger pattern has been observed, and, therefore, no diagnosis can be made, then it is meaningless to talk either of subtypes or of DSM-III's type of multi-axial classification. Given the lack of evidence that those called schizophrenic share important features, it is not surprising that the sub-division of schizophrenia into various subtypes has not proved particularly useful (McGlashan and Fenton, 1991; Flaum and Andreasen, 1991).

## DSM-IIIR and DSM-IV

In 1987 the APA published a revision of DSM-III (DSM-IIIR), and in 1994 a fourth edition of the Manual. Although I will examine the changes made in DSM-IIIR, I will focus mainly on DSM-IV, partly because the 1987 revisions to schizophrenia's diagnostic criteria were claimed to be minor (Kendler *et al.*, 1989; Andreasen and Flaum, 1991; Andreasen and Carpenter, 1993) but mainly because it is DSM-IV which is currently in use, with a new edition not planned until around 2006, and most of the changes made in the 1987 revision were retained in DSM-IV. There are also various changes in wording across the three sets (III, IIIR and IV) which do not significantly affect the implied meaning; DSM-IV's diagnostic criteria can be seen in Table 5.3.

*Table 5.3* DSM-IV diagnostic criteria for schizophrenia

A  *Characteristic symptoms:* Two (or more) of the following, each present for a
significant portion of time during a one-month period (or less if successfully
treated):

  1  delusions
  2  hallucinations
  3  disorganised speech (e.g. frequent derailment or incoherence)
  4  grossly disorganised or catatonic behaviour
  5  negative symptoms (i.e. affective flattening, alogia or avolition)

  Note: Only one Criterion A symptom is required if delusions are bizarre or
  hallucinations consist of a voice keeping up a running commentary on the person's
  behaviour or thoughts, or two or more voices conversing with each other.

B  *Social/occupational dysfunction:* For a significant portion of the time since the onset of
the disturbance, one or more major areas of functioning such as work,
interpersonal relations, or self-care are markedly below the level achieved prior to
the onset (or when the onset is in childhood or adolescence, failure to achieve
expected level of interpersonal, academic, or occupational achievement).

C  *Duration:* Continuous signs of the disturbance persist for at least six months. This
six-month period must include at least one month of symptoms (or less if
successfully treated) that meet Criterion A (i.e., active-phase symptoms) and may
include periods of prodromal or residual symptoms. During these prodromal or
residual periods, the signs of the disturbance may be manifested by only negative
symptoms or two or more symptoms listed in Criterion A present in an attenuated
form (e.g., odd beliefs, unusual perceptual experiences).

D  *Schizoaffective and mood disorder exclusion:* Schizoaffective disorder and mood
disorder with psychotic features have been ruled out because either (1) no major
depressive, manic, or mixed episodes have occurred concurrently with the active-
phase symptoms; or (2) if mood episodes have occurred during active-phase
symptoms, their total duration has been brief relative to the duration of the active
and residual periods.

E  *Substance/general medical condition exclusion:* The disturbance is not due to the direct
physiological effects of a substance (e.g., a drug of abuse, a medication) or a general
medical condition.

F  *Relationship to a pervasive developmental disorder:* If there is a history of autistic
disorder or another pervasive developmental disorder, the additional diagnosis of
schizophrenia is made only if prominent delusions or hallucinations are also present
for at least a month (or less if successfully treated).

*Classification or longitudinal course* (can be applied only after at least one year has elapsed
since the initial onset of active-phase symptoms):

*Episodic with interepisode residual symptoms* (episodes are defined by the re-emergence of
    prominent psychotic symptoms); also specify if:
*With prominent negative symptoms*
*Episodic with no interepisode residual symptoms*

*Table 5.3* continued

---

*Continuous* (prominent psychotic symptoms are present throughout the period of
   observation); also specify if:
*With prominent negative symptoms*
*Single episode in partial remission;* also specify if:
*With prominent negative symptoms*
*Single episode in full remission*
*Other or unspecified pattern*

---

Source: Reprinted with permission from *Diagnostic and Statistical Manual of Mental Disorders,* Fourth
Edition. Copyright 1994 American Psychiatric Association.

### Changing the diagnostic criteria: rationale and a critique

As I have emphasised, the publication of diagnostic criteria involves the fundamental and implicit claim that the criteria reflect a previously observed pattern
of phenomena which is 'held together' by an underlying process and which justified the inference to a concept which is now invoked at diagnosis. The devisers
of the DSM do not explicitly have to make this claim for it to hold; it is simply
that without it their work is meaningless, at least in terms of the medical/sci-
entific framework they claim to adopt. It follows that the changes made to
DSM-III, and the criteria finally published in DSM-IV, should have been based
on research which supported this fundamental claim. It must be emphasised
that the fact of changing diagnostic criteria does not invalidate the claim that
the original criteria referred to a meaningful pattern. As I pointed out in
Chapter 1, diagnostic criteria change when an assumed pattern is shown to be
reliably associated with another event which can be reliably measured or measured at an earlier point in the pattern's development. For example, the assumed
pattern of distinctive appearance and slowness in learning which led to the concept of Down's syndrome was found to be reliably associated with chromosomal
abnormalities which can be detected before birth and have now become the
diagnostic criterion for 'Down's syndrome'. We should therefore expect that any
changes made in the diagnostic criteria for schizophrenia from DSM-III to
DSM-IV should bear at least some resemblance to this process. At the very least,
we should expect that the criteria for 'schizophrenia' published in DSM-IV
refer to some kind of meaningful pattern regardless of what was claimed for
DSM-III. The following sections will consider each of the main changes made
to the criteria between DSM-III and IV, in terms of the extent to which they
conform to the claims implied by the publication of diagnostic criteria.

### The duration criterion

DSM-III included one duration criterion which I discussed in detail earlier:
that a person had to show 'continuous signs of the illness' for six months

before a diagnosis of schizophrenia would be given. These 'continuous signs', however, could include what were called prodromal or residual symptoms (i.e. some deviation from 'normal' functioning such as social isolation and withdrawal) which did not amount to one of the 'full symptoms' listed in the diagnostic criteria, such as delusions, hallucinations or incoherence. DSM-III had not specified any time period for which these 'full symptoms' (called the active phase) had to be shown. DSM-IIIR retained the general six-month requirement, but specified that the active phase of 'characteristic psychotic symptoms' had to be present for at least one week, or less 'if the symptoms are successfully treated'.

Kendler *et al.* (1989) briefly justified this change on the grounds that 'the clinical concept of schizophrenia required sustained psychotic symptoms' (954), but they offered no clarification of this statement or of why one week was an appropriate choice. The issue of the duration of 'characteristic symptoms', however, became much more significant in the development of DSM-IV because the 10th edition of the *International Classification of Diseases* (WHO, 1992) included for the first time its own diagnostic criteria for the psychiatric concepts included in Chapter V. The ICD criteria for schizophrenia – devised by different people from those involved in the DSM – specified a one-month duration of these 'characteristic symptoms' before a diagnosis of schizophrenia could be made. This placed the devisers of the schizophrenia section of DSM-IV in a difficult position. They had committed themselves to an empirical approach to DSM-IV (Andreasen, 1991), yet by their own admission there were no empirical data which would guide them in choosing between one week or one month or, indeed, any duration of 'characteristic symptoms' (Keith and Matthews, 1991). At the same time, concern was expressed over the possible consequences of producing two quite different sets of diagnostic criteria for 'schizophrenia' in the DSM and ICD. Keith and Matthews (1991) tried to resolve the problem by tracing the origins of the one-month duration chosen for the ICD. Unfortunately, it seemed to have been justified only through its use in the Present State Examination (Wing *et al.*, 1974) as a 'comfortable period to keep in mind' when asking people to recall their or their relatives' behaviour (cited in Keith and Matthews, 1991: 56). In other words, it was justified in terms of the fallibility of human memory rather than empirical evidence. In the absence of any studies 'designed to evaluate whether 1 week . . . or 1 month of psychotic symptoms was a "better" length of time' (ibid.: 57), it is clear that the eventual decision to change DSM's diagnostic criteria to 'one month of characteristic symptoms' was made to avoid disagreement with ICD-10. Keith and Matthews (1991), for example, stated that 'our general recommendation . . . is to use diagnostic criteria that are consistent with the international diagnostic system' (51), while First *et al.* (1994) claimed that 'DSM-IV increases the required duration of active phase symptoms from DSM-IIIR's one week to one month . . . to increase compatibility with ICD-10' (19). Some attempt was made, however, to introduce a seemingly empirical element into the process. First *et al.* (1994) claimed that the change was also being made to 'reduce false positives', a statement which has no meaning unless we assume that independent evidence exists to show that DSM-IV's criteria provide a more accurate diagnosis of schizophrenia than DSM-III's. In other words, the notion of 'false positives' begs the very questions being addressed. Flaum and Andreasen (1991) also tried to create an impression of empirically based decisions when they claimed that the 'field trials' which preceded the publication of DSM-IV '[would] compare the overall diagnostic reliability of criteria sets that employ a 1-week or a 1-month threshold' (134). Whether or not this was done hardly matters, as the reliability of a set of diagnostic criteria tells us nothing about whether it refers to a meaningful pattern.

The six-month duration criterion, which in DSM-III and IIIR could include 'prodromal' or 'residual' symptoms, raised a different set of problems. The ICD criteria for schizophrenia did not include this six-month duration or the idea of prodromal or residual symptoms. The devisers of DSM-IV certainly considered deleting these aspects of the criteria, again to ensure agreement with ICD-10. In the end, however, the six-month duration requirement was retained. Flaum and Andreasen (1991) claimed that this was done because 'the literature reviews offered clear support for the 6-month duration threshold as a predictor of a schizophrenic outcome' (137). This statement is not true. My earlier analysis of the literature cited in support of including 'six months of symptoms' in DSM-III showed that the evidence simply did not support this conclusion. Indeed, even the authors of the literature reviews mentioned by Flaum and Andreasen concluded, in a considerable understatement, that 'the 6-month criterion suffers from less support than we would like'; they were able to justify its continued inclusion only on the grounds that 'the established use of this time period at least in American psychiatry may make its retention useful' (Keith and Matthews, 1991: 64).

The problem for the devisers of DSM-IV was that specifying in the diagnostic criteria some reasonably lengthy time during which the person had been behaving strangely, did appear to have some link to future behaviour or 'outcome', presumably for some of the reasons I discussed earlier which suggest that the link was likely to have been a self-fulfilling prophecy.

### Delusions and bizarre delusions

In DSM-III, provided certain subsidiary requirements were met (see Table 5.1), a diagnosis of schizophrenia could be given simply on the basis of 'delusions' In DSM-IIIR, only 'bizarre delusions' could themselves lead to a diagnosis; 'non-bizarre delusions' had to be accompanied by another 'symptom', such as prominent hallucinations or flat affect. No clear justification was provided for this change, far less any empirical evidence (see Kendler *et al.*, 1989), although it may have had something to do with the continuing importance attached to

Schneider's claims about 'first rank symptoms', as definitions of bizarre delusions and first-rank symptoms tend to overlap. The definition of 'bizarre' was also changed in DSM-IIIR, from 'content which is patently absurd and has no possible basis in fact' (DSM-III) to '[beliefs] involving a phenomenon that the person's culture would regard as totally implausible'.

The issue of bizarre versus non-bizarre delusions was raised again during the development of DSM-IV because it appeared that most of those who would receive a diagnosis of schizophrenia using DSM-III, but not using DSM-IIIR, were excluded by the absence of what were assumed to be bizarre delusions. There were, however, a number of studies which suggested that the reliability of judgements of bizarre and non-bizarre delusions was unsatisfactorily low (Kendler et al., 1983; Flaum and Andreasen, 1991; Spitzer et al., 1993), a finding which has received further support since the publication of DSM-IV (Mojtabai and Nicholson, 1995). This latter study reported inter-rater reliability (Kappa) of 0.38 using a definition close to that adopted by DSM-IV. Ironically, in Flaum et al.'s study, a group of participants who were also members of the DSM-IV Work Group on Schizophrenia and Related Psychotic Disorders, had the lowest agreement of all groups of participants. In spite of these problems, and the lack of any evidence to support its inclusion, the bizarre/non-bizarre distinction remained in DSM-IV.

## Deletion of the age criterion

DSM-III stipulated that the 'onset of the prodromal or active phase of the illness' had to occur before age forty-five. This criterion was deleted in DSM-IIIR and this change was maintained in DSM-IV. Kendler et al. (1989) provided three reasons for the change, each of which is problematic.

The change was justified, first, on the ground of lack of historical precedent for an age tradition. Clearly, this appeal to tradition has nothing to do with evidence: historically, there was no evidence for or against such a restriction. The second reason for the change concerned sex differences in 'age of onset'. Because women tend to receive a first diagnosis of schizophrenia at a later age than men, Kendler et al. claimed that any age restriction in the diagnostic criteria 'preferentially eliminated females' (955). But there is no a priori reason why women – or men – should not be 'eliminated' by an age criterion provided there is independent evidence to support such a restriction. There was, of course, no evidence either way, but such 'elimination' cannot simply be declared wrong in principle in order, it appears, to provide a diagnosis which is more evenly distributed between the sexes.

Kendler et al. finally quoted research which, they claimed, does not support 'an etiological discontinuity between early and late onset schizophrenia' (955). Given that evidence about the aetiology of schizophrenia is lacking, this claim needs to be reworded as referring to research which might cast light on whether people who show particular behaviour or have particular experiences early or later in life can be thought of as belonging to one continuous or two distinct populations on the basis of some other variable. For example, Kendler *et al.* claimed that 'age of onset curves in schizophrenia do not consistently show bi-modality with a second peak above 45' and that '[f]amily studies suggest that relatives of individuals with late-onset schizophrenia are at considerably higher risk for schizophrenia than the general population' (955). But there is a serious conceptual muddle here. According to DSM-III, there can be no such disorder as 'late onset schizophrenia'. Kendler *et al.* are therefore quoting research which used a wide variety of diagnostic criteria which pre-dated DSM-III. This raises the questions of 'age of onset of what?' 'Family resemblance in what?' And, if these 'old' criteria can accurately diagnose both early and late-onset schizophrenia, then why are new criteria being sought? Or, if they are unsatisfactory, how can the use of research based on them be justified? But the fundamental problem with this deletion of the age criterion does not lie entirely in the inadequacies of research used to support it; it lies also in Karl Popper's point that it is axiomatic that when an element is removed from the definition of a concept, then evidence must be presented that *what is left* forms a meaningful pattern.

### Changes in the subsidiary requirements about affective disorder

In DSM-III, a diagnosis of schizophrenia could be made only if '(i) the full depressive or manic syndrome, if present, developed after any psychotic symptoms or (ii) was brief in duration relative to the duration of the psychotic symptoms in A' (the active phase, see Table 5.1). The wording of this requirement was changed in DSM-IIIR to delete the first part (i) and to emphasise the requirement for a brief total duration of 'all episodes of a mood syndrome'. These changes were maintained in DSM-IV.

No evidence was offered for these changes. Instead, Kendler *et al.* (1989) invoked Kraepelin, who had claimed that depression frequently precedes schizophrenia and then fades. In drawing on Kraepelin's authority, Kendler *et al.* again begged the question they were addressing of trying to find correspondence rules for schizophrenia: if Kraepelin could make this statement he must already have identified 'schizophrenia' according to valid criteria, in which case why were the devisers of DSM-IIIR having to search for them – why not use Kraepelin's? Of course, Kendler *et al.* also overlooked the highly dubious links between Kraepelin's work and the modern population of 'schizophrenics'.

Kendler *et al.* also supported the changes by describing a hypothetical case which would not be diagnosed as schizophrenic with the old DSM-III wording on affective disorder, but would be diagnosed as schizophrenic with the new wording. This case was apparently so obviously schizophrenic that changing the wording on affective disorder was a 'logical step'. But this is simply argument by assertion as well as by question-begging. It makes no sense to develop official criteria for inferring schizophrenia, as in DSM-III, and then to claim by fiat that obvious cases of schizophrenia lie outside them.

## The place of 'negative symptoms' in diagnostic criteria

A number of writers had suggested that 'symptoms of schizophrenia' could be divided into positive (e.g. hallucinations, delusions) and negative (e.g. poverty of speech, flat affect). Crow's (1980) paper, however, focused clinicians' and researchers' attention on the topic. Crow's model was based on two dichotomies: positive and negative symptoms and Type 1 and Type 2 schizophrenia. The potential importance of this model lay in the claim that Type 1 and Type 2 schizophrenia were associated with other variables: Type 1 with a good response to neuroleptic medication, absence of intellectual impairment or abnormal movement and with normal brain structure. Type 2 was claimed to be associated with a poor response to neuroleptics and possibly with abnormal movements and brain structure and with intellectual deterioration.

But in line with Schneider's emphasis on 'positive symptoms' – discussed in Chapter 3 – DSM-III paid little attention to 'negative symptoms': virtually all the 'symptoms' mentioned in the diagnostic criteria are 'positive', although not labelled as such. And, although it is possible in DSM-III for a diagnosis of schizophrenia to be given on the basis of two co-occurring negative symptoms (poverty of speech and flat affect) such diagnoses are likely to be far outnumbered by those based on 'positive symptoms'. This bias in favour of 'positive symptoms' was maintained or even intensified in DSM-IIIR, and with very little discussion of the issue.

The discussions surrounding DSM-IV, however, were very different, with much more emphasis on the role of 'negative symptoms'. This change was at least partly due to the fact that the Chair of the DSM-IV Work Group on Schizophrenia and Related Psychotic Disorders – Nancy Andreasen – was a prominent researcher on 'negative symptoms'. But although the Work Group recommended that these should be given more prominence in DSM-IV, the actual changes were more linguistic than substantial: the phrase 'negative symptoms' was used in the criteria and two further 'symptoms' – avolition (severe lack of motivation or 'drive') and alogia (marked poverty of speech) were added to the 'negative symptoms' already mentioned in DSM-IIIR. The changes may have been minimal in terms of explicit emphasis on 'negative symptoms', but the discussions surrounding this issue merit more detailed consideration for two reasons. First, they reveal a great deal about the arguments which the Work Group saw as justifying changes in the diagnostic criteria. Second, the issue of 'negative symptoms' in the criteria is unlikely to go away, not least because of the claim that they are linked in some way with brain abnormalities and so appear to hold out the hope of showing that 'schizophrenia' really is a brain disease. We might also argue that the insertion of the phrase 'negative symptoms' into the diagnostic criteria is more significant than it seems, that it gives credence to the idea of negative symptoms as more than a descriptive label and paves the way for greater emphasis on them in future editions of the DSM. The next sections will therefore examine first the arguments and theoretical framework put forward by the Work Group in support of giving 'negative symptoms' more prominence, and, second, the extent to which the Group met even the demands of their own framework. Finally, I will discuss the adequacy of this framework for making decisions about diagnostic criteria.

### Giving more prominence to 'negative symptoms': a justification

A number of arguments were made in support of giving 'negative symptoms' more prominence in DSM-IV, although the exact form this prominence might take was never made explicit (see Andreasen and Flaum, 1991; Flaum and Andreasen, 1991; Andreasen and Carpenter, 1993). These arguments included the fact that both Kraepelin and Bleuler had emphasised 'negative symptoms'; that these 'symptoms' could now be reliably measured; that their prevalence in people diagnosed as schizophrenic was high; that scales which measured 'negative symptoms' had high internal consistency; and that 'negative symptoms' were associated with other variables, including 'independent validators' such as cognitive impairment, differential treatment response and motor abnormalities (Andreasen and Flaum, 1991). It was argued, finally, that 'negative symptoms' should be given more prominence because medical insurers would expect it, given that treatment often had to focus on those 'symptoms' which prevented the person leading a productive life (Andreasen and Carpenter, 1993).

Putting aside for the moment the adequacy of these arguments for determining diagnostic criteria, I shall focus on the claims themselves and on how far the Work Group's interpretations of data appear to be justified. The point is important because, as we have seen, the devisers of DSM-III not only used problematic, though reasonable seeming, frameworks for choosing diagnostic criteria, they compounded their error and created a doubly false impression by failing to meet even their own declared standards.

The first problem which the Work Group failed to confront was the *idea* of negative symptoms. Instead, they used the term as if it were an agreed and straightforward representation of particular 'schizophrenic' behaviours. Yet as Peralta *et al.* (1992) have pointed out, there has been marked variability in definitions of positive and negative symptoms, while only one 'symptom' – flat affect – is common to all negative symptom scales (de Leon *et al.*, 1992). Perhaps not surprisingly, claims about the internal consistency of negative symptoms scales – suggesting that they form a meaningful cluster – have also been challenged. Peralta *et al.* (1992) reported a corrected internal consistency coefficient (Cronbach's Alpha) of 0.41 for the Scale for the Assessment of Negative Symptoms (SANS). Even this score may have been inflated by overlap in the criteria used to make judgements about the presence of different 'symptoms': someone who is emotionally unresponsive or shows little pleasure in life may more easily be judged to be lacking in drive or motivation.

The Work Group also argued that negative symptoms should be given more prominence because they were possibly more descriptive or more characteristic of schizophrenia than positive symptoms, and especially the first-rank symptoms favoured by DSM-III and IIIR. Andreasen and Flaum (1991) and Flaum and Andreasen (1991) argued that the prevalence of first-rank symptoms in samples of people diagnosed as schizophrenic was relatively low and that 'the notion that these symptoms are pathognomic for schizophrenia has been disputed by several studies that demonstrate their appearance in other psychotic disorders' (Flaum and Andreasen, 1991: 136). It was implied that 'negative symptoms' performed better in these respects, although no data were offered about their occurrence in other diagnostic categories. Klosterkötter et al. (1995), however, have shown that 'negative symptoms', as defined by various Negative Symptoms Scales, are frequently found in diagnostic categories other than schizophrenia and at rates not significantly lower than 'schizophrenia'. This raises serious problems for any arguments about negative symptoms being 'characteristic of schizophrenia'. Klosterkötter et al. also claimed that positive symptoms were more able than negative symptoms to discriminate amongst diagnostic categories; that is, they were more likely to be found in 'schizophrenia' than in other categories. Thus the Work Group's implication that 'negative symptoms' may be 'more characteristic of schizophrenia' is difficult to justify.

The Group argued that the reliability with which 'negative symptoms' could be measured also justified giving them more prominence in DSM-IV. Unfortunately, the data quoted (Andreasen and Flaum, 1991) are difficult to interpret: two of the studies are unpublished and none of them appear to use the Kappa correlation statistic which controls for chance agreement between raters and which was strongly recommended by the devisers of DSM-III (Kirk and Kutchins, 1992). One piece of data for one 'negative symptom' is quoted which does use Kappa (Endicott et al., 1982), but the result is not promising: the reliability of ratings of 'flat affect' was 0.13.

But even if we did have good evidence that 'negative symptoms' could be reliably assessed, there is a further problem which the Work Group did not emphasise. It has been acknowledged (Peralta et al., 1992; de Leon et al., 1992; Harrow et al., 1994) that negative symptoms may be produced by factors such as unstimulating environments, attempts to cope with 'positive symptoms' such as hearing voices and by neuroleptic medication. Within the Work Group's framework, therefore, a crucial question is how far researchers and clinicians can distinguish 'primary' negative symptoms (said to be caused by schizophrenia) and secondary 'negative symptoms' caused by other factors, including drug treatment for 'schizophrenia'. Flaum and Andreasen (1995), however, reported a median reliability coefficient (Kappa) of only 0.38 from a sample of independent raters who rated 'negative symptoms' as primary, sec-ondary or of unknown origin. Flaum and Andreasen suggested that the primary/secondary distinction should therefore not be incorporated into the use of 'negative symptoms' in diagnostic criteria, a suggestion which not only overlooks the implications of their own data but also encourages the impres-sion that 'negative symptoms' are somehow intrinsic to 'schizophrenia', rather than behaviours produced by a variety of factors, including drug treatment.

The Work Group argued, finally, that negative symptoms should be given more prominence in DSM-IV because they have been 'shown to be associated with a number of independent validators . . . including cognitive impairment, a differential treatment response and poor outcome' (Andreasen and Flaum, 1991: 37); 'negative symptoms' were also claimed to be associated with motor abnormalities, while a relationship with structural brain abnormalities was implied. But these claims are seriously problematic even within the Work Group's own framework because of the failure to establish the antecedents of whatever behaviours are said to be negative symptoms. It is well established, for example, that traditional neuroleptic medication is associated both with 'negative symptoms', such as severe lack of pleasure in life (anhedonia) (Harrow et al., 1994), and with motor abnormalities (Breggin, 1990; Day and Bentall, 1996). Implications of a relationship between 'negative symptoms' and brain abnormalities are equally problematic, not simply because a reliable association has not been established (Marks and Luchins, 1990; Andreasen et al., 1990a) but also because where such abnormalities are found they may be attributable, for example, to obstetric complications directly and indirectly associated with non-specific life disadvantage but with no direct relationship to 'negative symptoms', and to prescribed major or minor tranquillisers or to other drugs such as alcohol (Lader et al., 1984; Schmauss and Krieg, 1987; Breggin, 1990, 1993). Arguments about the reliability or validity of 'negative symptoms' were therefore not only unsupported by the available data, they also risk obscuring the possible consequences of treatment for those same 'symptoms'.

The previous section considered the Work Group's arguments about nega-tive symptoms in terms of their own framework: in other words, it examined how far the Work Group's own claims about negative symptoms were justified by the available evidence. I have argued that the claims were not justified, but this still leaves the question of the framework itself: how adequate in princi-ple were the arguments put forward by the Work Group for increasing the prominence of 'negative symptoms' in DSM-IV's criteria for inferring 'schiz-ophrenia'? The question is important because otherwise it can look as if the devisers of the next DSM simply need to find 'better' data to support their arguments. This section will therefore look critically at the arguments put for-ward by the Work Group in support of giving more prominence to 'negative symptoms'.

The Work Group put forward four main arguments (apart from claiming that insurers would expect to see 'negative symptoms' in the diagnostic criteria): (1)

Kraepelin and Bleuler had emphasised negative symptoms; (2) negative symptoms could be reliably assessed; (3) they were associated with 'independent validators'; and (4) they performed better than positive, first-rank symptoms in terms of their specificity to schizophrenia and their frequency of occurrence in schizophrenia.

The first, historical, argument is clearly spurious. The fact that Kraepelin and Bleuler emphasised 'negative symptoms' a century ago tells us nothing about what should be done now. As we saw in Chapter 3, Kraepelin and Bleuler were dealing with a population whose most likely diagnosis was post-encephalitic Parkinsonism, so that whatever they emphasised may have little relevance to today's 'schizophrenia', with one exception: the standard intervention for 'schizophrenia' – neuroleptic drugs – can produce similar changes in brain chemistry and possibly structure, and changes in motor behaviour, to those observed in post-encephalitic Parkinsonism (Breggin, 1990, 1993). Thus there *is* a possible link between Kraepelin's and Bleuler's emphasis on 'negative symptoms', and the behaviours observed in today's 'schizophrenics' – but not the link implied by the Work Group.

The second argument, about reliability, is not so much spurious as partial. It is not that reliability is unimportant, although its importance in the context of 'symptoms' may be overemphasised, a point I shall return to later; the more relevant point here is that the mere fact that a phenomenon can be measured reliably does not tell us whether it should be included in any particular set of diagnostic criteria. Weight loss, for example, can be measured very reliably but this conveys nothing about its meaning or its association with other symptoms or signs.

The third argument concerned the association of 'negative symptoms' with 'independent validators'. We have already seen the problems of claiming an association with cognitive impairment, movement disorders and brain abnormalities. It must be said, however, that if 'negative symptoms', as an agreed and specific set of phenomena, could be shown to be reliably associated with another, independently measurable phenomenon, without the many confounding variables known to be involved, then this would be of interest, but not in dictating diagnostic criteria for 'schizophrenia'. The Work Group also claimed that negative symptoms were associated with poor outcome (Andreasen and Flaum, 1991). I have already discussed the problems of using 'outcome' as a validating criterion for any diagnostic category, and the same problems surround 'negative symptoms'. For example, it would hardly be surprising if someone judged to show lack of persistence or motivation turned out to be unemployed or socially isolated when 'outcome' was measured, or if these circumstances did not lead to further 'negative symptoms' such as flat affect. As I emphasised in the discussion of DSM-III, the 'outcome' of a diagnostic category often amounts to no more than a statement about the persistence of various odd, troublesome and distressing behaviours and to statements about their understandable associations with other social and personal difficulties. None of this can enlighten us as to whether 'negative symptoms' form a meaningful pattern when combined with other phenomena such as strange beliefs or hearing voices.

A final argument put forward by the Work Group for giving 'negative symptoms' more prominence in the diagnostic criteria was that they performed better than positive, first-rank symptoms in terms of frequency of occurrence in 'schizophrenia' and specificity to 'schizophrenia'. This argument is extremely problematic and will be discussed in more detail and more generally later, in the context of 'base rates'. For the moment, however, it is worth noting that the argument is based entirely on question-begging: if the Work Group was able to establish to their satisfaction what the frequency of negative and positive symptoms was in schizophrenia, then they must have assumed that it was already possible validly to infer schizophrenia using particular diagnostic criteria. And they clearly did assume this, as they quoted research using various diagnostic criteria as if it told us something definite about 'schizophrenia'. But if this was the case, why did they need to seek new criteria? Or, if they needed to seek new criteria, how could they interpret the results of research using 'old' criteria? In fact, research on the frequency of what are called positive and negative symptoms of schizophrenia tells us a good deal about the practices of clinicians and nothing about how or whether 'schizophrenia' ought to be diagnosed. It is obvious that diagnostic criteria which favour 'positive symptoms' will tend to produce groups of 'schizophrenics' who show a high frequency of at least one 'positive symptom', and the same will be true for 'negative symptoms'. The latter, however, seem to be relatively common in psychiatric populations (Klosterkötter et al., 1995) and, as we have seen, may be associated with neuroleptic medication. They are therefore likely to be noted in any group diagnosed as schizophrenic.

Clearly, then, neither the empirical evidence nor the types of arguments used by the Work Group were of much use in reaching specific decisions about 'negative symptoms'. It is perhaps not surprising, then, that the final decision about negative symptoms in DSM-IV – to use the term and to list extra exemplars – should have been made without any clear justification being given (see First et al., 1994).

## Changing DSM-III to DSM-IV: an overview

None of the changes made to the diagnostic criteria for schizophrenia from DSM-III to DSM-IV were based on the kind of evidence I discussed earlier: that a previously observed cluster is found to be reliably associated with another observable phenomenon. Instead, the changes were based on a number of spurious arguments and on evidence which was often misrepresented or irrelevant. This approach, of course, had also typified the development of DSM-III and was almost inevitable given that the task itself – of finding correspondence rules for an existing concept – was deeply problematic. DSM-III,

IIIR and IV were, then, more or less doomed to failure or to rely on spurious arguments to support whatever correspondence rules or diagnostic criteria they 'found' for schizophrenia. There are, however, important differences between the context and process of the development of DSM-III and DSM-IV which merit detailed examination, for two reasons. First, they illuminate the ways in which the devisers of the DSM managed the failure of DSM-III to fulfil the hopes invested in it for 'schizophrenia'. Second, the DSM and the process of revising it are likely to play a major role in the theory and practice surrounding 'schizophrenia' – discussions are already underway on DSM-V. Critical examination of the DSM as the criteria change is therefore important in both anticipating and responding to future developments.

## DSM-III to IIIR to IV: the management of a failed project

The atmosphere surrounding the publication of DSM-III in 1980 can best be described as triumphalist. As I described in Chapter 4, the philosopher of science Carl Hempel had pointed to the problem that none of psychiatry's concepts was clearly tied to observables; DSM-III, with its lists of criteria for inferring each concept, seemed to represent a problem solved and was claimed to have brought psychiatry into the ranks of the scientifically respectable. Although there was opposition to DSM-III (see Kirk and Kutchins, 1992), it was not on this issue and, in any case, it was difficult to oppose the principle that diagnostic concepts should be tied to observables.

Ten or so years later, the situation surrounding the development of DSM-IV was rather different in at least two important ways. First, the 10th revision of the ICD was due for publication at around the same time as DSM-IV and, for the first time, Chapter V of the manual – and only Chapter V, on 'mental and behavioural disorders' – would contain specific criteria for inferring diagnostic concepts. As I mentioned earlier, however, in the case of 'schizophrenia', these criteria were being developed by different people from those involved in the DSM. And, as the Chair of the Work Group on Schizophrenia noted, 'The definition of schizophrenia in the draft ICD-10 is quite different from that in DSM-IIIR' (Andreasen, 1991: 25). This was potentially very problematic. As Andreasen and Flaum (1991) pointed out, 'the research community that studies schizophrenia is truly international and it is important that investigators be able to conduct cross-national attempts to validate one another's findings' (29). There was another issue which was not discussed but which was potentially more embarrassing than threats to international research: DSM-III had partly been developed in an attempt to confer scientific respectability on psychiatric diagnosis and this appearance was largely achieved through the listing of specific criteria for inferring the diagnostic concepts. This scientific veneer would clearly be threatened by the existence of two very different sets of criteria for schizophrenia, both supposedly based on scientific evidence and both endorsed by experts. It is not surprising, then, that 'consonance with the ICD was seen as an important goal for DSM-IV' (Andreasen and Flaum, 1991: 45).

A second important difference between the contexts of DSM-III and DSM-IV was in the nature of the opposition to the projects. Opposition to DSM-III had come, for example, from psychoanalysts who objected to what they saw as a return to an atheoretical Kraepelinian system and from those who objected to racist and sexist biases. There had also been opposition from psychologists who objected to what they saw as psychiatric 'colonisation' of behaviour and psychological problems (see Kirk and Kutchins, 1992, for detailed discussion of these points). Much of the opposition to DSM-IV, however, came from within the traditional psychiatric community and centred on the frequency of revisions to the DSM. Flaum and Andreasen (1991), for example, noted that '[t]he development of DSM-IV has been controversial. Critics suggest that frequent changes in diagnostic "fashions" are counterproductive for both clinical and research activities' (133). The revisions seemed to create two problems for users of the manual. First, clinicians had scarcely become competent in applying one set of often complex criteria before they had to learn a new and equally complex set. Second, research using the 'old' criteria quickly became obsolete, while longitudinal studies could be out of date before they were completed. These points were forcefully made by Zimmerman (1988, 1990), who argued that the very basis of the DSM – its claim to be based on scientific research – was threatened by frequent revisions: how could revisions of the manual be based on research when there was not sufficient time to carry out the research needed to inform the next revision? Unfortunately, critics did not make the point that the entire basis of the DSM – searching for correspondence rules for existing concepts – was a travesty of scientific research, so that it scarcely mattered how often it was revised. But in a context where it was assumed that it *was* reasonable to search for correspondence rules, these criticisms had some force, particularly given DSM's claim to be a research-based manual. Worse, both Zimmerman and another highly respected supporter of psychiatric diagnosis, Robert Kendell, suggested that financial rather than scientific considerations might have become more important in the revision process, given the profits to be made from each new edition.

The devisers of the DSM took these criticisms seriously; indeed they could hardly do otherwise, given, as Kendler (1990) had pointed out, that frequent changes to diagnostic criteria ran the risk of 'undermining the credibility of the entire nosological process' (970). But abandoning the fourth edition of the DSM was never seriously considered. In any case, ICD-10, with its own, and different, criteria, would still be published. Yet it was essential to maintain the co-operation of clinicians and researchers and to ensure that they used the new manual. The alternative might be a return to the past when clinicians and researchers used their own preferred criteria for making diagnoses, the very situation that DSM-III was supposed to have ended.

The DSM-IV Work Group on Schizophrenia and Related Psychotic Disorders responded directly to critics' concerns in two ways. The first was by emphasising their aim of producing criteria which were 'user friendly'. By this they meant criteria which were 'easy to learn and remember' and 'easy to apply in clinical and education settings' (Flaum and Andreasen, 1991: 141). Indeed, being 'simple enough to remember' was listed as one of the characteristics of the 'ideal criteria set for schizophrenia and related disorders' (ibid.: 140). Clinicians were assured that ratings of 'user-friendliness' would be made in the 'field trials' of draft criteria for schizophrenia and that these ratings would be given 'careful consideration' in the selection of the final criteria for schizophrenia (ibid.: 141). But this concern for 'user-friendliness' is obviously absurd from a scientific point of view – rather like suggesting that the equations surrounding relativity theory should be revised because they are difficult to learn and remember.

The second way in which the Work Group responded directly to critics' concerns was by trying to minimise the reclassification rates of schizophrenia which might result from revising the diagnostic criteria. In other words, as few people as possible who had been diagnosed as schizophrenic by DSM-IIIR should be classified as not schizophrenic by DSM-IV and as few 'new cases' as possible should be added by the use of DSM-IV. In addition, there should be very little difference in the classification rates for schizophrenia using DSM-IV and ICD-10. These points were strongly emphasised by the Work Group. For example, 'maintaining continuity of diagnosis and classification' of 'schizophrenia' was described as a 'high priority', while evaluating the relative classification rates of draft criteria sets for DSM-IV and ICD-10 for 'schizophrenia' was said to be one of the 'primary goals' of the DSM-IV field trials (Andreasen and Flaum, 1990: 956). In additional, the first-mentioned characteristic of an ideal set of diagnostic criteria for schizophrenia was that it 'would classify patients in a manner not significantly different from both DSM-IIIR and ICD-10' (Flaum and Andreasen, 1991: 140). To do otherwise, it was argued, would be 'detrimental to research and confusing to clinicians' (Andreasen and Carpenter, 1993: 204).

The problem with these arguments is that it is impossible to specify in advance what effect research should have on classification rates. Medical research not infrequently results in reclassification when important differences are demonstrated amongst people once thought to belong to the same diagnostic category, as for example in the separation of diabetes mellitus and diabetes insipidus. Equally, if strong evidence were presented tomorrow that half of those diagnosed as suffering from diabetes mellitus had a parasitic infection which destroyed the pancreas, then another reclassification would be called for, regardless of the sensibilities of clinicians or their reluctance to learn new diagnostic criteria. Thus, far from being detrimental to research as the Work Group claimed, reclassification is an important *result* of successful medical research. In fact, the Work Group's goal of minimum reclassification came perilously close to an admission that they would ignore research which suggested that a major reclassification was necessary. It is difficult to avoid the conclusion that the Work Group were able to placate clinicians and researchers with talk of minimum reclassification because they knew that no research existed which would clearly have a bearing on reclassification one way or the other. Given this, then the Group might as well choose those diagnostic criteria which would arouse least opposition.

### But what about science?

Reassurances about user-friendliness and reclassification might have met the concerns of some critics, but they sat uneasily with DSM-IV's commitment to science. Certainly, they fell far short of a convincing demonstration of the scientific framework which was claimed to inform DSM-IV:

> Both to provide the necessary stability and to gradually increase the scientific basis for our nosological system, an increasingly rigorous and data based revision process is needed.
>
> (Kendler *et al.*, 1989: 960)

> More than their predecessors, the committee charged with the development of DSM-IV have been instructed to emphasise scientific criteria in the evolution of proposed nosological changes.
>
> (Kendler, 1990: 970)

> The guiding principle behind the development of DSM-IV has been that proposed changes in the current criteria be clearly supported by empirical evidence.
>
> (Andreasen, 1991: 25)

There were, however, a number of serious problems in implementing this scientific framework, apart from maintaining 'user-friendliness' and minimising reclassification, and apart, of course, from the fact that searching for correspondence rules for an existing concept was itself highly questionable. It might, then, be more accurate to say that there remained serious problems in *appearing* to implement a scientific framework.

The Work Group believed that searching for correspondence rules for an existing concept – schizophrenia – was a reasonable thing to do. But even if they were thus able to ignore the first rule of concept development – that observation of patterns precedes inference of concepts – they could not entirely ignore the second: that a concept's correspondence rules, or in this case, diagnostic criteria, are supposed to refer to a meaningful pattern. As we have seen, the preferred way of trying to ensure this in medicine is to show that a postulated cluster of subjective complaints or symptoms is reliably associated with another, reliably measurable event (sign) which can reasonably be thought of as an antecedent of the symptoms. Given this, then the first problem in appearing to implement a scientific framework was researchers' persistent failure to show a reliable association between a diagnosis of schizophrenia and any biological event or process (Jackson, 1990; Ross and Pam, 1995; Chua and McKenna, 1995; McGrath and Emmerson, 1999; Moncrieff, 2000). In a considerable understatement, Andreasen and Flaum (1990) suggested that 'it would be premature to incorporate biological markers into the [diagnostic] criteria [for schizophrenia]' (955). But since abandoning the concept of schizophrenia was clearly never considered as an option, the Work Group were faced with resorting to what might be called second-rate standards for arguing that a particular cluster of behaviour and experience actually formed a meaningful pattern and therefore justified inferring 'schizophrenia'. These standards included 'outcome', 'course', 'age of onset' and 'familial pattern' and were, of course, exactly the kind of criteria used, for want of better, by Kraepelin; they also formed the basis of DSM-III's justification for its correspondence rules for schizophrenia. I have already discussed the considerable problems they present and the extent to which neither Kraepelin nor the devisers of DSM-III met even their own problematic standards.

But a decade after the publication of DSM-III, the problems associated with the use of 'age of onset', 'outcome', and so on, were becoming more difficult to ignore. It had, in any case, been argued in DSM-IIIR that 'schizophrenia' was *not* associated with any particular age group; it was, then, no longer possible to invoke 'age of onset', however inappropriately, as evidence that the diagnostic criteria for schizophrenia formed a meaningful pattern. There was also very little discussion of 'course' or 'family resemblance', perhaps in the face of persistently variable research results. This left 'outcome', the standard on which DSM-III had placed considerable emphasis. In other words, the devisers of DSM-III had argued that their criteria for inferring schizophrenia formed a meaningful pattern by virtue of the fact that they defined a group homogeneous for 'outcome'. As we saw in the earlier discussion of DSM-III, this claim was false in 1980; by the early 1990s, however, its problems were even more apparent. The most the DSM-IV Work Group could claim was that a DSM-III diagnosis of schizophrenia 'demonstrated reasonably good prediction of long-term outcome' and that 'there appears to be some support for the predictive validity of [DSM-III criteria for schizophrenia]' (Andreasen and Flaum, 1991: 35). In fact, the authors of the literature review which had informed the Work Group's discussions had reached a less generous conclusion: 'We are faced with several excellent studies that amply demonstrate the heterogeneity of outcome of schizophrenia after many years of established illness' (Keith and Matthews, 1991: 62). Indeed, Davidson and McGlashan (1997) later suggested that the most consistent conclusion from follow-up studies reviewed in a special issue of *Schizophrenia Bulletin* in 1988 was the heterogeneity in long-term outcome of 'schizophrenia'.

It was not just this heterogeneity, though, which made reliance on 'outcome' as a way of justifying particular correspondence rules so problematic for the DSM-IV Work Group. Heterogeneity had, after all, always been present but was simply glossed over. There were two further, potentially more embarrassing problems. First, commentators were increasingly pointing out the tautology which had always been inherent in the DSM-III and IIIR diagnostic criteria: the criteria claimed validity partly through their ability to identify a group homogeneous for 'poor outcome'. As we have seen, the criteria did not actually do this, but to the extent that some DSM-III or IIIR 'schizophrenics' did have a poor outcome, this could be explained as a self-fulfilling prophecy because the criteria also required at least six months of 'disturbance' before the diagnosis could be made. And since the longer you were 'disturbed' the longer you were likely to be 'disturbed', a clear tautology was created. As Keith and Matthews put it in their review paper for the Work Group:

> At issue is that the current criterion [of six months of symptoms] essentially establishes a tautology: the longer one has an illness, the more likely one is to have it for a long time.
>
> (1991: 60)

A second problem created by emphasising 'outcome' was the increasing evidence that the outcome of 'schizophrenia' was more favourable in non-Western countries. Davidson and McGlashan (1997) have described this as 'one of the most striking and unexpected findings of the World Health Organisation [International Pilot Study of Schizophrenia]' (38). And several studies completed or nearing completion during the Work Group's deliberations offered further support for this 'unexpected' conclusion (e.g. Leon, 1989; Leff et al., 1992; see also Warner, 1994). Although these studies did not use DSM-III criteria, their results had the potential to shift our attention sharply from the 'neurobiological substrate' which the Work Group claimed for 'schizophrenia' (Andreasen and Flaum, 1990: 955) and to lead to questions about the role of social and economic factors in the maintenance of bizarre behaviour as well as to awkward questions about the appropriateness of Western methods of intervention. Overall, then, it must have seemed that a continuing emphasis on 'outcome' as evidence that the diagnostic criteria for schizophrenia formed a meaningful pattern, could create more problems than it solved.

The issue of outcome, however, was not the only problem which the Work Group faced in maintaining an appearance of scientific rigour. The issue of reliability which had been given such prominence in DSM-III (see Kirk and Kutchins, 1992) had apparently not been solved. For example, the Work Group noted that no reliability data were available on the 'deterioration' criterion of DSM-III or IIIR (i.e. the requirement that people should show a deterioration in social or occupational functioning as well as 'psychotic symptoms') (Andreasen and Flaum, 1991). It was also noted that the reliability of 'individual symptoms' of 'schizophrenia' was largely unknown and that 'the more ambitious goal of the current field trial is to quantify reliability at the level of individual symptoms' (Flaum and Andreasen, 1991: 141).

Clearly, then, DSM-IV would need to adopt a rather different approach to the science question from that taken in DSM-III in producing correspondence rules for 'schizophrenia'. But given that the ideal solution of showing a reliable association between schizophrenia's correspondence rules and an antecedent biological event was not available, then whatever approach was taken would inevitably have more to do with appearance than substance. But because of the importance of appeals to science in maintaining the credibility and authority of the DSM, these attempts to deal with the science question merit detailed examination. The next sections will therefore discuss three papers by members of the Schizophrenia Work Group in which they attempt, directly and indirectly, to deal with this issue.

### DSM-IV and 'schizophrenia': maintaining a scientific veneer

The first paper, by Kenneth Kendler, was published in 1990 and appeared to have three aims: (1) to set the scene for discussions of the DSM-IV diagnostic criteria; (2) to warn its audience that the diagnostic system was likely to fall short of a scientific ideal; (3) to make clear where the blame for this lay.

Kendler began by reminding us of the 'emerging consensus' that psychiatric nosology 'should become more scientific' (969). He then argued that 'the essence of the scientific method is hypothesis generation and hypothesis testing' and that 'scientific nosology would thus involve the generation of hypotheses about the reliability and validity of competing diagnostic schemas' (970). Kendler may well be correct in saying that hypothesis generation and testing is part of what we think of as science but he neglected to make the crucial point that the *content* of these hypotheses is also important: there is no logical connection between the general activity of hypothesis generation and testing and *which* hypotheses are reasonable to test. To put it bluntly, scientists do not test any old hypotheses. The word 'thus' in Kendler's quote creates a false impression that comparing the reliability and validity of 'competing diagnostic schemas' (i.e. diagnostic criteria) is intrinsically scientific. But on the contrary, researchers who compare different sets of correspondence rules for a psychiatric concept in an attempt to find the 'best' are only (inappropriately) doing so because previous researchers invented concepts without following the first rule of scientific research: that hypothetical concepts must be tied to an observable pattern. And, interestingly, Kendler does not say what would be the null hypothesis in this situation. It would, of course, be that there were no differences in reliability or validity between two sets of diagnostic criteria for the same concept. But what if both were equally poor? Or suppose the two sets were significantly different but one was very poor and the other mediocre. Would the concept then be abandoned? This kind of research, where several sets of diagnostic criteria are compared, is very frequent in 'schizophrenia'. Experience shows, however, that the option of abandoning the concept is virtually never considered. Instead, the 'least bad' set of diagnostic criteria may be favoured.

Having thus given us a highly misleading view of science, Kendler then outlined the advantages of a scientific nosology. These took up little space – less than one column of an eight-column paper – and included protection against 'fashion'; keeping psychiatry honest and increasing the 'credibility and prestige' of its classification system (970). By contrast, discussion of the 'limitations of a scientific nosology' was much more extensive, taking up almost three times the space of the advantages. These limitations included the exclusion of historical tradition and experience; the undesirability of complex criteria, even if they are more valid, because they are difficult to learn and remember, and the exclusion of areas such as intra-psychic factors which are less amenable to scientific study. In a conclusion of breathtaking arrogance, Kendler summarised the limitations of a scientific approach to psychiatric nosology by claiming as the fundamental problem that 'the scientific method can only answer "little questions"' whereas 'in nosology, we need answers to "big questions"' (972). In fact, these 'big questions' turn out to be the meaningless questions posed by psychiatric nosologists trying to pick up the pieces behind their predecessors who invented concepts without demonstrating their links to observable patterns ('What is the best criteria set for the diagnosis of . . .?': 972). In other words, the 'big questions' reflect nosologists' failure to confront their question-begging, back-to-front approach and their failure to appreciate that you cannot simply take an invented concept like 'schizophrenia', assume it to be valid, and then search for a set of referents that will 'prove' that it is.

I am not suggesting here that the methods of the natural sciences, which have informed the development of classification systems in medicine, can necessarily provide answers to all important questions we might ask about problematic behaviour and experience; the point, however, is that psychiatric nosologists have claimed to be working within this natural sciences framework and have claimed authority and status as a result. When the methods appear not to be producing the desired result, we can reasonably expect better arguments than this about the reasons for failure; we should also expect an alternative epistemological framework which would justify our paying attention to psychiatric nosology or giving credence to any statements from nosologists about the content of their systems. Kendler offers no such alternative. Instead, he suggests that the most useful conceptual framework 'within which to incorporate the scientific process into nosology . . . is the *advisory model*'. In this model, 'scientific information . . . is objectively evaluated . . . [and] used to advise and inform the [DSM] committee' (972; emphasis in original). Kendler compares this model with that used by Congressional committees deciding, for example, whether to pass bills restricting the growth or sale of tobacco. In other words, Kendler wishes to keep parts of the scientific model he has discredited, presumably to deal with the 'little questions', but to leave the 'big' questions (what are the best correspondence rules for 'schizophrenia'?) in the hands of a group (the DSM committee) whose framework for decision-making remains obscure. And the overall message of the paper is clear: psychiatric nosologists have done their best to work within a scientific framework. If the results have not repaid the effort, if we are still awaiting reliable and valid correspondence rules for 'schizophrenia', then the blame cannot be laid at the nosologists' door: it is science itself which is inadequate.

Perhaps not surprisingly, this 'advisory model' was not enthusiastically taken up by other members of the Work Group. It was, perhaps, quickly perceived that it might lead to awkward questions: if the 'big' questions are to be dealt with by panels analogous to Congressional committees, then who elects them? To whom are they accountable? What interests and values will inform their judgements? How can they be replaced if those affected by their conclusions do not like them? From where does their authority derive? And so on. It was, however, still necessary to maintain a scientific veneer for DSM-IV, but perhaps in a less obviously contentious way than that suggested by Kendler. The next two sections will examine two further papers which attempt to deal with this problem more indirectly, led by the Chair of the Work Group, Nancy Andreasen.

### Science through biometrics

Andreasen and Flaum's 1991 paper suggested some 'principles and approaches to guide the development of DSM-IV' in relation to 'schizophrenia' (27). Because the suggested approach was new, it had to be made to look superior to the 'old' approach of DSM-III/IIIR in terms of its links with science. This was achieved in three main ways: first, by denigrating the approach used in DSM-III; second, by using technical and prestigious-sounding language to describe the new approach and, third, by claiming that the new approach was based on up-to-date data not available to the devisers of DSM-III. Andreasen and Flaum claimed, for example, that previous diagnostic criteria had been selected on the basis of 'common sense and clinical experience' (29), whereas DSM-IV could be based on 'modern biometric methods' or on 'more empirical, data-based, biometric approaches' (29, 33). The existing diagnostic criteria for 'schizophrenia' apparently did 'not make optimal use of modern biometric approaches', while the availability of new data 'can be used to provide a more data-based and empirical approach to developing diagnostic criteria' (44).

But what were these 'modern biometric methods'? Andreasen and Flaum suggested two 'basic biometric principles' which should guide the selection of diagnostic criteria for 'schizophrenia'. The first was reliability. It is, in fact, rather disingenuous to imply that reliability was not a consideration for DSM-III, given the efforts made to present DSM-III as having faced and solved the 'reliability problem' (see Kirk and Kutchins, 1992). Andreasen and Flaum, however, were talking here about the reliability of 'individual symptoms' rather than the reliability of diagnostic judgements, and it appears that few data, new or otherwise, were available because 'the more ambitious goal of the current field trial is to quantify reliability at the level of individual symptoms' (Flaum and Andreasen, 1991: 141) then, 'other things being equal, symptoms that have demonstrated high rates of reliability are preferable' (Andreasen and Flaum, 1991: 29).

The problem with this 'biometric principle', however, is that observers' judgements of 'symptoms' or subjective complaints *are* often rather unreliable; it is almost one of the defining features of phenomena which are called symptoms. As I pointed out in Chapter 1, it is partly because judgements of symptoms are known to be potentially unreliable that 'signs' – that is, antecedent events found in association with symptoms and which can be reliably observed – are so important in the identification of medical patterns. And it is precisely the absence of any event which could be called a sign in any cluster from which 'schizophrenia' is inferred which has reduced Andreasen and Flaum to this focus on the reliability of individual 'symptoms' – that, and an unwillingness to confront the implications of this lack. Quantifying the reliability of every phenomenon said to be a symptom of schizophrenia is therefore, to put it bluntly, a waste of time: it is not simply that observers' judgements will show varying reliability, but the level of reliability will tell us nothing about whether the 'symptom' forms part of a meaningful pattern which would justify inferring 'schizophrenia'. In other words, quantifying the reliability of individual 'symptoms of schizophrenia' begs the prior question: how do you know which phenomena to study?

The second 'biometric principle' suggested by Andreasen and Flaum was 'an adequate base rate [for each symptom]' (29). It must be said that it is not immediately obvious what Andreasen and Flaum are talking about here. Base rates *are* an important issue in psychometrics and medical screening but they are not usually discussed in relation to pattern identification or in relation to individual symptoms. Base rates are defined as the rate of occurrence of a condition or phenomenon in a particular setting and their importance in psychometrics or screening can be seen from the following example:

Suppose I work in a unit where 90 per cent of residents are known to be brain damaged. The base rate of brain damage *in that setting* is 90 per cent. My best prediction about the next person referred is that they will be brain damaged – the probability of a correct prediction is 0.9 using the base rates alone. Suppose, however, that I have a cognitive test whose overall efficiency in classifying people as brain-damaged or not, according to valid and independent criteria, is 80 per cent (i.e. 80 per cent of classifications made by the test are correct). If I were to use the test to 'discover' whether the next referral to my unit were brain damaged, I would actually be more likely to be wrong than if I simply used the base rate, because the probability of a correct classification with the test is only 0.8. But suppose now that I transfer to a unit where only 10 per cent of the residents are known to be brain damaged and that we need to identify those people. The cognitive test might now be better than a base rate prediction in identifying brain damage. To complicate matters further, however, the efficiency of a test in making correct classifications can change, sometimes quite dramatically, if the base rate of a particular condition is very different in the setting where the test is used from that in the setting in which the test was developed.

It is for these reasons that base rates are such an important issue in psychometrics and screening and have to be taken into account in judging the usefulness of tests and screening devices in particular settings. Andreasen and Flaum, however, were using the term in a quite different way and in a way which has nothing to do with its use in psychometrics. The problem they were trying to solve is this: studies of people diagnosed as schizophrenic by various criteria have charted the frequency of what are said to be particular 'symptoms' in the study sample. Mellor (1970), for example, studied a group of people diagnosed as schizophrenic and reported that 21.4 per cent showed 'thought broadcasting'; 19.7 per cent 'thought insertion', and so on. The problem is that different studies, using different samples, often produce very different frequencies for the same 'symptom', and some of the frequencies are relatively low. Andreasen and Flaum claimed, however, that the frequency of what they called negative symptoms in samples of people diagnosed as schizophrenic was relatively high and argued that '[diagnostic] criteria should be limited to those symptoms which occur relatively frequently, and an ideal [base] rate would probably be greater than 30 or 40 percent' (30).

This argument is extremely problematic and is based on a complete misrepresentation of the idea of base rates and of the diagnostic process. First, when useful medical concepts are applied in diagnosis (i.e. when new exemplars of well-established patterns are identified), this produces groups of people who share important features – important in the sense that they may signify other, as yet unobserved, shared features. Thus, people who receive a diagnosis of diabetes mellitus share blood-glucose abnormalities; 'cancer' means sharing cells of certain types; 'Down's syndrome' means sharing certain chromosomal patterns, and so on. We could then say that the base rate of a certain chromosome pattern in Down's syndrome was 100 per cent. But we do not say this because it is a tautology: the figure is produced because the diagnosis is not made except in the presence of this feature. On the other hand, the frequency of 'symptoms' will vary within a diagnostic category. Some people with cancerous tumours will experience pain or nausea or fatigue and others will not, depending on the site of the tumour, its stage of development, the person's sensitivity to bodily cues, and so on. If we were to talk about the 'base rates' of each of these symptoms in 'cancer' we would probably be greeted with some puzzlement and questions about relevance. This kind of variability in frequency, then, is common at the level of symptoms or subjective complaints regardless of diagnostic category. In the case of 'schizophrenia', however, with its varying sets of diagnostic criteria and its diagnostic dependence on subjective complaints, the problem is compounded by clinician preferences: those who follow Schneider in believing that positive, 'first rank symptoms' are important in 'schizophrenia' will tend to produce groups of 'schizophrenics' with relatively high rates of at least one of these; the same applies to 'negative symptoms'. The problem, of course, is embarrassing, but it cannot be solved by invoking 'base rates' or by suggesting arbitrary frequencies for the 'symptoms' which are included in the diagnostic criteria for 'schizophrenia'.

A second problem with invoking 'base rates' in this context concerns the fact that the idea of base rates is meaningless except with reference to a specific setting: the base rate of joint pain in an office is very different from the rate in a rheumatology clinic. Surprisingly, Andreasen and Flaum did not make this point about setting, so that we are left with the impression that 'base rate' is somehow an intrinsic property of a 'symptom'. It is clear, however, that they were talking about base rates in relation to people already diagnosed as schizophrenic. In other words, they were arguing that DSM-IV criteria for 'schizophrenia' should only contain 'symptoms' which occur relatively frequently in 'schizophrenia'. This kind of argument, already discussed in Chapter 3 in relation to Schneider, is, of course, based entirely on question-begging: its unstated assumption is that there already exists a valid means of diagnosing 'schizophrenia'; otherwise, how would it be possible to calculate the frequency of particular 'symptoms' in 'schizophrenia'? It is, then, another example of the devisers of the DSM beginning their task of finding diagnostic criteria for schizophrenia while implicitly assuming that the task has already been successfully completed.

Given all of these problems, it is not surprising that Andreasen and Flaum (1991) should be reduced to invoking 'common sense' (30) as the basis of their choice of base rate for including 'symptoms' in the DSM-IV criteria for schizophrenia – on this 'common-sense' criterion, base rates of less than 10–15 per cent are too low; more than 30–40 per cent would be 'ideal' (30). It is ironic that Andreasen and Flaum should earlier have derided this same common sense as the basis for DSM-III's diagnostic criteria (29), a common sense which was to be superseded by 'modern biometric methods'.

Andreasen and Flaum briefly discussed a third aspect of 'biometrics' which was claimed to be useful in making decisions about diagnostic criteria: discriminant function analysis. When it is used in relation to diagnostic classification, the starting point of this statistical technique is two or more groups who have already been given a diagnostic label, e.g. schizophrenia, affective disorder, delusional disorder, etc. Each person, regardless of diagnostic label, is rated on a list of items or 'symptoms' chosen by the researcher, and one aim of the technique is to identify which items or 'symptoms' best discriminate the groups. Put another way, discriminant function analysis helps answer the question of whether, although we have assigned these people to separate groups, the categories really are statistically separate, or whether they overlap to such an extent that we might think of them belonging to one population. If the categories do seem to be statistically separate, then we can ask which items or 'symptoms' seem to be achieving this separation. The technique is complex, is based on a number of assumptions and is useful for investigating certain questions (see Kendell, 1975b). It is, however, of no use for the purpose to which Andreasen and Flaum wish to put it – selecting items for DSM-IV criteria for schizophrenia, by trying to identify which 'symptoms' best discriminate groups already diagnosed as schizophrenic and groups with a 'related' diagnosis such as affective disorder. There are several reasons for this. First, as Kendell (1975b) has pointed out, because the starting point of discriminant function analysis is always already diagnosed groups, the method is only capable of testing existing classifications, not of generating new ones. A second problem is that even if certain 'symptoms', say 'hallucinations', *did* appear to discriminate the categories of schizophrenia and affective disorder, this statistical discriminating power is entirely relative to all the other 'symptoms' included in the analysis. As Kendell has pointed out, the apparent discriminating power of a particular 'symptom' can alter dramatically and unpredictably if the discriminant function analysis is repeated using a different mix of items/'symptoms'. In other words, discriminant function analysis cannot tell us about the discriminating power of individual 'symptoms'.

Thus, Andreasen and Flaum's suggestion of using this kind of analysis to identify which symptoms are more 'powerful in achieving [a] classification [of schizophrenia]' (1991: 29) makes limited statistical sense. It also makes no theoretical sense because even if we could identify specific symptoms which discriminated different diagnostic groups, this tells us nothing about whether or how these 'symptoms' form part of a pattern; it may simply tell us about clinicians' diagnostic preferences or about their adherence to particular diagnostic systems.

It is clear, then, that the 'modern biometric methods' suggested by Andreasen and Flaum as the basis for selecting DSM-IV's criteria for 'schizophrenia' are both irrelevant to the problem and involve extensive misrepresentation of the techniques. It has to be said that this misrepresentation was necessary, otherwise the irrelevance of 'biometrics' to the problem of finding correspondence rules for 'schizophrenia' would have been obvious. What Andreasen and Flaum have done, in effect, is to borrow the credibility and status of established ideas and techniques which have relevance in specific contexts, in order to give scientific credence to an activity – searching for correspondence rules for 'schizophrenia' – in which it is entirely lacking.

In pursuing the use of 'modern biometric methods', the Schizophrenia Work Group promised that 'the base-rate, sensitivity and specificity [discriminating power] for each symptom included in each of [five alternative draft] criteria sets [for schizophrenia] will be quantified [in the DSM-IV field trials]' (Flaum and Andreasen, 1991: 141). But the data obtained from this exercise would inevitably vary from research centre to research centre and, in any case, there were no rules, except arbitrary ones, or 'common sense', which might guide the application of the data to the choice of DSM-IV criteria for 'schizophrenia'. These arguments about biometric methods, however, were made in the preparatory period of DSM-IV; they were accounts of what was desirable or was going to happen and clearly functioned to surround the process with an air of technical and scientific authority. But given the arguments' lack of substance, it is interesting to examine how this scientific veneer was maintained when DSM-IV was actually published. The next section will therefore look at a third paper which (indirectly) addressed the science question. It was written by the Chair of the Work Group and another prominent 'schizophrenia' researcher (Andreasen and Carpenter, 1993) and published just before the publication of DSM-IV; this section will also look at the introduction to DSM-IV itself.

### Presenting the DSM-IV criteria

Andreasen and Carpenter's paper presented the draft DSM-IV criteria for 'schizophrenia', which were very similar to the final version. It also described some of the process of developing DSM-IV and reported that the field trials had recently been completed. Perhaps all the trial data had not yet been analysed, but readers of this paper would still be entitled to expect a detailed examination of how the 'modern biometric methods', discussed so extensively in 1991, had been used to inform the development of the DSM-IV criteria for 'schizophrenia'. Surprisingly, however, the term 'biometric methods' was not mentioned in the 1993 paper. Instead, readers were merely told that 'DSM-IIIR criteria for schizophrenia have been evaluated to determine whether they have a high enough base-rate to be useful and serve a gate keeping function (i.e. are relatively specific)' (204). How exactly this related to the development of DSM-IV criteria was not explained. It appears that the emptiness of the promise held out by 'modern biometric methods' had become too obvious to ignore, or at least too obvious for the same prestigious-sounding language to be used in 1993 as had been employed in 1991. Not only that, but on the eve of publication of DSM-IV, the Work Group clearly felt obliged to acknowledge the issue of 'user-friendliness' which had featured in previous discussions. Thus, the 'overall goal has been to produce a new set of criteria [for schizophrenia] that provide a more complete coverage of symptoms, to re-emphasise the breadth of the characteristic symptoms of schizophrenia and to simplify the criteria to enhance user friendliness' (204).

But this mix of question-begging (how could they know what were the characteristic symptoms of schizophrenia unless they already had valid diagnostic criteria?) and reassurance that the criteria would not be too difficult to learn and remember, hardly amounted to a robust defence of their scientific basis, particularly when it was admitted that the criteria were 'arbitrary' (210). Andreasen and Carpenter achieved this defence, or more accurately a defence of the criteria's *lack* of a scientific basis, by the subtle but powerful device of embedding their very brief discussion of DSM-IV within two much longer sections on the past and the future.

The paper opened with the statement that 'Schizophrenia is a clinical syndrome of extraordinary complexity. The care of persons afflicted with schizophrenia is challenging, fascinating and frustrating' (199–200). But this is perplexing: the paper was written for a highly specialist journal with a specialist and experienced readership who did not need to be told this. The only possible function of such a statement in this context was to warn the audience not to expect too much of DSM-IV. The section continued with further statements about problems which would already be well known to readers; for example, '[t]he student of schizophrenia pursues a moving target. Manifestations of this disorder are varied' (200), followed by a detailed discussion of the history of the concept of schizophrenia and of Kraepelin's, Bleuler's and Schneider's unsuccessful attempts to define its 'features'. The implicit message was clear: if the founding fathers of psychiatry could not agree on a definition of this complex disorder, how can we be expected to do any better? There was further discussion of attempts to validate 'schizophrenia' which had been no more successful than attempts to define its features. Again the message was clear: many have tried to solve the nosological problem of schizophrenia and been defeated by its complexity, so do not expect too much from DSM-IV.

This kind of discussion, however, is clearly rather unsatisfactory as a way of introducing the publication of new diagnostic criteria for 'schizophrenia'; it is obviously little more than an apologia for failure. But unlike Kendler's paper, which I discussed earlier, Andreasen and Carpenter's paper lays the blame not on science – a tactic, which, I suggested, might raise too many awkward questions – but on the complexity of 'schizophrenia' itself. This is a more hopeful stance, for it is the task of scientists to persevere and to solve complex problems. The final section of the paper, and the longest, therefore focused on the future, a tactic which both diverts attention from the failures of the present and provides an illusion of progress. This future will involve not 'modern biometric methods', but 'clinicopathologic correlational validation using the new techniques of neuroscience' and using methods which attempt to find the 'neural substrates' of diagnostic categories, or subcategories or even 'symptoms', in order to identify the 'underlying mechanisms and causes of schizophrenia' and thus to develop definitions of it (205, 206). We have returned here to prestigious and technical language, so necessary if a scientific veneer is to be maintained. These 'neural substrates', however, have never been identified, so the remainder of the paper is taken up with a non-specific discussion of the difficulties of *that* process in the face of the well-known complexities of 'schizophrenia'. The implicit message in this discussion is that although the future of 'schizophrenia' is bright, it may take some time for success to be achieved. But, since DSM-V is some years away, Andreasen and Carpenter will not immediately be called to account.

These authors thus draw on the very powerful theme of 'progress through science' in attempting both to justify and divert attention from the shortcomings of DSM-IV's diagnostic criteria for schizophrenia. But although this focus on the future is likely to be at least partly effective for these purposes, it is not entirely satisfactory because it still leaves potentially difficult questions about the present: if DSM-IV's criteria for 'schizophrenia' are 'arbitrary', why should we pay any attention to them or, indeed, to the diagnostic category of schizophrenia? Andreasen and Carpenter's final comments are clearly intended to address this problem: the diagnostic criteria for 'schizophrenia' might be arbitrary, but they are also 'robustly valid for many clinical, research and demographic purposes' (210). Quite how this extraordinary conjunction of arbitrariness and robust validity – certainly unique in the history of science – has been achieved is not explained.

Andreasen and Carpenter's paper was published in the year before the publication of DSM-IV. Perhaps not surprisingly, the manual itself does not refer to 'arbitrary criteria'; this may have been permissible in a specialist journal and in the context of discussions of past and future, but it is more risky in the manual itself. Instead, DSM-IV returns to the language of science. It claims, for example, that 'more than any other nomenclature of mental disorders, DSM-IV is grounded in empirical evidence' (xvi) and that it 'reflects the best available clinical and research literature' (xix). In addition, the decision-making process is described in technical language:

> The domains considered in making decisions [about diagnostic criteria] included clinical utility, reliability, descriptive validity, psychometric performance characteristics of individual criteria and a number of validating variables.
>
> (xviii)

There is, however, a later 'cautionary statement' which claims that '[t]he specified diagnostic criteria for each mental disorder are offered as guidelines for making diagnoses because it has been demonstrated that the use of such criteria enhances agreement among clinicians and investigators'. And if this seems to contradict the elaborate claims made earlier about validity, then the reassurance is offered that 'The proper use of these criteria requires specialised clinical training that provides both a body of knowledge and clinical skills' (xxvii). The implication here is that there exists a separate body of knowledge and expertise, presumably derived from science, which inexplicably could not be incorporated into DSM-IV but which still informs its use. Thus, regardless of criticisms which might be made of DSM-IV itself, the veneer of science is maintained and protected..

## The DSM: an overview

In discussing the development of DSM-III, IIIR and IV in relation to schizophrenia, I have emphasised the futility of the task of trying to 'find' correspondence rules or a set of regularities for an existing concept and, moreover, for one with such a problematic history. Not surprisingly, DSM-IV, like its predecessors, failed in this task. The process of developing diagnostic criteria for schizophrenia in DSM-IV, however, was more fraught and more complex than for DSM-III or IIIR. I have suggested that one of the reasons for this was that the relatively straightforward if misguided approach adopted by DSM-III of trying to identify a cluster of 'symptoms' which were associated with particular onset and outcome had clearly not worked. This was, of course, the same approach adopted, with equal lack of success, by Kraepelin. In the face of this lack of success, the devisers of the DSM could either abandon schizophrenia diagnoses, which appeared to be unthinkable, or demonstrate that the 'symptoms' from which schizophrenia was inferred were reliably associated with brain abnormalities. This option was simply unavailable and apparently unlikely to be available in the foreseeable future. The alternative, then, was to construct new, elaborate and plausible-seeming frameworks for making decisions about 'schizophrenia' in DSM-IV which maintained an impression of science while allowing decisions to be made on a range of grounds which owed nothing to relevant research evidence.

One further point deserves emphasis and that is the extent to which the development of DSM-III, IIIR and IV is based on question-begging. Like Kraepelin, Bleuler and Schneider, the devisers of the DSM did not appear to doubt the validity of 'schizophrenia': it might be complex, it might have many subtypes and many causes; we might not yet have a clear definition, but it *is* a diagnosable disorder which clinicians know when they see. This cognitive starting point is crucial both in maintaining the plausibility of the task of 'finding' diagnostic criteria and in making failure seem like a temporary aberration; I shall discuss it further in Chapter 7.

For the moment, however, I want to return to the issue of the theoretical network of 'schizophrenia'. I emphasised in Chapter 1 that correspondence rules which denote a set of regularities are a prerequisite, a necessary condition, for examining the fate of predictions from a concept and, therefore, for developing its theoretical network. But if the conclusions drawn here are valid – that the official correspondence rules for 'schizophrenia' do not denote and never have denoted a set of regularities – then it is extremely difficult to understand how a concept without, so to speak, this benefit could have developed the kind of rich theoretical network said to surround 'schizophrenia'. Central to this network is the persistent claim that schizophrenia has a genetic basis; in other words, that the construct has enabled researchers to make predictions and to gather supporting data which imply genetic antecedents of a particular cluster of behaviour. Kendell (1975b), for example, claimed that there is 'incontrovertible evidence that genetic factors are involved in the transmission of [schizophrenic illness]' (185) and that the evidence that genetic factors play a major role in its aetiology is already 'beyond challenge' (1991: 61); an editorial in *The Lancet* (14 January 1989) declared that '[a]n impressive body of evidence . . . suggests that inheritance plays an important part [in schizophrenia]' (79), and ten years later, in the same journal, Schultz and Andreasen (1999) seemed to take this 'important part' for granted in claiming that 'current research seeks to detect causal mechanisms in schizophrenia through . . . models of genetic transmission such as polygenic models of inheritance in genetic research'; Michael Rutter claimed that 'twin and adoption studies [of schizophrenia] show that there is a substantial genetic influence' (BBC Radio 4; *The World Tonight*, 20 February 1997), while Tsuang *et al.* (2001) argued that '[d]ata from family, twin and adoption studies show overwhelming evidence of a substantial genetic component in schizophrenia' (18). Finally, DSM-IV claims that 'much evidence suggests the importance of genetic factors in the etiology of schizophrenia' (1994: 283). This paradox – of a construct without, apparently, an empirical base, nevertheless being surrounded by a strong theoretical network – will be examined in the next chapter.

# Chapter 6

# Genetic research

It is notable that before any empirical literature existed, the belief that 'schizophrenia' or 'dementia praecox' had a genetic basis was already well established. Kraepelin (1899) claimed, without providing any supporting evidence, that '[a]n inherited predisposition to mental disturbances was apparent in approximately seventy per cent of those cases in which data could be evaluated' (203). Some clues as to how he reached this conclusion were provided by Kraepelin's comment that '[b]odily signs of degeneracy were often found – a small or deformed skull, childlike appearance, defective teeth, misshapen ears, strabismus, masses of warts on the chest, general feebleness and indications of an easily excited brain' (203). Bleuler shared Kraepelin's beliefs, and his lack of evidence:

> [I]f an adherent of an 'infectious theory' of this disease should choose to say that there is no hereditary factor in schizophrenia but merely an infection from some common source . . . we would be unable to produce any proof to the contrary. Such skeptics could observe that in many cases, even after the most thorough study, no evidence of any hereditary *anlage* and no individual predisposition has ever been proven. And yet heredity does play its role in the etiology of schizophrenia . . .
>
> ([1911] 1950: 337)

Thus, before any attempt at systematic research was ever made, the two most prominent users of the concepts of dementia praecox and schizophrenia were disseminating the view that whatever phenomena they included under these terms were largely inherited.

The subsequent empirical literature can be divided into three parts. The first consists of studies of unseparated families; of particular interest here is a series of twin studies in which the prevalence of schizophrenia diagnoses in the monozygotic and dizygotic co-twins of 'schizophrenics' has been examined. The second set of studies is usually referred to as the adoption studies. Their major aim was to study the prevalence of schizophrenia diagnoses in the biological relatives of adopted children who had been diagnosed as schizophrenic and in the 'adopted-away' children of 'schizophrenic' mothers. The third type of research is known as genetic linkage and this examines the relationship between family patterns of genetic markers (biochemical products of gene loci) and particular psychiatric diagnoses. Each of these will be considered in turn.

## Twin studies

Although a variety of methods have been used to study 'schizophrenics' and their twins, the aim of all studies is to locate a reasonable number of people diagnosed as schizophrenic who are also members of a twin pair. The zygosity of the twin pairs is then investigated and the prevalence of 'schizophrenia' in identical and same-sex fraternal co-twins is examined. It is assumed that monozygotic (MZ) twins are genetically identical and that dizygotic (DZ) twins, like siblings, share, on average, half their genes. It is apparently taken for granted (Gottesman and Shields, 1972, 1982) that if the prevalence of schizophrenia diagnoses is significantly different in the MZ and DZ co-twins, and if no plausible environmental factors are suggested to explain this, then we can assume that genetic factors are important in schizophrenia. The extent to which a group of MZ and DZ twins resemble each other in terms of diagnoses of schizophrenia is usually expressed by a concordance rate. There are a number of ways of calculating and interpreting these rates which will be discussed in more detail later. Table 6.1 presents rates derived from a number of twin studies using what is usually known as pairwise concordance. This rate expresses the proportion of the MZ or DZ group in which both twins have received a diagnosis of schizophrenia (or probable schizophrenia or schizoaffective disorder, etc., depending on the diagnostic criteria used). It is, in fact, virtually impossible to present the results of twin studies in tabular form without giving a misleading impression of what actually went on. Table 6.1, however, simply presents the pairwise concordance rates reported by researchers using broad criteria for inferring schizophrenia. Some recent studies are not presented here because they have not reported pairwise rates. Onstad *et al.* (1991), however, used the possibly narrower criteria of DSM-IIIR and reported pairwise rates of 33 per cent MZ and 4 per cent DZ; Franzek and Beckmann (1998) reported eighteen pairwise rates using different combinations of diagnostic criteria, but their rates of 67 per cent MZ v. 17 per cent DZ or 78 per cent MZ v. 27 per cent DZ would seem the most appropriate for comparison.

The question of interest here is how this disparate set of results, from studies with, as will be seen, considerable methodological and conceptual problems, has come to be presented as part of the 'incontrovertible evidence' that schizophrenia has a genetic basis. Clearly, in order to support this view two points must be argued: first, that the data can be interpreted as support for a genetic view rather than being interpretable in other ways; second, that the

Table 6.1  Reported pairwise concordance rates from some earlier and later twin studies using broad diagnostic criteria

| Author | Date | MZ rate (%) | DZ rate (%) |
|---|---|---|---|
| Luxenburger | 1928 | 58 | 0 |
| Rosanoff et al. | 1934 | 61 | 13 |
| Essen-Möller | 1941 | 71 | 17 |
| Kallmann | 1946 | 69 | 11 |
| Slater | 1953 | 65 | 14 |
| Kringlen | 1966 | 38 | 10 |
| Allen et al. | 1972 | 27 | 5 |
| Gottesman and Shields | 1972 | 50 | 19 |
| Hoffer and Pollin | 1970 | 14 | 4 |
| Fischer | 1973 | 48 | 20 |
| Tienari | 1975 | 15 | 7.5 |

results are consistent across studies and thus lead to similar and reliable conclusions. The devices by which writers on this topic have succeeded in drawing conclusions from twin data which support the genetic hypothesis can be roughly divided into two types. The first involves ignoring or underemphasising serious methodological and conceptual problems which cast doubt on the validity of the data. The second involves presenting, or re-presenting data in such a way as apparently to achieve some conformity to genetic theory and to give an impression of consistency across studies. I shall consider these two issues separately although they are not, of course, independent: it is in part by ignoring methodological and conceptual problems that the data can be made to seem consistent.

## Methodological and conceptual problems

The type of study which I will review here is usually conducted over a number of years and can be divided into several stages. First, the sampling frame is selected; that is, the geographical and residential confines within which the 'schizophrenic' twins will be sought. Second, when this group has been selected, efforts are made to trace their co-twins. Third, the twins' zygosity is investigated. Fourth (or concurrently) information is collected from the twins themselves and from other sources, and diagnoses are made. Fifth, concordance rates are calculated and interpreted. Problems can – and do – arise at any or all of these stages.

### Sample selection

Participants initially selected for study are usually called probands or index cases. They must satisfy two criteria: they must conform to the researchers' idea of a schizophrenic and they must be a twin. Rosenthal (1962a) has discussed some of the problems which might arise in trying to find people who belong to both these relatively infrequent groups. In those studies which begin with hospitalised samples, then only those who have come to psychiatric attention can become probands. It is not unreasonable to suppose that two people whose behaviour is disturbing are more noticeable, and more of a burden to their family, than is one and that one or both are more likely to be admitted to hospital. Thus, the use of a hospital population may result in an excess of concordant pairs. Leonhard (1980) has suggested that both twins are more likely to be admitted in a concordant MZ than in a DZ pair, thus spuriously heightening the MZ concordance rate of a hospital sample. Of course, once admitted, MZ twins are extremely striking, so that some early twin researchers' practice of asking staff to find twins for study would exacerbate this bias.

Kringlen (1976) has clearly demonstrated another way in which concordance rates may be inflated by the use of hospitalised participants and in particular by the use of a small and unrepresentative sampling frame. His argument runs as follows:

> If the probability of being hospitalised and reported to a twin researcher is 80 per cent, and members of a concordant pair are admitted and reported independently, then the probability of being included in the sample = 0.8 for a discordant pair.
>
> For a concordant pair, $p$ = 0.96 (the probability that either of two outcomes will occur equals the sum of their independent probabilities minus the probability that both will occur together).
>
> If the probability of being hospitalised and reported = 50 per cent (i.e. the sampling frame is smaller) then:
>
> $p$ (discordant pair) = 0.5
> $p$ (concordant pair) = 0.75
>
> If the sampling frame is reduced further, and the probability of being hospitalised and reported = 10 per cent, then:
>
> $p$ (discordant pair) = 0.1
> $p$ (concordant pair) = 0.2

Thus with a very small sampling frame, using hospitalised participants, the probability of concordant pairs being reported may be double that of discordant pairs. This bias should, of course, influence both MZ and DZ pairs unless, as Leonhard has suggested, concordant MZ pairs are more likely to be admitted or more likely to be noticed by hospital staff.

With the exception of Gottesman and Shields' research, ironically often used to make the strongest claims about twin study data, the later studies listed in Table 6.1 and more recent studies by Onstad et al. (1991) and Cannon et al. (1998) have avoided some sampling biases by beginning not with a hospital population but with a twin register. Unfortunately, comprehensive registers exist only in Scandinavian countries but they have enabled researchers to conduct twin studies with far more representative samples than was ever the case with the older twin studies. Hoffer and Pollin's (1970) US study also began with a twin register – the National Academy of Science/National Research Council's Panel of all Veteran Twins. Some of these studies have cross-referenced twin registers with records of psychiatric hospitalisation (again, central registers exist only in Scandinavian countries).

### Determining zygosity

Having chosen a proband sample and traced their partners, it is relatively easy to decide whether a same-sex pair is fraternal; it is much more difficult to know if they are identical. Even reports that the twins shared one chorion (the membrane surrounding the foetus) cannot be taken as strong evidence of identity; it appears that some pairs, which by other criteria are obviously fraternal, were monochorionic (Tienari, 1963). Similarly, a number of apparently MZ pairs were reportedly dichorial (Price, 1950). It is, however, generally agreed (see, e.g. Tienari, 1963; Fischer, 1973) that identity can be established with a satisfactorily high probability by comparing twins on eight or nine serological systems. Although blood comparisons are more common in later twin studies, and one or two recent studies have used some form of genetic matching, it is notable that none of the twin studies discussed here applied biological matching systems to all twins eventually called MZ, and some did not employ such methods at all. In the early studies, e.g. Luxenburger (1928), as Kringlen (1966) has pointed out, decisions as to zygosity were often made only by supposed similarity of appearance. Kallmann (1946) also appears to have used this method: he claimed that zygosity was decided by personal investigation and by extended observation by the author. Essen-Möller (1941) also used personal examination supplemented 'if possible' by blood groupings and fingerprinting.

It is not difficult to see how such methods could lead to inaccurate conclusions. Researchers' judgements as to similarity of appearance may have been influenced by personal biases, not the least of which was their opinion about diagnoses and knowledge of whether one or both twins had been hospitalised. If twins were not seen simultaneously (and this apparently was the rule rather than the exception; Essen-Möller, 1941, for example, saw only fifteen out of sixty-nine pairs simultaneously) then judgements might have been influenced by poor or biased memory of the first twin's appearance. In MZ pairs where only one twin had been hospitalised, the appearance of the pair may have become dissimilar. Thus, discordant MZ pairs might have been judged to be DZ, and the MZ concordance rate inflated.

Personal observation was often supplemented or replaced by questioning twins' relatives about confusion of identity, similarity of appearance, etc. Hoffer and Pollin (1970) made extensive use of this method and themselves presented data which queries its accuracy. They noted that in a number of cases only one twin of a pair returned the questionnaire; they commented that when this was the schizophrenic twin, a much higher number claimed to be monozygotic than when the non-schizophrenic co-twin answered. And when other relatives were asked about twins, it is not unreasonable to suppose that similarity or dissimilarity in behaviour might have led to overestimations or underestimations of similarity in appearance. Franzek and Beckman (1998), however, reported 97.4 per cent agreement between molecular genetics and their questionnaire methods in a sub-sample of their participants.

Nevertheless, Slater's (1953) account highlights problems with the similarity method of which he made extensive use. He also, however, took fingerprints from 62 per cent of pairs eventually called MZ, but reported that he used a method of quantifying similarity which had never been used before and whose accuracy was therefore unknown. The only evidence he produced as to its accuracy were data demonstrating greater print similarity within MZ than DZ pairs, *but where similarity scores had already been used as one of the criteria for the zygosity decision.* Slater did provide more, albeit sparse, detail than did the authors of some of the other older twin studies about the information on which zygosity decisions were based. Rather than reassuring the reader, the information in fact emphasises the apparent arbitrariness of some decisions and the fact that they may have been influenced by knowledge of diagnoses. All the participants described below were included by Slater, and by those who have reported his study, in the concordant MZ group:

> The family told them apart by a difference about the eyes, but they were often mistaken by others . . . It was not possible for me to make contact with M owing to family obstruction . . . In hospital records, M's eyes are recorded as hazel, C's as blue but no great reliance can be placed on this and it does not appear that any direct physical comparison between the twins was made. Their past history strongly suggests uniovularity. Their psychotic states bear many resemblances . . .
>
> (1953: 150–151)

> They were not mistaken at school as L was fatter and not clever . . . M says she is the taller by 1 or 2 inches . . . Despite the history of no close resemblance, either physically or in personality in early years, there can be little doubt that these twins are uniovular. Both have paranoid illnesses coming on at the time of the menopause and within two years of one another, and with many clinical resemblances . . .
>
> (1953: 127–129)

> A photograph taken of the twins at about fourteen shows close but not startling facial resemblance. P's hair looks rather darker.
>
> (1953: 144)

The problem of establishing zygosity is compounded by the fact that some of the research sample may actually be dead at the time the research is carried out. For example, 43 per cent of Fischer's sample were dead; one partner was already dead in 27 per cent of Slater's MZ group; 29 per cent of Kringlen's sample had either died, left the country, could not be traced or refused to co-operate in zygosity determination; 15 per cent of Kallmann's sample were dead, while Hoffer and Pollin reported that 1.5 per cent of their sample had committed suicide, but not how many had died from other causes.

## Collecting information about the twins

The ways in which data have been collected by twin researchers have at times been as haphazard and incomplete as the methods used to determine zygosity. The methods used have included talking to twins and their relatives (sometimes for only short periods and sometimes only after considerable pressure had been exerted on the reluctant), searching case records and asking questions of family doctors, relatives or even family friends. Each of these methods could clearly result in inaccurate reporting whether through biases or problems in recall. There is, moreover, no twin study in which those who collected the information were definitely blind as to the twins' possible zygosity or to the diagnoses of the proband participants. Nor are there any reports of the reliability or accuracy of the information. The methods used by twin researchers to obtain information, and the problems they present, can perhaps best be illustrated by quoting from the accounts which some of them have provided and which, apparently, contain the total amount of information on which a diagnosis was based:

> X (co-twin) replied to an enquiry, but he died before a follow-up examination could be made. He stated that he was well. A friend of the family related that X was 'eccentric', living entirely alone in a small house, but no further details were known.
> (Fischer, 1973: 123; diagnosis: nervous, odd, neurotic or ? normal; MZ group)

> [Co-twin] had no psychiatric history. Family unwilling for him to be contacted . . . neither twin was seen by us.
> (Gottesman and Shields, 1972: 140; diagnosis: normal; DZ group)

> [Co-twin] refused to be seen for the Twin Investigation, remaining upstairs out of sight, but his wife was seen at the door and an MMPI form left for B. He did not consider completing the MMPI and his wife reported, 'once his mind is made up, nothing will make him change.' He was regarded as a healthy, level headed, solid, happy person who got on well with others, had few close friends and was something of a home bird.
> (Gottesman and Shields, 1972: 170; diagnosis: normal; DZ group)

[Co-twin] had a nervous breakdown at 27 in which she could not concentrate and could not work. She is said to have had periods of confusion
and to have thought she would go mad. She did not have any hospital
treatment . . . after the birth of her third child in 1938 her husband . . .
was killed in an accident. D developed mental symptoms and was transferred to a mental hospital in the West Country which it has proved
impossible to trace . . . She was seen again (by a psychiatric social worker)
for a few minutes in 1948, when she refused all information. She spoke of
the past with little feeling. She said she suffered badly with her nerves, but
would not say more about them than that she felt so tired. She seemed
withdrawn and apprehensive.

(Slater, 1953: 135, 136; diagnosis: psychosis/?schizophrenia;
MZ group)

About 20 [co-twin] started to lie late in bed in the mornings and was so
often late at the office that he was eventually fired . . . He joined the
army as a private, went to India and about 3 years later his uncle heard
that he had committed suicide, by swallowing poison. No other details
were provided by the authorities but some unposted letters found at his
death were returned to the family and showed no suicidal intention or possible reason for such an act.

(Slater, 1953: 143; diagnosis: ?schizophrenic; MZ group)

## Making a diagnosis

It is worth noting that no twin researcher apparently doubts the validity of the
concept of schizophrenia, even if its boundaries are uncertain. There are occa-
sional references to validity (e.g. Gottesman and Shields, 1972, 1982) or to low
reliability (e.g. Fischer, 1973; Onstad et al., 1991), but the implications are
rarely pursued. Twin studies have used a wide range of diagnostic criteria and
many of the studies listed in Table 6.1 did not even state what criteria were
used. Slater, for example, simply reported that '[o]ur material divides itself
conventionally into four main diagnostic groups. By far the largest of these is
formed by the schizophrenic psychoses' (1953: 33). In some of those studies
which have provided criteria, they are at times so vague as to make it impossible to know what specific phenomena were used to infer schizophrenia.
Fischer, for example, stated that:

The criteria used were: A psychiatric disorder with disintegration of personality and affect, associated with impaired relation to reality, disturbance
of thought, hallucinations and/or delusions. There should be no clouding
of consciousness, no marked disturbance of mood and no major signs or
symptoms of organic defects.

(1973: 11)

Kallmann did not provide any diagnostic criteria in his 1946 paper, but did so elsewhere in 1950:

> [O]ur diagnosis of schizophrenia rested on the constellative evaluation of basic personality changes observed in association with a whole group of possible psychopathological mechanisms, rather than on the presence of any particular type of symptomatology. As a general principle, greater diagnostic importance was attached to the demonstrable effect of a 'bending' curve of personality development than to any surface similarities to pathognomic textbook descriptions, especially when this bend was found in conjunction with such malignant features as xenophobic pananxiety, loss of capacity for free-association, inability to maintain contact with reality (autistic and dereistic attitude towards life), or a compulsive tendency to omnipotential thought generalisations.
>
> (quoted in Kringlen, 1964: 22)

With such non-specific, or with no stated, criteria it might be supposed that researchers would at least report on the reliability of their inferences. Reliability has, in fact, been reported in only one of the studies listed in Table 6.1 – that of Gottesman and Shields. This study differs from the others in having had diagnoses made by a panel of six judges, from written material. Each judge was asked 'to apply his personal criteria in his own way' (211). Of those participants eventually called 'schizophrenic' by consensus, 66 per cent had been independently called this by six judges and 90 per cent by five or six. Some recent studies have reported reliability using the more appropriate Kappa statistic which controls for chance agreements, but the figures are not high: 0.75 for DSM-IIIR schizophrenia (Cardno et al., 1999); 0.65–0.67 for ICD8/DSM-IIIR schizophrenia (Cannon et al., 1998). The problem of reliability is compounded by the fact that in many twin studies the diagnoses were made by the researchers who had themselves collected the sometimes extremely limited information on which they were based, and who apparently knew, or at least suspected, the twins' supposed zygosity. Even in those studies where zygosity judgements were made quite independently of the researchers, it is difficult to believe that in the course of collecting information the researchers did not pick up strong clues as to zygosity. Similarly, in those studies where diagnosis appears to have been made independently of researchers' information collection, problems remain. Cannon et al.'s (1998) study, for example, was based on diagnoses recorded in hospital and other official sources, with no way of knowing whether these were influenced by knowledge of zygosity or the psychiatric status of a co-twin. In Gottesman and Shields' (1972) study, the written material on which diagnostic judgements by a separate panel were based was prepared by the authors, who reported that '[o]f course, when we prepared the summaries, we knew about both twins and tried to do justice to both similarities and differences' (210). It can only be assumed here that they were referring to zygosity, as well as to other details; certainly, they did not reassure readers to the contrary. Given that Gottesman and Shields' bias in favour of genetic explanations of twin data is so strong as to invite chastisement from a fellow twin researcher (Kringlen, 1976), it is difficult completely to share their confidence. In Hoffer and Pollin's (1970) study, diagnoses were made by a variety of army doctors. There is, however, no way of knowing to what extent they were aware of whether their patients' MZ or DZ twins had also been diagnosed as schizophrenic. In the later extension of this research (Allen *et al.*, 1972), these diagnoses were accepted or rejected by the authors after examination of case material. Unfortunately, the case material was arranged in twin pairs and included details of assumed zygosity.

Once diagnoses, however problematic, have been made, it is a relatively simple matter to calculate the concordance rates which are generally presented as data in primary and secondary sources. As will be seen in the next section, however, the ways in which these data have been calculated and reported have served to obscure the considerable methodological and conceptual problems presented by the twin studies.

## The presentation of twin studies and their data

It is clear that the inadequacies both of the concept of schizophrenia and of twin researchers' methods make the conversion of their subjective judgements into numerical data and the interpretation of such data very problematic. Nevertheless, the conversion and interpretation have both been achieved and in such a way as apparently to leave beyond doubt the fact that schizophrenia has a genetic basis. The two most prolific commentators on twin studies have been Irving Gottesman and James Shields. They have also produced a textbook (1982) devoted to reviewing genetic research on 'schizophrenia'. Although post-1982 studies could obviously not be included, Gottesman and Shields' comments will be considered in some detail because of their extensiveness and for several other reasons. First, recent studies have not resolved the methodological problems highlighted here; second, the results from these studies are still very inconsistent, so that examining ways in which an impression of consistency has been created for earlier research remains important; third, some of the studies discussed in Gottesman and Shields' review, and the review's conclusions, are often cited in secondary sources as part of the established evidence that schizophrenia has a genetic basis; finally, Gottesman and Shields' review was arguably very influential in encouraging the use of the problematic probandwise method (see pp. 166–168) of calculating twin concordance for 'schizophrenia'.

### The uncritical road from judgements to numbers

Gottesman and Shields (1982) presented the results of twin studies apparently as a series of straightforward 'findings', in two tables (here Tables 6.2 and 6.3).

Table 6.2 Simple pairwise concordance in older schizophrenic twin series (reported by Gottesman and Shields, 1982)

| Investigator | MZ pairs | | SS DZ pairs | |
|---|---|---|---|---|
| | Total | Concordance (%) | Total | Concordance (%) |
| Luxenburger | 19 | 58 | 13 | 0 |
| Rosanoff | 41 | 61 | 53 | 13 |
| Essen-Möller | 11 | 64 | 27 | 15 |
| Kallmann | 174 | 69 | 296 | 11 |
| Slater | 37 | 65 | 58 | 14 |
| Inouye* | 58 | 59 | 20 | 15 |
| Total | 340 | 65 | 467 | 12 |

Note: *Updated with 1972a final report and using schizophrenic plus schizophrenic-like psychotic disorders in co-twins.

Table 6.3 Concordances* in newer schizophrenic twin series (reported by Gottesman and Shields, 1982)

| Investigator/ locus | MZ pairs | | | SS DZ pairs | | |
|---|---|---|---|---|---|---|
| | Total | Pairwise† concordance (%) | Proband-wise (%) | Total | Pairwise† concordance (%) | Proband-wise (%) |
| Tienari‡/Finland | 17 | 0–36 | 35 | 20 | 5–14 | 13 |
| Kringlen/Norway | 55 | 25–38 | 45 | 90 | 4–10 | 15 |
| Fischer/Denmark | 21 | 24–48 | 56 | 41 | 10–19 | 27 |
| Pollin et al.‡/USA | 95 | 14–27 | 43 | 125 | 4–8 | 9 |
| Gottesman and Shields/UK | 22 | 40–50 | 58 | 33 | 9–19 | 12 |
| Weighted total | | | 46 | | | 14 |

Notes:
*At the level of functional schizophrenic-like psychoses in co-twins.
†Value or range reported by investigators.
‡Only male twins were studied. Results for 1971 tabled for Tienari because 1975 summary data adding three MZ and twenty-two DZ new pairs lack details; he reports MZ rate 15 per cent, DZ 7 per cent.

Indeed, they had earlier (1972) referred to some of these as forming part of a 'network of basic facts'. There was no detailed discussion of the problems described here, although they did mention some of them: Kallmann's concordance rates, for example, might have been rather high because he used a resident hospital population; it was reported that 35 per cent of Fischer's sample were dead; that Rosanoff's series was obviously incomplete and that he made no personal investigations. In general, however, the problems were either overlooked or, in some cases, mentioned and then excused. Kallmann, apparently, laid himself open to criticism because he unfortunately never found the time to report the details of his study (Shields *et al.*, 1967). Similarly, it was admitted that methods of establishing zygosity often left much to be desired but, although Gottesman and Shields cannot possibly know, they claimed that '[early researchers'] clinical judgements, when based on the simultaneous examination of both twins were not likely to be much in error' (1972: 24). Unfortunately, they omitted to mention that even this crude method was not routinely used by early twin researchers.

## The search for consistency

Gottesman and Shields' major concern appears to be with the creation of an impression of consistency amongst the twin research data. It is, of course, important that such an impression be created if the research is to look credible. A consistent impression demands, first, that concordance rates for MZ twins be relatively high and obviously higher than those for DZ twins and, second, that the rates be roughly similar across studies. It seems obvious, however, that MZ rates ranging from 69 per cent to nought per cent are neither consistent nor always particularly high. The question of interest is therefore how Gottesman and Shields have presented the data in order that it should appear to support their conclusion. The methods discussed in the next section, together with an examination of Tables 6.2 and 6.3, will show some of the ways in which this goal has been achieved.

## The use of the 'schizophrenia spectrum'

Gottesman and Shields report two sets of pairwise rates obtained using narrow and broad criteria for inferring schizophrenia; that is, less or more relaxed criteria for calling twins concordant. The use of broad criteria will tend to inflate concordance rates. The rates may be inflated unequally in MZ and DZ groups: it appears, from the small amount of information available, that more effort may have been expended in gathering information about MZ than about DZ co-twins (for example more of them were personally interviewed) or, at least, that judgements about MZ co-twins were based on more detailed information. Given that various eccentricities appear to have been labelled as 'schizophrenia' or '?schizophrenia', then these are more likely to show up in the group for which more information is available. When this problem is considered together with the fact that the criteria for '?schizophrenia' are extremely vague and that the researchers may have known or suspected the twins' zygotic status, then it seems not unreasonable to suppose that the inflation of rates may be unequal. The extent to which concordance rates may be changed by broadening diagnostic criteria is shown in Table 6.4. As we can see, 'schizophrenia' can apparently be changed from a genetic to a non-genetic disorder simply by altering the criteria used to infer it.

*Table 6.4* Pairwise concordance rates for MZ twins using the authors' broad and narrow criteria

| Author | Narrow criteria (%) | Broad criteria (%) |
|---|---|---|
| Essen-Möller (1941) | 14 | 71 |
| Tienari (1963) | 0 | 19 |
| Kringlen (1968) | 27* | 38† |
| Fischer (1973) | 24 | 48 |

Notes:
*Based on 'registered hospitalised cases'.
†Based on 'personal investigations'.

The use of broad criteria has been justified by the concept of the schizophrenia spectrum (Gottesman and Shields, 1972). This concept, in turn, has been justified by the claim that, although some relatives of schizophrenics have not behaved in such a way as to earn the label themselves, they nevertheless deviated from normality in ways that were more or less similar to the proband group. It is thus assumed that there is a spectrum of schizophrenic disorders and that those who are genetically related to a schizophrenic may show not full-blown schizophrenia but some lesser variant. At first glance, this argument may appear reasonable and, indeed, in principle it is reasonable. Applied to 'schizophrenia', however, it has two major problems. First, there is, not surprisingly, no agreement about the referents of the spectrum. This means that there is no way of knowing just how similar – or dissimilar – are the twins who are called concordant. It also makes comparisons across studies, already a difficult task, virtually impossible. In their tables, Gottesman and Shields present a misleading picture of orderliness by implying that the figures are comparable across studies.

The second, more important, problem stems from the status of the parent concept of schizophrenia. The problem is perhaps best understood by drawing an analogy with the familiar concept of diabetes, particularly as this is a comparison favoured, in another context, by Gottesman and Shields. There have been a number of studies of concordance for diabetes in MZ and DZ twins (e.g. Cerasi and Luft, 1967; Pyke *et al.*, 1970). These, however, have looked at concordance for signs and symptoms and for *signs* only. If we found a twin pair where one had an abnormal response to a glucose tolerance test, sugar in the urine, severe thirst, weight loss, tiredness, etc., while the other had recently lost some weight or sometimes felt 'a bit tired', it would be absurd to call them concordant for diabetes in the absence of signs in the second twin and because weight loss and tiredness are so overdetermined. But this is exactly how twin researchers have proceeded, but without, of course, the presence of any phenomena in the proband twin which would merit the term 'sign'. It will be recalled that the variable cluster from which schizophrenia is inferred contains no sign, but only a number of presumably overdetermined behaviours called 'symptoms' and which have never been shown to be meaningfully related in the ways required by the use of 'schizophrenia'. To use another analogy, if we call a pair of twins who share one or two of these 'symptoms', concordant for schizophrenia, it is almost like calling concordant for cancer a pair of twins where both report that they sometimes get headaches or feel nauseous. There is, in fact, no exact analogy for the absurdities of the schizophrenia spectrum; the major point to be made is that it is impossible to have 'lesser varieties' of a non-existent pattern. The behaviour of twin researchers who use the spectrum concept is, in fact, not dissimilar to that of medieval medical men who tried to group physical complaints in ignorance of their antecedents and who created classificatory chaos. It must be added that in 'schizophrenia' research the error is compounded because concordance is not judged by degree of similarity between twins but by the extent to which each twin independently satisfies the researchers' criteria for 'schizophrenia' or the 'schizophrenia spectrum'. Because these criteria are so broad and subjective it is quite possible to call concordant a twin pair who have none or very few of the behaviours of interest in common, and this is as true of recent studies using 'official' criteria as of earlier research. Given this, it is perhaps not surprising that Onstad *et al.* (1991) should have commented that 'the results [of studies of the genetic relationship between schizophrenia and spectrum disorders] are contradictory and which disorders are to be included in the spectrum is still a matter of dispute' (395–396) – a situation which has not been clarified by more recent studies (e.g. Cannon *et al.*, 1998; Franzek and Beckmann, 1998).

## The presentation of concordance rates

Once diagnostic judgements have been made, then the pattern of concordance across pairs can be expressed in a number of ways. Initially, the most popular way of expressing concordance was by the pairwise method. As I mentioned earlier, this expresses the percentage of pairs where both twins have received a schizophrenia or schizophrenia spectrum diagnosis. Later, however, Gottesman and Shields showed a marked preference for concordance rates calculated in a different way – by the proband method; indeed, in their 1982 text they talked of this as the 'standard, appropriate method' (107), although it must be said that it was they who set the standard and who argued most volubly for its appropriateness.

The use of the term 'proband method' reflects the fact that it depends on counting not pairs but *probands*. Probands are those 'schizophrenic' twins found independently, usually in the original search for participants rather than during the later process of tracing co-twins. It is possible that some of these proband participants will actually be each other's twins. If this were true of five pairs in a sample of thirty pairs, then the researcher would talk not of thirty probands and their co-twins but of thirty-five probands and their co-twins. Thus, the use of the pairwise and probandwise methods implies different questions. The pairwise

*Table 6.5* Methods of calculating concordance in twin studies

| Pairwise | Probandwise |
|---|---|
| 100 pairs | 100 pairs |
| 30 with both 'schizophrenic' | 30 with both 'schizophrenic', but 10 of the 30 'schizophrenic' co-twins found in the original search |
| Concordance = 30/100 = 30% | Concordance = 30+10/100+10 = 36.4% |

method asks: in what proportion of pairs are both called schizophrenic? The probandwise method asks: in what proportion of probands is there a 'schizophrenic' co-twin? It is obvious that the use of the proband method will result in some participants being counted twice, because if twin A and twin B are both found during the original search for subjects, then A will be said to be concordant with B and B with A, making, in effect, two concordant pairs. The way in which these rates are calculated is shown in Table 6.5.

Clearly, the probandwise rate will vary depending on the number of 'schizophrenics' who are found independently of their twins. At first glance, the use of a 'counting twice' method might appear suspect. It is, however, not so *provided certain sampling requirements are met and the appropriate conclusions are drawn*. If the sampling is exhaustive – if a researcher, in the original search for participants, managed to trace every person in a very large population who was a twin and who fulfilled criteria for inferring schizophrenia, and if the diagnostic judgements on the twins were in no way dependent, then it follows that every participant would have been located independently. If the researcher again produced 100 twin pairs, in thirty of whom both partners were called schizophrenic, then the probandwise concordance rate would be 30 + 30/100 + 30 = 46.1 per cent. This rate, however, equals what is known as the *casewise* rate, which is calculated in answer to the question: How many cases in the sample have a 'schizophrenic' co-twin? In calculating this, every member of concordant pairs is counted twice – the term 'casewise' reflects the fact that all 'cases of schizophrenia' are counted, regardless of how they were found. Thus, when all 'cases' are found independently, the probandwise and casewise rates are identical. Marshall and Pettit (1985) have demonstrated that the casewise rate is in fact not an expression of concordance as the term is usually understood, but of the prevalence of the diagnosis of schizophrenia amongst the co-twins of 'schizophrenics'. It can thus only be compared meaningfully with the *population* prevalence of schizophrenia diagnoses.

If the pairwise rate expresses the proportion of concordant pairs and the casewise rate is comparable to a population statistic, where does this leave the probandwise rate as a measure of concordance? The simple answer is nowhere or, as Marshall and Pettit point out, as an arbitrary and uninterpretable figure somewhere between pairwise and casewise rates. Probandwise rates are arbitrary because they are completely dependent on the vagaries of sampling, the extent of which is usually unknown. Neale and Oltmanns (1980), following Slater and Cowie, have noted that the probandwise method is appropriate *'only if the probability of ascertaining an index case (proband) is independent of the condition of the co-twin'* (182; my emphasis). It is extremely unlikely that this condition could be met by any twin study of 'schizophrenia' or that it could ever be possible – short of investigating every twin in an exceptionally large population – to know whether it had been achieved. It is challenging credulity to suggest that, if both partners in an MZ twinship are behaving strangely, and one has been reported, then the other has no more chance of being noticed (and therefore ending up as an index case) than has a single person. Whether or not both twins are noticed may depend on such factors as the attitude and tolerance of the family, the curiosity of the psychiatrist, the age gap between the twins becoming deviant, the age at which one was reported, and the geographical mobility of the population. These last two are important because twins living close together or even in the same house are surely more likely both to be reported than are twins who live far apart. It may be that any bias towards joint reporting is greater for MZ than for DZ twins in the same way that concordant MZ pairs may be more likely both to be admitted to hospital. Allen *et al.* (1967) have argued that probandwise rates can be used provided the twin sample is representative of a defined population. They have suggested that, if this condition is met, then the 'double ascertainment' of concordant pairs in a hospital sample will be balanced by pairs in which neither twin is ascertained as an index case. The problem with this argument is that it is virtually impossible to demonstrate that such a research sample *is* representative of the population of interest – in this case MZ and DZ twins where one or both are behaving strangely – because the parameters of the population are unknown. It may be that some twin researchers believe that a sample is representative if its ratio of MZ to DZ pairs approximates the population rate. But this is not the only criteria which must be fulfilled here. It must also be shown that twin study samples – many of whom are drawn from *hospital* populations, are the same samples which would result from a representative selection of the appropriate ratio of MZ and DZ pairs from the total population of all deviant twins whose behaviour – whether reported or not – might earn them the labels 'schizophrenia' or 'schizophreniform', or whatever.

It can be seen from Table 6.3 that probandwise rates are higher than pairwise rates in all later twin studies. The use of probandwise rates will almost certainly inflate concordance rates. Double ascertainment may also be more likely for MZ than for DZ pairs because MZ pairs are more remarkable, because physical identity may heighten an impression of behavioural identity, and because MZ twins *may* live closer together. Thus, at a stroke, concordance rates may be inflated, MZ and DZ groups made to look less similar and 'schizophrenia' made to look 'more genetic'. Given these problems, it is dismaying that some of the most recent studies (e.g. Cardno *et al.*, 1999; Cannon *et al.*, 1998) should have omitted pairwise rates in favour of probandwise rates.

*Selective criticism of low-rate studies*

The two studies which have obtained the lowest pairwise rates are those by Tienari and by Hoffer and Pollin. These rates have been inflated by the use of the probandwise method, but Gottesman and Shields have further inflated the rates from these studies by the selective presentation and criticism of their data.

In 1975, in an extension of his 1963 study and using broad diagnostic criteria, Tienari reported an MZ pairwise concordance rate of 15 per cent. This low figure, however, did not appear in Gottesman and Shields' table because, they claimed, the report lacked case details. To be fair, Tienari's results were mentioned in a footnote, but it is curious that they were not tabled because studies whose (higher) rates *were* tabled also lacked case detail. Kallmann (1946), for example, presented no case detail; Fischer reported information only for MZ twins and Slater only for concordant MZ pairs and for DZ pairs which he considered to be of special interest. Gottesman and Shields were also peculiarly critical of Tienari's sample, in claiming that his 1963 nought per cent concordance rate '[was] mitigated by the fact that some of the pairs seemed to us to be organic psychosis from the detailed case histories Tienari provided' (1982: 103). It is not clear why Tienari's research should be singled out in this way, given the haphazard and often unreported information on which other researchers based their diagnoses. In addition, Fischer mentioned clear organic problems in some of her sample and the fact that some cases had had head injuries; Allen *et al.* (1972) apparently included participants with histories of chronic alcoholism, head injuries, febrile convulsions and tuberculosis, while Gottesman and Shields themselves admitted of one of their probands that 'The role of organic factors in A's personality development and eventual somewhat atypical schizophrenia is unclear' (1972: 179). Nevertheless, A remained in the sample as part of a discordant DZ pair. Tienari's supposedly organic discordant MZ participants were, however, omitted in Gottesman and Shields' presentation of the maximum pairwise concordance rate, and they later explicitly drew attention to the fact that Tienari's study had now been 'brought into the fold':

> The possible use of some kind of age correction together with the probandwise method of calculating rates makes the Finnish study no longer so much of an odd-man-out in the literature.
>
> (1982: 105)

Although Gottesman and Shields did not make this age correction (i.e. take into account that not all participants in a twin study might have passed the risk age for being diagnosed as schizophrenic) it is strange that they should even suggest it, given that they had earlier rejected the idea for Kallmann's data, that they have not suggested it for other studies and that Tienari's later figures were derived from a sample all of whom were forty and over, thus virtually eliminating the need for any age correction. If, however, Gottesman and Shields wished to be consistent themselves, they could have applied age corrections to some older studies and compared Tienari's results with those. Had they done so, however, they would have been forced to compare Tienari's age-corrected (and probably little changed) 15 per cent with, for example, an age-corrected rate of 86 per cent for Kallmann and 76 per cent for Slater.

Gottesman and Shields' treatment of Hoffer and Pollin's (1970) study offers further support to the idea that they have tried to create an impression of consistency where none exists. Using a very large sampling frame, one of the largest samples in this research area, and diagnoses made independently of the authors, Hoffer and Pollin reported a pairwise MZ concordance rate of 13.8 per cent. Two years later, Allen *et al.* (1972) reported a rate of 27 per cent obtained by presenting themselves with Hoffer and Pollin's case material *but arranged as twin pairs of known zygosity* and by widening diagnostic criteria. Clearly, these two studies, carried out in very different ways by different people, should have been presented separately. As can be seen from Table 6.3, however, Gottesman and Shields have presented them as one study by Pollin *et al.* The way in which the data have been presented could create the impression that Hoffer and Pollin's 13.8 per cent was obtained using narrow criteria and Allen *et al.*'s using broad. But this was not the case. Hoffer and Pollin's sample had been diagnosed by military psychiatrists who apparently used the broad and rather vague criteria of DSM-I or DSM-II, and it is impossible to know how far the rise to 27 per cent was a result of Allen *et al.*'s broad criteria or of their extremely flawed methodology. Nevertheless, Hoffer and Pollin's data were effectively ignored, while Allen *et al.*'s were apparently used to calculate the probandwise rate. Gottesman and Shields merely commented that Allen *et al.*'s results are 'not very different from other samples but quite different from the first reports of these data by the investigators' (1982: 101).

Although Gottesman and Shields have thus created some impression of consistent results across later studies, the problem remains of the discrepancies between the results of older and later studies. Gottesman and Shields have dealt with this partly by offering comparisons between the *pairwise rates* from older studies with the *probandwise* rates from the later work and declaring them to be similar. They made no attempt to perform the appropriate (from their point of view) comparison between the *probandwise* rates of earlier and later studies. This is curious because not only are pairwise and probandwise comparisons meaningless even within their framework, but they have in another context (Shields *et al.*, 1967) provided estimated figures which easily allow the calculation of a likely probandwise rate from Kallmann's data: for his MZ twins, the figure is around 77 per cent, which is hardly consistent with their figure of 35 per cent for Tienari's study or 43 per cent for Allen *et al.*'s. Rosenthal, too, has published figures showing the number of twins in each of the older studies who were independently ascertained (1962a). Although his figures are for MZ + DZ pairs, he presumably had separate figures for the two groups and would, if asked, have made these available to Gottesman and Shields. Instead, having compared pairwise and probandwise rates, they reached the conclusion that:

> Allowing as we have for the small sample sizes in some of the twin studies and for certain key dimensions, many of the alleged discrepancies among all twin studies are attenuated. We feel quite comfortable in concluding that the twin studies of schizophrenia as a whole represent variations on the same theme and are, in effect, sound replications of the same experiment.
>
> (1982: 115)

This questionable conclusion appears to have been reached by three simple devices: first, by the use of probandwise rates for the later studies which both inflated concordance rates and possibly blurred the reduction in concordance rates produced by improved sampling; second, by the comparison of early studies' pairwise with later studies' probandwise rates; third, by the claim that these consistent results must be taken note of because the newer data, which replicate the old, were obtained using improved sampling techniques. What Gottesman and Shields did not mention was that those studies with the most sophisticated sampling techniques – and this does not include their own study – have produced the lowest concordance rates. It is also clear that, in spite of their claim, Gottesman and Shields made no allowances for small sample sizes. And, since the highest and lowest pairwise rates come from the two largest samples – Kallmann's and Hoffer and Pollin's – it is difficult to know what allowances could be made.

## Interpreting the results of twin studies

It was assumed virtually without question, and particularly following the publication of the later twin studies reviewed by Gottesman and Shields, that the research reported here supported the idea that schizophrenia had a strong genetic component. Obviously, this conclusion was partly based on a disregard for the considerable conceptual and methodological problems discussed here. It was also based, however, on the assumption that any difference in the concordance rates between MZ and DZ twins must be explained by invoking genes. It was apparently assumed, in other words, that the environments of MZ twins are, on average, no more similar than are those of DZ twins. Gottesman and Shields, for example, commented that:

> MZ and DZ co-twins of schizophrenic probands *despite sharing virtually the same ecology with their twin siblings* . . .
>
> (1972: 9; emphasis added)

But not only is there no evidence to suggest that MZ and DZ twins are usually exposed to highly similar environments, there are good reasons to suggest that they are not. Any greater similarity in the environments of MZ pairs may be the result of many factors, but two of the more important are likely to be the greater amount of time they apparently spend together (Rose *et al.*, 1984) and their striking physical similarity; indeed, they may have their identity fostered by being dressed alike. There is abundant evidence that appearance is an important factor in the ways in which others react to us. When we add to this the fact that MZ twins are frequently mistaken for each other, it becomes highly likely that they will be 'behaved towards' in very similar ways by others. Sarbin and Mancuso (1980) have highlighted one aspect of this process. They point to the strong evidence that the age at which boys reach puberty is an important determinant of when and whether they are seen as leaders. Boys who mature early are apparently more likely to be seen as behaving like adult males and to be given more responsible tasks, and assigned more authority, by their peers. Because MZ twins reach puberty at roughly similar times, this series of roles and expectations is likely to be more similar for them than for DZ twins. By contrast, Gottesman and Shields appear to see 'the environment' in a simplistic and one-dimensional way, as being rather like the decor – something that is there and reacted to, rather than a complex series of interactions (see Ross and Pam, 1995, for more detailed critical discussion of the 'equal environments' issue).

### An afterword on the twin studies' population

I suggested in Chapter 3 that Kraepelin's and Bleuler's descriptions of 'cases of dementia praecox/schizophrenia' were often virtually identical to von Ecomono's later descriptions of encephalitis lethargica and its Parkinsonian sequel. I also suggested that considerable diagnostic confusion followed von Economo's research, not least because of the erroneous assumption that 'schizophrenia' had been described as a separate and valid pattern. We can reasonably argue, for two reasons, that this confusion is reflected in the data provided by twin researchers, i.e. that at least some of their participants were undiagnosed cases of the sequelae of encephalitic infection. First, the majority of participants in these studies lived at a time when encephalitis lethargica and other infectious diseases were, apparently, much more common than is the case today; indeed many of the participants lived through the great European epidemic of encephalitis lethargica: all but two of those for whom Slater (1953) and Fischer (1973) give birth dates, for example, were born before the epidemic began in 1916–17; the remaining two were born during it. Many participants in the most recently published studies were born during the 1930s, 1940s and 1950s so that their mothers would have lived through the great epidemic and may have transmitted the virus *in utero*, a mode of infection noted by von Economo and possibly more likely to affect both foetuses in MZ pairs who shared a placenta. The second and more direct reason for questioning the nature of twin studies' populations is that parts of many descriptions of participants show a strong similarity to von Economo's descriptions of post-encephalitic Parkinsonism. The descriptions of Slater, Gottesman and Shields, and Fischer, for example, contain references to phenomena said by von Economo to be the result of infection. These include jerky movements of the limbs, dramatic weight changes, sleep disorders, profuse sweating, cyanosis of the extremities, convulsions, 'attacks' of total rigidity, chronic constipation, difficulties in swallowing, peculiarities of gait, tics and facial twitches. In addition, most of Slater's and Fischer's sample, and some of Gottesman and Shields', are described as slipping into stuporous or semi-stuporous states from which they might sometimes 'awake' only to indulge in 'maniacal' behaviour such as smashing windows and crockery, screaming, howling, running, jumping, turning somersaults, etc. Again, these two contrasting patterns are similar to von Economo's descriptions. It is interesting to note that Slater appears to have used the virtually identical motor and other physical phenomena shown by some twin pairs (including, in one pair, cyanosis of the extremities) to support a few of his more uncertain judgements of monozygosity. He also mentions one case in which a shuffling gait and (unspecified) ocular symptoms suggested a diagnosis of post-encephalitic Parkinsonism. This, however, was apparently rejected in favour of schizophrenia because tremor and other (unspecified) ocular neurological signs were absent. Sacks (1982), however, has pointed out that tremor was very often absent as a sequel to the infection, while von Economo commented on the variability of ocular disturbances. It is unfortunate that recently published studies have not provided case information, although, interestingly, Cardno et al.'s (1999) study included the twin pairs who were participants in Gottesman and Shields' (1972) study.

It is obviously impossible to know in retrospect whether many of these participants should have received diagnoses of post-encephalitic Parkinsonism, or of some other organic disorder, but the detailed case material and the historical context certainly suggests that this diagnosis was plausible. If we add to this the twin studies' inconsistent results and their methodological and conceptual problems, then the idea that they provide strong evidence that schizophrenia is a genetic disorder is clearly seriously problematic.

## Adoption studies

It is not simply that twin studies are flawed in the ways described here; it is also obvious that in unseparated families the genetic endowment and a large part of the rearing environment are provided by the same people. It was in an attempt to avoid this problem that Kety, Rosenthal and their colleagues in Denmark, and Tienari and his colleagues in Finland, designed what have become known as the adoption studies of schizophrenia. Kety et al. claimed that:

Studies of adopted individuals and their biological and adoptive families offer a means of disentangling the genetic and environmental contribution to a disorder such as schizophrenia and permit an examination of the effects of one type of influence while the other is randomised or controlled.

(1976: 413)

(As with twin studies, the complexities of the nature/nurture debate and the naivety of assuming that it is ever possible to disentangle the effects of genes and environment on behaviour, are not issues here. What is of interest, again, is how these studies have come to be seen as supporting the view that schizophrenia has a genetic basis.)

Very soon after the publication of the first adoption studies, the claims made for them were, if anything, even stronger than those made for twin studies. Gottesman and Shields (1976), for example, called them 'the straw that broke the environmentalist's back' (364). Neale and Oltmanns (1980) claimed that they '[have] provided almost irrefutable confirmation of the importance of genetic factors' (142); Revely and Murray (1980) called their methodology exemplary, while Crowe (1982) claimed that the studies' findings resolved the nature–nurture controversy.

The adoption studies have been designed in three ways. First, there is a series where the focus of interest is the biological and adoptive relatives of a group of adoptees who had been diagnosed schizophrenic; second, a series where the focus was on the adopted-away children of mothers who had been diagnosed schizophrenic and, third, a study of the adopted children of 'normal' mothers but one of whose adoptive parents had been diagnosed schizophrenic. This last type is known as the 'cross-fostering' strategy.

### Studies with 'schizophrenic' adoptees as the index group

The first of these studies was reported by Kety *et al.* (1968). The research was made possible by the existence in Denmark of excellent records, not only of the general population and its geographical movements but also of all adoptions granted by the state, including details of biological mother, putative father and adoptive parents. Records are also kept of admissions to psychiatric hospitals and of diagnoses. Participants were drawn from the records of all adoptions in Copenhagen between 1924 and 1947. Cross-referencing of the adoption and psychiatric registers yielded 507 people whose hospital records were examined by two Danish psychiatrists, one of whom knew the purpose of the research. One of them classified these people as 'definitely schizophrenic', 'definitely not schizophrenic' or 'probably schizophrenic'. A summary was also prepared by the second psychiatrist, who was ignorant of the purpose of the research, giving details such as 'symptoms', judgements of work performance, 'sexual adjustment', 'intellectual ability', 'age of onset', marital status and most probable diagnosis. This summary was sent to the US collaborators – Kety and

Wender – who independently rated each person as 'definitely', 'definitely not' or 'probably' schizophrenic. Where all three psychiatrists rated an adoptee as definitely schizophrenic, the adoptee became a potential participant. Those unanimously called definitely not schizophrenic were dropped. Where there was disagreement, the first Danish psychiatrist prepared and forwarded a summary from the hospital records. Where a consensus on 'definitely schizophrenic' was reached by the Danish and two American psychiatrists, the adoptee was included. By this method, thirty-three participants (called index cases) were selected. No information was provided on the reliability of these judgements. The control group was selected from a pool of adoptees who had no record of admission to a psychiatric hospital or unit. Index and control groups were matched for age, age at transfer, social class of adoptive parents and time spent with biological relatives, in institutions or with foster parents.

Having selected index and control groups, Kety *et al.* began the daunting task of searching for their relatives, both biological and adoptive. The searches were made by people who did not know which were index and which control participants. Relatives were traced through the population register – 150 and seventy-four biological and adoptive relatives respectively for the index group and 156 and eighty-three for the controls. Information about these relatives was gathered from psychiatric registers, police and military records and the Mothers' Aid organisation. The records of those relatives with a psychiatric history were obtained and summarised, mainly by a psychiatrist unaware of the research design; some (the exact number was not given) were summarised by one of the authors. The summaries were then edited to delete diagnostic opinions and any information which might have indicated whether the relative 'belonged' to an index or control adoptee. Unfortunately, although Kety *et al.* concede the importance of this strategy, they made no check on its success by, for example, asking independent raters to guess the group to which relatives belonged. An edited summary for each relative was given to the four authors who independently 'diagnosed' the relative. Kety *et al.*, like the twin researchers, made use of the concept of the schizophrenia spectrum; the concepts they included in this term, and the criteria for inferring them, are shown in Table 6.6.

## Interpreting the results

Kety *et al.* (1968) analysed their data in several ways. They showed, first, that 8.7 per cent of biological relatives of index adoptees (i.e. those called schizophrenic) had been assigned a spectrum diagnosis, while the figure for control participants was 1.9 per cent. Second, they showed that this significant difference remained when only biological relatives of 'early separated' index and control participants were compared (10 per cent versus nought per cent). They showed, third, that there was a significant difference in the number of biological families of index and control participants in which at least one member

*Table 6.6* Diagnostic classification system used in adoption studies

| | |
|---|---|
| A | Definitely not schizophrenia (specify diagnosis). |
| B | Chronic schizophrenia (chronic undifferentiated schizophrenia, true schizophrenia, process schizophrenia). *Characteristics:* (1) Poor prepsychotic adjustment; introverted; schizoid; shut-in; few peer contacts; few heterosexual contacts; usually unmarried; poor occupational adjustment. (2) Onset: gradual and without clear-cut psychological precipitant. (3) Presenting picture, presence of primary Bleulerian characteristics; presence of clear rather than confused sensorium. (4) Post-hospital course; failure to reach previous level of adjustment. (5) Tendency to chronicity. |
| B2 | Acute schizophrenic reaction (acute undifferentiated schizophrenic reaction, schizoaffective psychosis, possible schizophreniform psychosis, (acute) paranoid reaction, homosexual panic). *Characteristics:* (1) Related good premorbid adjustment. (2) Relatively rapid onset of illness with clear-cut psychological precipitant. (3) Presenting picture: presence of secondary symptoms and comparatively lesser evidence of primary ones; presence of affect (manic-depressive symptoms, feelings of guilt); cloudy rather than clear sensorium. (4) Post-hospital course good. (5) Tendency to relatively brief episode(s) responding to drugs, electroshock therapy, and so on. |
| B3 | Borderline state (pseudoneurotic schizophrenia, borderline ambulatory schizophrenia, questionable simple schizophrenia, 'Psychotic character', severe schizoid individual). *Characteristics:* (1) Thinking: strange or atypical mentation; thought shows tendency to ignore reality, logic and experience (to an excessive degree) resulting in poor adaptation to life experience (despite the presence of a normal IQ); fuzzy, murky, vague speech. (2) Experience: brief episodes of cognitive distortion (the patient can, and does, snap back, but during the episode the idea has more the character of a delusion than an ego-alien obsessive thought); feeling of depersonalisation, or strangeness, or unfamiliarity with or towards the familiar; micropsychosis. (3) Affective: anhedonia – never experiences intense pleasure – never happy; no deep or intense involvement with anyone or anybody. (4) Interpersonal behaviour: may appear poised, but lacking in depth ('as if' personality); sexual adjustment – chaotic fluctuation; mixture of heterosexuality and homosexuality. (5) Psychopathology: multiple neurotic manifestations that shift frequently (obsessive concerns, phobias, conversion, psychosomatic symptoms, etc.); severe widespread anxiety. |
| C | Inadequate personality. *Characteristics:* A somewhat heterogeneous group consisting of individuals who would be classified as either inadequate or schizoid by the APA (1968) Diagnostic Manual. Persons so classified often had many of the characteristics of the B3 category, but to a considerably milder degree. |
| D1, 2 or 3 | Uncertain B1, 2 or 3 either because information is lacking or because even if enough information is available, the case does not fit clearly into an appropriate B category. |

Source: Kety et al. (1968).

had received a spectrum diagnosis. Kety *et al.* commented that 'this study found little to support the importance of environmental transmission of schizophrenia between family members' (359).

A closer analysis of their data, however, suggests that both their analyses and their conclusions are questionable. Before a reanalysis of their data is presented, two points must be emphasised. First, some of the criticisms centre on Kety *et al.*'s use of the 'schizophrenia spectrum'. This is not to suggest that there is some proper usage or that their B1 and B2 (non-spectrum) diagnoses were more accurate. Second, part of the reanalysis involves comparing Kety *et al.*'s data with studies of family resemblance for schizophrenia diagnoses. Again, it is not being suggested that data from these family studies are accurate. What is of interest here is the way in which Kety *et al.* have analysed and presented their data and the extent to which they have ignored analyses which, within these authors' own framework, would have been more appropriate. Kety *et al.*'s analyses and conclusions ignore four major factors which could influence the results and their interpretation. First, there is the issue of the type of adoptive homes in which participants were reared and the extent to which they were matched; second, the weakness of their diagnostic concepts and in particular their spectrum concept; third, the different genetic loadings which must be given to first- and second-degree relatives and, fourth, the fact that a significant difference in the prevalence of spectrum diagnoses between index and control biological relatives could arise in different ways. Two of these ways are of particular interest here: if the index biological relatives had a higher than expected prevalence of schizophrenia diagnoses and the control relatives were indistinguishable from the general population *or* the index relatives resembled the general population and the control relatives were exceptionally free from diagnoses, then significant differences, but carrying very different interpretations, could appear.

## THE ADOPTIVE HOMES OF INDEX AND CONTROL SUBJECTS

Kety *et al.* have apparently assumed that index and control groups' adoptive family homes were virtually identical and that any supposed similarity between participants and their biological relatives was mediated by genetic factors. In order to foster similarity amongst adoptive families, index and control groups were matched in various ways, but this does not indicate how well individuals were matched; Kety *et al.* reported only that out of four possible controls who matched each index on age and sex, one was chosen 'who matched best in respect of socio-economic status of adoptive family and time spent with biological mother or father, in a children's home or with foster parents' (1976: 422).

Rose *et al.* (1984), however, have presented data which suggest that this matching process may have been inadequate. Using unpublished data supplied to them by Kety *et al.*, Rose *et al.* demonstrated that in 24 per cent of the adoptive families of index participants, an adoptive parent had been in a psychiatric hospital, while not one adoptive parent of a control participant had been admitted. It is interesting to note also that the rate of admission of a parent (6 versus 24 per cent) was significantly lower ($\chi^2$ = 6.9 df 1 $p$ < 0.01) in the biological than in the adoptive families of index participants. It is of course possible that the adoptive parents were driven to the psychiatric services by the behaviour of their child, but it remains interesting that Kety *et al.* did not publish this potentially important data, although it was apparently easily retrievable from data sheets. Rose *et al.* have suggested that this apparently greater deviance amongst index participants' adoptive families might reflect the operation of 'selective placement', and thus have created a spurious impression of similarity between adoptive participants and their biological relatives. It is common practice to attempt to match the backgrounds of biological and adoptive families. Obviously, the matching must be limited because adoptive parents have to conform to certain standards. But a selective placement effect does seem to have operated in the Danish samples, because Kety *et al.* (1976) and Wender *et al.* (1973, 1974) have reported a significant correlation between the social class of the biological and adoptive families. More seriously, Kety *et al.* have never satisfactorily demonstrated that their choice of index participants was not influenced by knowledge of some characteristics of biological relatives. (They have, apparently, satisfied themselves that this was not the case, but that is not quite the same thing.) If selective placement factors were operating, and if the biological parents of index participants were known 'deviants', then, within limits, so too might have been the adoptive parents.

## DIAGNOSES AND THE SCHIZOPHRENIA SPECTRUM

Some of the problems of the spectrum concept were discussed in the previous section, but they are sufficiently important and so often ignored as to justify brief repetition here. Kety *et al.* made no attempt to justify their spectrum concept empirically; rather, they appear to have fallen into the same trap as the twin researchers of assuming that just because some relatives show behaviours which seem vaguely similar to those of the index participants, then they must be 'suffering from related disorders'. (And the sheer breadth of Kety *et al.*'s concept emphasises just how tenuous this similarity may be.) Some of the problems of Kety *et al.*'s use of the spectrum concept can be highlighted by drawing a similar analogy to that used in the previous section. If their strategy were to be used by, say, cancer researchers, we should hardly consider them justified in including in a 'cancer spectrum' biological and adoptive relatives who had ever complained of nausea, abdominal pain, or of passing blood or even of 'growths' such as warts, bunions or cysts. If the analogy seems absurd, it does so only because it is known *in advance of the research* that the antecedents and characteristics of the phenomena of interest, in this case malignant tumours, are quite different from those of warts, etc., and that there are many antecedents of nausea, etc. apart from cancerous tumours. It was, however, in total ignorance of the antecedents or of any other aspects of the long and disparate list of phenomena in Table 6.6, and in ignorance of whether any of them form a meaningful pattern, that Kety *et al.* decided on their criteria for their schizophrenia spectrum. The arbitrariness of their spectrum classification is suggested by Kety *et al.*'s own (1968) report that it 'was worked out largely by Dr. Wender' (353). In the face of criticism of the width of their spectrum concept, Kety *et al.* (1976) protested that it had merely been a 'hypothesis or group of hypotheses on which we hoped our continuing studies might cast some light' (417). But Kety *et al.* made no such reservations in their earlier reports of this work and, as will be seen, have relied heavily on some or other version of their spectrum concept in their attempts to secure apparently significant results. But it is not simply the width and arbitrariness of Kety *et al.*'s spectrum which should give cause for concern. The criteria for inferring many of its concepts are extremely vague. Nor have Kety *et al.* indicated how many of the characteristics on the list people must show in order to be called borderline schizophrenic or whatever.

No data were provided on the reliability of diagnoses made from these criteria. Kety *et al.* stated simply that:

> those cases in which there was a disagreement among the raters were discussed at a conference of all four authors where an effort was made to review additional edited information which it was possible to obtain and to arrive at a consensus diagnosis.
>
> (1968: 351)

Unfortunately, Kety *et al.* did not say what this additional information was, where it had been obtained and whether it was likely to 'identify' a relative. It is notable also that some of the diagnoses were apparently made on the basis of very little information, as Kety *et al.* pointed out. Some of those for whom information was lacking were assigned to one of the D (uncertain) groups. These presumably already highly heterogeneous categories were therefore made up of those who were not assigned to a B category because information was lacking and of those for whom a good deal of information was available but who did not, in the raters' opinions, match the B groups.

## ANALYSING THE DATA: GENETIC WEIGHTING OF RELATIVES AND POPULATION COMPARISONS

The major analyses carried out by Kety *et al.* involved grouping together all biological relatives (parents, sibs and half-sibs) of index and control participants and comparing the frequency of spectrum diagnoses in the two groups. As Benjamin (1976) has pointed out, however, this kind of analysis assumes that all relatives stand in the same genetic relationship to the index and control participants. It fails to acknowledge that the predictions made about the occurrence of any genetic phenomena in biological relatives will depend on their degree of closeness. Half-sibs, of whom there were many in Kety *et al.*'s study, are particularly problematic because predictions depend, as Lidz and Blatt (1983) have noted, on whether the common parent shows the phenomena of interest, whether the other parent is known and 'affected', and on the genetic model used. Similarly, as I mentioned earlier, a simple comparison of two groups of biological relatives does not indicate how similar each is to the general population. In the case of the 'schizophrenic' adoptees, it would be predicted from a genetic theory that the prevalence of schizophrenia diagnoses in their first- and second-degree relatives should be higher than that in the general population and similar to that of unseparated relatives, although even this latter finding would not preclude non-genetic explanations.

A much clearer picture of Kety *et al.*'s data could therefore be obtained by separating first- and second-degree relatives and comparing the prevalence of schizophrenia diagnoses with population rates. (And see also Lidz and Blatt, 1983.) Kety *et al.* (1976) in fact claimed that they 'toyed with the idea of giving [half-siblings] half the weight as soon as we recognised how many were being identified but rejected it as being too pretentious' (416). It is difficult not to wonder whether the idea was also rejected because it leads to a quite different set of conclusions but, to Kety *et al.*'s credit, they have made it easy for others to perform a more appropriate analysis.

Kety *et al.*'s data for first- and second-degree relatives can be compared both between experimental and control groups and with two sets of population figures: the prevalence rates for diagnoses of schizophrenia in the general population and the rates for unseparated relatives of those already diagnosed as schizophrenic. There are, of course, problems with these population comparisons. As would be expected, the prevalence rates for the general population vary from study to study, even when the same measure is used (e.g. lifetime risk or prevalence at a particular point). So too do the rates for relatives. For example, as Rosenthal (1970) has shown, the risk for parents of 'schizophrenics' in one study is sixty times that in another, while the risk for sibs in one study is twenty-eight times larger than that for parents but in another the risk for parents is 1.5 times larger than that for sibs. One of the reasons for this is presumably that researchers have used different criteria for inferring schizophrenia and that they have gathered different kinds of information, sometimes about people who had been dead for many years. It has been acknowledged, moreover, (see, e.g., Gottesman and Shields, 1972, 1982; Cooper *et al.*, 1972) that the criteria used by European psychiatrists were generally narrower (sometimes much narrower) than are those used by North American psychiatrists. Many of the studies for which prevalence rates have been derived are European and would almost certainly have excluded Kety *et al.*'s D3 and C categories and possibly their B3. To add to the difficulties the rates quoted for relatives or for

*Table 6.7* Estimated risk of being diagnosed schizophrenic in the general population and in relatives of 'schizophrenics'

| General population (%) | Parents (%) | Second-degree relatives (%) |
|---|---|---|
| 0.7–1.5 | 0.2–12 | 0.3–6.5 |

Sources: Rosenthal (1970); Gottesman and Shields (1982).

*Table 6.8* Prevalence of B, D1 and D2 diagnoses in first-degree relatives of index and control schizophrenics*

| | Biological (%) | Adoptive (%) |
|---|---|---|
| Index | 1.5 | 0 |
| Control | 2.9 | 2.4 |

Note: *Because so few sibs were traced, the figures for parents and sibs have been combined. The figures for biological parents only are 1.5 per cent and 1.6 per cent.

*Table 6.9* Prevalence of B, D1 and D2 diagnoses in second-degree relatives of index and control schizophrenics

| | Biological (%) | Adoptive (%) |
|---|---|---|
| Index | 8.2 | 0 |
| Control | 0 | 0* |

Note: *None identified.

the general population are sometimes for an age-corrected lifetime risk of being diagnosed schizophrenic, and different researchers have used different risk periods. Kety *et al.*'s data do not allow such calculations, although it can reasonably be assumed that many of the biological parents, who make up almost the whole sample of first-degree relatives, were close to or had passed the so-called risk age of around forty-five. Because of the difficulty of determining an appropriate numerical base for the population figures, direct statistical comparison of these with Kety *et al.*'s data will not be attempted. The best that can be done is to offer a range of figures obtained for the general population and for relatives of 'schizophrenics' and to compare these with Kety *et al.*'s figures for first- and second-degree relatives (see Tables 6.7–6.9). The comparisons may be made somewhat more meaningful by taking only the B (definite and borderline schizophrenia) categories and, so as to give Kety *et al.* the benefit of the doubt, the D1 and D2 categories, which may resemble the 'probable schizophrenia' of European psychiatrists. Even so, these criteria may be broader than those used in many population and family studies.

These figures reveal patterns in Kety *et al.*'s data which were obscured by their 'unpretentious' analysis. They show, for example, that the rates of B, D1 and D2 diagnoses in the first-degree biological relatives of index participants are not clearly different from the population rate and that the rates for index and control relatives are not significantly different from each other ($\chi^2 = 0.004$ df 1). The comparison remains non-significant even when D3 and C categories are included; that is, when the full width of the spectrum is used and when only data from parents is analysed. Kety *et al.*'s statistically significant results appear to be derived from the relatively high rate of spectrum diagnoses in biological half-sibs of index participants combined with their non-existence in the half-sibs of control participants. Unfortunately, Kety *et al.* have provided no information on the backgrounds of these half-sibs, whether they were from 'broken homes', institutions, or what. It is notable that the rate of spectrum diagnoses is higher – though not significantly so – in the second-degree than in the first-degree relatives of the index subjects, a result which even genetic researchers have called 'genetically meaningless' (Gottesman and Shields, 1976; Kringlen, 1976).

### An extended study, using interviews

In a later report, Kety *et al.* (1975) described an extension of this study in which some biological and adoptive relatives were interviewed. Diagnoses were then based on interview data rather than on hospital records. Kety *et al.* reported that the results of this extended study 'confirm results previously obtained only from institutional records' and that their data are 'strongly suggestive of the operation of genetic factors' (163). As with the previous study, however, closer inspection of their methods and data shows that these conclusions are untenable. There are three major problems with this extension study: first, the methods by which the interview data were collected; second, the criteria used to assign spectrum diagnoses and, third, the data analyses.

#### DATA COLLECTION BY INTERVIEW

Kety *et al.* secured the co-operation of an independent psychiatrist to conduct interviews with as many biological and adoptive relatives as could be traced and agreed to be interviewed. Because the interviewer knew the design and purpose of the study, and because clues to participants' status may have been given during the interview, Kety *et al.* asked the interviewer to guess the status of his interviewees. His guess was correct for 17 per cent of interviews. Although Kety *et al.* then reanalysed their data to exclude these interviews, this hardly amounts to a demonstration that the data collection was completely uncontaminated. The interviewer, after all, knew why he was being asked to guess the participants' status. It is not unreasonable to suppose, and without accusing him of lying, that his guesses might not have been an accurate reflection of what actually took place during the interview. Of more concern, however, is the way in which some of the interviews were conducted. Kety *et al.* reported that about 10 per cent of relatives refused to co-operate and that:

> Even though a subject refused initially, Dr. Jacobsen would telephone and try to persuade him and, occasionally, when he passed his door, would knock and attempt personally to obtain his co-operation, and with considerable success. In addition, in twelve instances, even though the individual persistently refused to give an interview, Dr. Jacobsen nevertheless obtained considerable information in the process.
>
> (1975: 150)

We are thus asked to believe that the diagnosis of a serious mental disorder can be based on the behaviour of someone either distressed or annoyed at being persistently asked, in spite of refusals, to give personal information to a stranger.

From the way in which Kety *et al.* described the data collection there is nothing to suggest that 'an interview' was not just that – a researcher talking to someone (however reluctant) and recording the results. Kety *et al.* then recorded the diagnoses in one of their data tables with a clear indication of whether this was based 'on an interview'. The term 'interview', however, was apparently used by Kety *et al.* in a quite different way from the usual usage. Rose *et al.* (1984) contacted the psychiatrist who had conducted the interviews and asked him what had happened when relatives were dead or unavailable. The psychiatrist reported that, in an unspecified number of these cases, he had prepared a 'pseudo interview' using hospital records. In effect, he had conducted an interview with himself by asking how (he thought) this person might have responded had he actually conducted a personal interview.

## MAKING A DIAGNOSIS

The procedure for making diagnoses in this extended study was similar to that of the earlier research: edited transcripts of the interviews and pseudo-interviews were read independently by Kety, Rosenthal and Wender and a diagnosis recorded. Later, the raters met and discussed each participant in order to reach a consensus diagnosis. As before, no information was given about reliability, although it was promised elsewhere. Kety *et al.* merely remarked that 'In formulating the consensus diagnoses we were constantly impressed with the agreement among our independent diagnoses' (157). It is difficult to know how the raters could have been impressed by their agreement if they did not know its extent or, if they knew enough about it to be impressed, why they did not share the information with their readers.

Although Kety *et al.* did not discuss the fact, they adopted different criteria for diagnosing the schizophrenia spectrum in this extended study. Previously, the spectrum had included the B, D and C categories described in

Table 6.6. Now, however, it included only the B and D categories because, on analysing their data, Kety *et al.* discovered that the C category diagnoses did not distinguish between the biological relatives of the index and control groups. At least we must assume that this was the reason, for none was given. Kety *et al.* thus behaved like a researcher who hypothesises that men are more intelligent than women but who refuses to accept as a test of intelligence any task on which men and women perform equally well.

This elasticity of the spectrum concept is particularly interesting when considered alongside the information which Rose *et al.* uncovered about the 'interviews'. They reported that one participant – a biological relative of an index adoptee – had twice been given a diagnosis of manic depressive psychosis by hospital doctors and that this had been recorded in the notes used by Kety *et al.* to make their diagnosis. In the first study, this woman had been given a 'C' diagnosis – inside the spectrum – and had therefore contributed towards the supposedly significant results. In the extended study she was recorded not, as would be expected, as outside the spectrum, now made up only of B and D diagnoses, but as still inside, with a diagnosis of 'uncertain borderline schizophrenia/severely schizoid individual' (D3) *based on an interview*. The woman, however, was dead and had never been interviewed; the interviewing psychiatrist had made up an interview from her hospital notes. The fact that a woman who had twice been called manic depressive should consistently be included in Kety *et al.*'s spectrum is interesting in view of their comment that '[m]anic-depressive illness was never thought to be in the schizophrenia spectrum by us' (417).

ANALYSING THE DATA

Once again, Kety *et al.* produced significant results by grouping together all biological relatives of index and control participants and showing a significant difference in spectrum diagnoses between the two groups. Again, however, a rather different picture emerges when the data are split into first- and second-degree relatives and comparisons made between them and with population rates. (The problematic D3 is again removed.) These figures can be seen in Tables 6.10 and 6.11.

Several important points emerge from this presentation of the data. First, the rates of B, D1 and D2 diagnoses are not significantly different for first-degree biological relatives of index and control groups ($\chi^2$ = 0.0004 df 1) and the differences remain non-significant when D3 diagnoses are included ($\chi^2$ = 0.76 df 1). Second, in these relatives, all but two of the diagnoses are B3 or D3 (borderline or uncertain borderline state) and the majority were reportedly obtained by interview. It will be recalled that the population rates are derived from studies which probably excluded D3 and possibly B3 behaviours from a schizophrenia category and which usually used hospital records, rather than population interviews. There is no known population rate for B and D diagnoses made by interview, but it is likely to be considerably higher than 1.5 per

*Table 6.10* Prevalence of B, D1 and D2 diagnoses in first-degree biological relatives*

| Index schizophrenics (%) | Control schizophrenics (%) |
|---|---|
| 5.8 | 4.3 |

Note: *Parents and sibs; figures for parents only are 4.5 per cent and 3 per cent. Diagnoses are counted if given after either interview or examination of hospital records.

*Table 6.11* Prevalence of B, D1 and D2 diagnoses in second-degree biological relatives*

| Index schizophrenics (%) | Control schizophrenics (%) |
|---|---|
| 11.5 | 1 |

Note: *See Table 6.10.

cent. Kety *et al.* (1978b) in fact claimed a prevalence of 4 per cent for B and D diagnoses from interview, using all adoptive relatives and biological control relatives. It cannot therefore be claimed confidently that the rate of spectrum diagnoses for first-degree biological relatives of index adoptees is above the expectation for the general population. Third, as with the previous study, it is the apparently high and difficult-to-interpret rate of B and D diagnoses in the second-degree biological relatives of index adoptees, combined with a very low rate in control relatives, which appears to have contributed most to Kety *et al.*'s significant result.

Kety *et al.* (1975) emphasised the fact that there was a significantly higher rate of spectrum diagnoses amongst the paternal half-sibs of index adoptees than amongst paternal half-sibs of controls. Because these people did not share an intra-uterine environment with the adoptees, Kety *et al.* considered this to be 'compelling evidence that genetic factors operate significantly in the transmission of schizophrenia' (1975: 156). But what Kety *et al.* did not mention, and which is very difficult to explain by their genetic theory, is that the frequency of spectrum diagnoses does not differ between *maternal* half-sibs of the index and control participants (for B, D1 and D2 diagnoses, $\chi^2 = 0.49$ df 1; for B and D diagnoses, $\chi^2 = 2.4$ df 1 $p > 0.05$).

Kety *et al.* also provided an analysis of their data by family, rather than individual. That is, they compared the number of index adoptees' biological families in which at least one member had been given a spectrum diagnosis, with the corresponding number for control adoptees. It was claimed, in a summary table derived from a more detailed table of data, that fourteen families of index adoptees contained someone given a B diagnosis (the spectrum criteria had apparently changed again) compared with only three for control adoptees. The difference was highly significant. In fact, the figure for index relatives is incorrect and should be *eight*. The difference between index and control families is then not significant ($\chi^2$ = 1.89 df 1 $p$ > 0.05). It is very difficult to understand how this mistake (acknowledged as such by Kety *et al.*; see Paton-Saltzberg, 1982) was made in the first place, but even more to understand why it has apparently not been corrected. Seven years after the wrong figures first appeared Gottesman and Shields (1982) reported and claimed significance for them. And thirteen years later these figures were quoted again (*The Mind Machine*; BBC2, 18 October 1988), although by now they had been transformed to the claim that 14 per cent of biological relatives and 3 per cent of adoptive relatives of schizophrenic adoptees had received a diagnosis of schizophrenia.

An extension of the adoption study to the whole of Denmark, in which the majority of biological relatives' diagnoses were made by interview, has been reported by Kety *et al.* (1994). Unfortunately, this 'Provincial' study is not easily compared to or combined with the Copenhagen study just discussed, because the diagnostic categories and possibly criteria appear to have changed. The provincial sample included twenty-nine index adoptees (adults with a diagnosis of schizophrenia who had been adopted as children) and twenty-four control adoptees (adults who had also been adopted as children but who were 'free of affective or schizophrenia spectrum disorders' (Kety *et al.*, 1994: 443)). Diagnoses, including 'classical/chronic' or 'latent' schizophrenia in the biological and adoptive relatives of index and control adoptees, were made independently and then by consensus by Kety and Wender, using hospital records, interview data and 'refusal reports' (researchers' observations on some of those who refused to be interviewed). It is not clear how these diagnoses were made, as Kety *et al.* noted that '[a] description of the criteria we used in making the global diagnoses remains to be made and incorporated into an operational form' (445). It is also notable that the reported inter-rater diagnostic agreement ($\kappa$ = 0.68) was not high.

Kety *et al.* reported a significant difference between the number of biological families of index and control adoptees with at least one member whom the researchers gave a diagnosis of either classical or latent schizophrenia. They also reported a significant difference in the proportion of classical schizophrenia in the first-degree biological relatives of index and control adoptees and a significant difference in this diagnosis between the full and half-siblings of index adoptees.

Once again, however, a more detailed analysis suggests a more complex picture, difficult to explain by any known genetic model. First, the use of 'latent schizophrenia' raises all the problems discussed earlier of the spectrum concept, and it is notable that no comparison of the prevalence of 'latent schizophrenia' diagnoses in index and control adoptees' biological relatives approached significance (first-degree relatives index versus control; second-degree relatives index versus control; full-sibs index versus full-sibs control; full-sibs index versus half-sibs index – not all of these comparisons were actually reported by Kety *et al.*). This is in spite of the fact that the spectrum concept was developed on the grounds that even if biological relatives did not show a significant excess of 'schizophrenia', they might show an excess of 'milder forms'.

Second, and not reported by Kety *et al.*, there is no significant difference in the proportion of 'schizophrenia' diagnoses in biological parents of index and control adoptees ($\chi^2$ = 1.01 df 1), although the small numbers involved obviously compromise analyses. It is not possible to compare Kety *et al.*'s rate of schizophrenia diagnoses in index and control adoptees' biological parents (5.2 per cent versus nought per cent) with population figures as many of the diagnoses appear to have been derived from interviews for which no population figures exist using Kety *et al.*'s criteria. Third, given the inevitably small numbers involved in such a research project, we might assume that the researchers would take every opportunity to combine their data in theoretically meaningful ways to increase the sample size. Yet in their crucial comparison of the proportion of schizophrenia diagnoses in first- and second-degree biological relatives of index adoptees, Kety *et al.* do the opposite by comparing only full and half-sibs, and reporting a significant result. But they do not comment on the rather curious fact that the entire total of schizophrenia diagnoses in index adoptees' full-sibs (three) is contributed by one family. When this bias is minimised by including biological parents in the comparison of index adoptees' first- and second-degree relatives, the comparison is not significant. Nor is the comparison, again not reported by Kety *et al.*, between the prevalence of schizophrenia diagnoses in biological parents and half-sibs of index adoptees ($\chi^2$ = 0.27 df 1).

It is not easy to construct a genetic model which would accommodate Kety *et al.*'s data (not all of which has been discussed here), and, perhaps not surprisingly, the researchers do not try. Nevertheless, they reach strong conclusions about the genetic transmission of 'schizophrenia' (see also Ingraham and Kety, 2000) by selective and partial analyses and by minimising the importance of their failure clearly to specify diagnostic criteria or to make highly reliable diagnoses. A final point is worth noting: the adoptees studied here were adopted between 1924 and 1947. This means that some adoptees and many biological relatives would have lived during the great epidemic of post-encephalitic Parkinsonism and its aftermath. As with twin studies, it is not possible to know how much any family resemblance in reported schizophrenia diagnoses could be attributed to infectious transmission, including from mother to foetus, combined with the kind of diagnostic confusion discussed in Chapter 3.

### Studies of adopted-away children of a 'schizophrenic' parent

Rosenthal *et al.* (1968) began with the same pool of adoptees as had Kety *et al.*, but their interest focused on their biological parents. (The biological father was

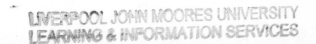

unknown in about 25 per cent of cases and may well have been incorrectly recorded in others.) As before, names were cross-referenced with psychiatric records in order to find those parents who had given a child up for adoption *and* who had received a psychiatric diagnosis. The records were read and summarised by psychiatrists, who then made a diagnosis according to the criteria used by Kety *et al.* and described in Table 6.6. The summaries and diagnoses were then reviewed by Rosenthal *et al.*, who also recorded diagnoses. No data on reliability were given, but Rosenthal *et al.* reported that 'In each case where we have a full consensus that the parent is in the schizophrenic range (coded B1, B2 or B3) the child he or she gave for adoption is selected as an index case' (379). Fifty-six parents (2.5:1 mothers to fathers) were selected by this method. Information about the children of each of the index parents was then recorded (name, sex, birth date, age of transfer to adoptive parents, age at formal adoption, adoptive parents' occupations, income and 'fortune'). To obtain control participants – that is, adopted children whose biological parents had no psychiatric record – Rosenthal and one other person ranked adoptees close to each index adoptee in the relevant characteristics. The person with the highest summed rank was chosen as a control. If any refused to participate, the adoptee with the next highest summed rank was chosen; if they refused, then the next highest, and so on. Fifteen potential control participants refused, but no information was provided on how well index and control adoptees were eventually matched. Information on index and control adoptees (i.e. those with and without a 'schizophrenic' biological parent) was sent to Copenhagen, but without identifying information. Index and control adoptees were then contacted by a social worker who, without revealing the purpose of the study, attempted to persuade them to participate.

The researchers were then faced with the problem of what to do with these people as, by their own admission, they lacked a clear-cut theory. Perhaps predictably, Rosenthal *et al.* again fell into the same trap as had the twin researchers in assuming that any vague similarity between adopted children of 'schizophrenics' and the researchers' idea of a schizophrenic meant that they were 'showing signs of the same disorder'. Indeed, their reasoning was, if anything, even more confused:

> [Our] strategy was based on the idea that we should find the same kinds of traits and aberrations in our index groups as in the premorbid personality of known schizophrenics. Of course, those who become schizophrenic must be different in some way from those who do not, and since we could expect only a few of our subjects to become schizophrenic, we might be focusing on the wrong traits. Moreover, the literature on the premorbid personality of schizophrenics was hardly exciting. It was based on retrospection, or on past clinical records in service settings for reasons not necessarily coinciding with ours. Formulations thus derived emphasised traits such as shyness, timidity, passivity, sex difficulties, introversion and

others. We would, of course, look for such traits, but we hoped for a more fine grained description of the inherited diathesis than that. We included a self-assessment procedure whose items were based on such literature and on our own clinical observations or impressions as well.

(1968: 380–381)

Rosenthal *et al.* also included three sets of test procedures. First, a 'conditioning procedure' and a 'habituation and a demandingness' procedure, claimed to discriminate between schizophrenic and control groups, though with what reliability and for what purpose was not discussed; second, an unnamed set of projective and cognitive tests based on the work of Singer and Østergaard and, third, 'a few tests' included on the basis of 'hunches' and 'which would take much too long to describe' (381). It is thus not at all clear what information was actually collected from participants, how reliable it was or even why some of it was collected.

Rosenthal *et al.* assessed a total of 155 adoptees (some of whose parents had been given a diagnosis of manic depressive psychosis). The assessors' impressions, which may or may not have included test data, were somehow converted to spectrum diagnoses, although no information was provided on how, by whom, with what reliability or using what criteria. Instead, readers were offered the information that 'Dr. Welner made a carefully formulated diagnostic evaluation of each case examined' and the claim that '[b]oth he and Dr. Schulsinger, who pinch hit for him when Dr. Welner was ill, have an appreciation of the nuances of diagnosis which is too often discounted in the United States. In addition, both have had training and supervision in psycho-analysis and both have been psychoanalysed' (386). Although the arbitrariness of Rosenthal *et al.*'s procedure means that it hardly matters, readers might be misled here into thinking that Welner and Schulsinger actually decided whether each participant was in or out of the spectrum. Private enquiries by Rose *et al.* (1984) however, have indicated that this was apparently not the case. Who made the decision, and how, remains unknown.

The number of adoptees investigated was 155 (sixty-nine index and eighty-six control). Eighty-six (thirty-nine index and forty-seven control) were examined in detail. Only one of the 155 had ever been hospitalised with a diagnosis of schizophrenia, a rate at the lower end of the expectation for the general population. This was an index adoptee, so that the rate for this group was 1.4 per cent. This contrasts sharply with a pooled rate of 12.8 per cent quoted by Gottesman and Shields (1982) for children of a parent diagnosed as schizophrenic. Rosenthal *et al.* in fact made no attempt to analyse their data on the distribution of spectrum diagnoses in index and control adoptees, but simply reported on the number of these diagnoses in index and control groups (thirteen versus seven). The thirteen, however, included two children whose parent had been given a diagnosis of manic depressive psychosis, which the same authors were later to state, as was pointed out earlier, was never thought by them to be in the schizophrenia spectrum (Kety *et al.*, 1976). In fact, these authors appear to be in some confusion about this as, two years earlier, Rosenthal *et al.* had claimed that they were 'tentatively including' manic depressive psychosis in the schizophrenia spectrum (1974: 153). It may be that Rosenthal *et al.* did not elaborate on the figures they presented because, with or without 'manic depressive' parents, there were no significant differences in the rate of spectrum diagnoses in index and control adoptees ($\chi^2 = 3.09$ df 1 $p > 0.05$; $\chi^2 = 1.89$ df 1 $p > 0.05$).

Rosenthal *et al.* also reported on the results of participants' self-assessments on supposedly pre-schizophrenic traits and on their MMPI scores. From a genetic point of view, the results of the self-assessments were extremely disappointing. Group means for both index and control adoptees were within the average range on all items. In between-group comparisons, three items differentiated groups in the predicted direction and three in the opposite direction. Without providing any evidence in support, Rosenthal *et al.* claimed that these latter scores suggested that index participants 'may have a distorted self-image or are over defensive with respect to these traits' (390). The MMPI results were equally disappointing: there were no significant differences between groups on any of the so-called pathology scales, including the schizophrenia scale. It is perhaps hardly surprising that Rosenthal *et al.* should have said that they '[did] not want to spend too much time with possible explanations of these findings' and that they '[did] not want to dwell on these findings' (390). They gave as their reason the fact that they intended to collect data from more participants, but it is difficult not to wonder whether the data would have been dismissed so readily had it been in line with their expectations. What happened to the data from the remaining tests was not reported.

### Adopted-away children of 'schizophrenics' – an extension

Ten years after the first report had been published, Haier *et al.* (1978) reported on the results of an MMPI assessment of a larger sample of adoptees: sixty-four index (i.e. from a 'schizophrenic'/spectrum biological parent) and sixty-four control. In this report, however, the analyses were more extensive. The authors first looked at the 'overall configuration' of scores on the MMPI but found no significant differences between index and control groups. It was noted also that no scale mean for either group exceeded seventy, the cut-off point for supposed psychopathology. Thus, both index and control groups appeared to be remarkably 'normal', according to MMPI criteria. The test data were then analysed scale by scale, using thirty-four univariate tests (seventeen scales × two sexes). Of these, four comparisons yielded significant differences: index males scored higher (but still within the 'normal' range) than did control males on scales purporting to measure masculinity/femininity and schizophrenia. Index females achieved higher scores (but still within the 'normal' range) on 'hysteria' and 'psychopathic deviance'. As the authors point out, however, 'these . . . differences are not powerful statistically and should be interpreted with the caution implied by the use of multiple univariate tests' (172).

Haier *et al.* conducted three further analyses, each looking at the scoring patterns of the index and control groups. It is notable that the concept of the schizophrenia spectrum had apparently been abandoned and that the authors were now arbitrarily searching for anything which would discriminate index and control groups. The search was unsuccessful: the number of index and control participants who had 'generally elevated MMPI profiles' (i.e. 4 or more T = >70 scales, either clinical or masculinity/femininity) was not significantly different. Nor were the 'profile types' for the two groups (this involves a comparison of the two highest scales). The final analysis involved combining various scale scores to derive what was claimed to be a composite index of psychological disturbance, psychotic signs and schizophrenia signs. These methods had been developed by other researchers and no details were provided by Haier *et al.* For reasons they did not explain, Haier *et al.* did not take the obvious step of comparing index and control group scores on each of these indices. Instead they conducted an apparently meaningless statistical analysis by calculating a mean score for index and control groups combined and then comparing the percentages of index and control subjects who scored more than one standard deviation (SD) above this mean. The analysis showed no significant differences between either male or female index and control groups on the 'psychotic' or 'schizophrenia' indices; on the 'psychological disturbance index', significantly more index than control adoptees scored one SD or more above the combined group mean. The problem with this technique is that it is easy to construct examples where the attainment of a significant or non-significant result depends on the criterion adopted for a high score. Figure 6.1 shows a possible distribution of high scorers, based on Haier *et al.*'s figures, in which the choice of one SD above the mean as the criterion would produce a significant result, but the equally arbitrary choice of 1.5 SD would not. And even if these authors could reassure us that their analysis was valid, the result would still be a long way from supporting their original genetic hypothesis.

It will be recalled that in their 1968 report, Rosenthal *et al.* did not say how or by whom the spectrum diagnoses had been made. Embedded in Haier *et al.*'s 1978 report are the results of consensus spectrum diagnoses of the index and control adoptees, but again with no information about criteria or reliability. There was no significant difference in the proportion of index and control children who were assigned spectrum diagnoses by consensus. It is interesting to note, as an indication of the breadth of the diagnostic criteria, that 25 per cent of *control* subjects were assigned spectrum diagnoses. Perhaps in the face of this weight of insignificant results, Haier *et al.* again lost sight of their original hypothesis and of the spectrum concept. Instead, they introduced another new criterion in an attempt to discriminate index and control groups – a spectrum diagnosis plus a score of T = >70 on any one of the nine

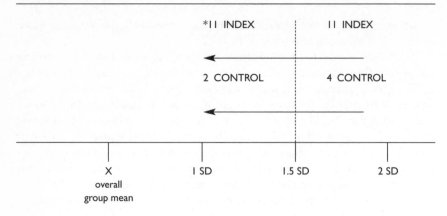

Scores on composite index

Note: *Haier *et al.* (1978) report that twenty-two index and six control subjects scored one SD or more above the overall group mean

*Figure 6.1* A hypothetical distribution of data from adopted-away children of 'schizophrenic' and 'normal' parents

MMPI clinical scales *or* the masculinity/femininity *or* the social introversion scale. But even criteria as lax as these still did not discriminate female index and control groups. In the male groups a higher proportion of index than control participants fulfilled one of the criteria. It is interesting to note that these arbitrary and *post hoc* 'anything will do' MMPI criteria described in the text had become 'MMPI criteria for schizophrenia spectrum disorders' by the time they reached the table of results (174).

In the face of this theoretical chaos, and lacking any systematic evaluation of the participants' backgrounds or information on the success of the matching procedures, Haier *et al.* still felt able to conclude that their combination criteria 'continue to support a genetic hypothesis' (175). Quite what, by now, this genetic hypothesis might be – given that both independent and dependent variables had been abandoned – they did not say.

### Cross-fostering studies

A further strategy which has been used by the adoption researchers is that of comparing the prevalence of schizophrenia diagnoses in groups of children said to have the characteristics shown in Table 6.12. The number of children adopted by someone who will later be diagnosed as schizophrenic is clearly small, because adoptive parents are screened. Wender *et al.* (1974) reported that they were unable to find a sufficiently large sample of adoptees whose

*Table 6.12* Sample characteristics of cross-fostering studies

| Biological parent | Adoptive parent |
| --- | --- |
| 'Normal' | 'Schizophrenic'* |
| 'Schizophrenic' | ?† |
| 'Normal' | ?† |
| 'Schizophrenic' | —‡ |

Notes:
*Cross-fostered group.
†Refers to the groups described earlier in the adoption studies.
‡Non-adopted group.

adoptive parents had received a diagnosis of chronic or borderline schizophrenia and so included participants whose adoptive parent had been called chronic schizophrenic; certain or doubtful acute schizophrenic or schizoaffective; borderline schizophrenic; doubtful schizophrenic or schizoaffective. They did not say how or by whom these diagnoses were made. These criteria produced twenty-eight 'cross-fostered' participants. As in the Haier *et al.* (1978) report, however, the concept of schizophrenia spectrum appears to have been abandoned by Wender *et al.* in favour of global ratings of psychopathology made from the recorded brief impressions of an interviewing psychiatrist. The global ratings were made from one to twenty. Wender *et al.* compared the percentage of participants in each of the three groups (cross-fostered; adoptee with 'normal' biological parent; adoptee with 'schizophrenic' biological parent) who had been assigned scores of sixteen and above. It was claimed, although there is no way of knowing if it was the case, that this corresponded to Kety *et al.*'s B and D categories. There were no significant differences amongst the three groups. Wender *et al.* then combined the cross-fostered and 'normal' parent adoptee groups and compared this group with that of the 'schizophrenic' parent adoptees. The justification for this *post hoc* comparison was that it represented a test of genetic versus non-genetic effects. In the absence of information on the success of matching procedures or on the participants' environments, not to mention the possibility of contaminated ratings and the obscurity of their meaning, it clearly may mean nothing of the sort. The final analysis also reflects a quite different prediction from that originally made by Wender *et al.* and it allows the combination of chance differences in the two groups and the inflated size of the new comparison group, to produce an apparently significant effect from data which was previously shown not to support the main hypothesis.

In the same year Paikin *et al.* (1974) published a report concerned with the personal characteristics of those who refused to participate in the adoption studies. Embedded in this paper, and neither analysed nor commented upon, is a table crucial from the adoption researchers' point of view. It shows not only the prevalence of spectrum diagnoses in the three adoptee groups but also their prevalence in a new group – of children reared with their biological 'schizophrenic' parent. No details were given of the procedures used to collect these data, of the diagnostic criteria or their reliability (the diagnoses were apparently made by Wender), or of where the considerable number of additional participants came from. But the table does show that there was no significant difference in the prevalence of spectrum diagnoses between the cross-fostered group, with their 'normal' biological but 'schizophrenic' adoptive parent, and the non-adopted group, reared by their 'schizophrenic' biological parent ($\chi^2 = 0.04$ df 1).

## Studies of adopted-away children of 'schizophrenic' mothers and their adoptive families

Tienari and colleagues' Finnish longitudinal study contains elements of the 'adopted-away' studies and of the 'cross-fostering' studies, where the focus is on the psychological characteristics of the adoptive parents (e.g. Tienari *et al.*, 1985a, 1985b, 1987, 1994; Tienari, 1991; Tienari and Wynne, 1994; Wahlberg *et al.*, 1997). Tienari (1991) noted that this series of studies was 'interested in assessing to what extent genetic variables and family relationships jointly contribute to psychopathology of adoptees' (460).

Tienari and his colleagues began with a nation-wide sample of all the women in Finland who had been hospitalised 'because of schizophrenia'. The sample included the resident population of 1 January 1960 and later consecutive admissions 'for schizophrenia' until the end of 1979. Various public registers were then used to identify which of these women had had children who had been adopted. Mothers were excluded from the study if their child had been adopted by relatives, adopted abroad or adopted after the age of four. Following the selection of the initial sample of mothers, 'two experienced psychiatrists reviewed the records to confirm the diagnosis of schizophrenia by using the diagnostic criteria that are traditional in Finland . . . Two additional raters applied the Research Diagnostic Criteria to the hospital records of the biological mothers' (Tienari, 1991: 460–461). Mothers were also interviewed 'when possible' and DSM-IIIR criteria were applied, as well as the Present State Examination, the Rorschach test and the MMPI. It is not clear, however, how the final categorisation of the women, or the final decision as to inclusion in the sample, was made or with what reliability. Tienari (1991) reported that 'a total of 179 offspring of 164 index schizophrenic women comprised the final sample of index cases' (460). In fact, this is rather misleading as the sample of mothers whose adopted-away children were assessed included women with diagnoses other than schizophrenia, and, for many of the analyses, the exact diagnostic status of the index adoptees' biological mothers is not clear. Not only that, but the number of biological mothers whose children and their adoptive families were included in the analyses varies from one analysis to another. This is perhaps inevitable in a large-scale study which depends on participants' consent to extensive assessment, but it does make interpretation of the results more difficult, particularly given the very small numbers of adoptees in some diagnostic categories.

Having identified a sample of adopted-away children of mothers given a hospital diagnosis of schizophrenia or paranoid psychosis (the index group) the researchers then sought a comparison group of children, also adopted, but born to parents who had not 'been treated for psychosis'. Some of these parents had 'received psychiatric help for reasons other than psychosis' (Tienari, 1991: 461) but, unfortunately, no details have been given about this. The adopted-away children of these parents (the control group) were approximately matched with the index children on a number of criteria, including age (to within a year); ages of adoptive parents (to within ten years); sex and age at adoption (to within six months). Tienari *et al.* (1987: 479) also reported that 'the two series [index and control groups] (were) also comparable in social status, residence of the family (town/country) and structure of the adoptive family (mother and father vs father or mother only)'. It is not clear from this whether this latter matching was done on an individual or group basis.

The most important feature of these studies concerns the extensive assessments which were then carried out, not only on the adopted-away children (as in the Danish studies) but also on their adoptive families. These included in-depth interviews with individuals, families and couples as well as individual and consensus Rorschach tests and the MMPI (see Tienari *et al.*, 1987, for details). These assessments were carried out by four psychiatrists who were not told whether the interviewees belonged to the index or control groups, although there were no checks on whether the assessors actually were blind as to group membership. Unfortunately, adoption agency rules meant that each family could only be seen by one interviewer, so that the same person assessed both the adoptive parents and family *and* the adoptee. As a partial check on potential bias, the four interviewers carried out inter-rater reliability studies from audiotapes of joint family interviews; although the results were reported to have been 'rather satisfactory' (Tienari, 1991: 463), the sparse details provided are not enough to allow readers to reach their own conclusions.

These assessments were then converted in three ways. First, adoptees and their adoptive parents were assigned to one of six categories: 1 = no diagnosis; 2 = mild eccentricities/symptoms which fall short of any diagnostic category; 3 = moderate and mild symptoms of non-psychotic disorders including less severe personality disorders; 4 = severe personality disorders; 5 = borderline syndrome; 6 = psychosis, including schizophrenia, paranoid psychosis and affective psychosis. It is not clear how this process was carried out and with what reliability. The second conversion involved assigning each adoptive family to one of five categories from 'healthy' to 'severely disturbed' based on judgements of, for example, conflicts and their resolution, and appropriateness of boundaries and family roles. Again, details have not been provided on exactly how this process was carried out or on its reliability. Finally, the researchers devised a 33-item family rating scale which dimensionalised the global ratings of family functioning. Tienari (1991) reported that only four of the thirty-three items gave poor reliability, but the reliability of each dimension, or of the scale as a whole, was not reported.

## The results

Tienari and his colleagues have analysed and reported their data in a number of ways. They reported that, overall, there was a significant difference in the distribution of diagnoses (or no diagnoses) between index and control adoptees, with index adoptees being more likely to receive a 'severe' diagnosis, including 'severe personality disorder' (Tienari, 1991). It is perhaps worth noting that 53 per cent of the index adoptees and 49 per cent of the control group were given some kind of diagnosis. Analysis of index adoptees and their families, however, showed a highly significant relationship ($p < 0.00005$) between the diagnostic status of the index adoptees and the degree of disturbance judged to be present in their adoptive families. No index adoptee who was raised in a 'healthy' family (category 1) was judged at that admittedly early point in the study to be psychotic, borderline, severe personality disorder or even neurotic (Tienari et al., 1987).

Further analyses involved dividing the adoptive families (both index and control) into those where both parents were 'healthy' (category 1 or 2) and those where at least one parent was 'disturbed' (categories 3–6). Within 'healthy' families, the majority of adoptees received no diagnosis (65 per cent of the index and 64 per cent of the control group) and there was no significant difference in the distribution of diagnoses (or no diagnosis) between the two groups. In 'unhealthy' families, however, there was a significant difference in the distribution of diagnoses, with the index adoptees (i.e. the children of 'psychotic' mothers) more likely to receive a 'severe' diagnosis. Tienari et al. also reported a number of multivariate analyses in which they examined the relationship between a number of independent variables (global ratings of family functioning; status of biological mother – index or control – adoptive mother's and father's mental health) and the dependent variable of adoptee mental health rating – categories 1–6. One of these analyses (Tienari, 1991) found that the strongest predictor of ratings of adoptees' diagnostic status was the global rating of adoptive family functioning ($p < 0.000$). The index or control status of the biological mother and the interaction of this with the family ratings also contributed significantly to adoptees' diagnostic status ($p = 0.016$; $p = 0.028$). A second set of analyses using different independent variables (Tienari et al., 1994) found that the strongest predictor of adoptees' diagnostic status was ratings of the adoptive mothers' mental health ($p < 0.000$). Adoptive fathers' mental health was also a significant but weaker predictor ($p = 0.021$), while the status of the biological mother did not significantly predict adoptees' diagnostic status ($p$ = 0.073). Finally, Tienari (1991) reported highly significant relationships between twelve aspects of adoptive family functioning which were rated with reliabilities between 0.68 and 0.84 (e.g. criticism; disrupted communication; rigid family hierarchy) and adoptees' diagnostic status.

## INTERPRETING THE RESULTS

These results have been interpreted as indicating the importance of the interaction of genetics and the environment in the development of 'schizophrenia' and other psychological 'abnormalities'; this interaction has been described in terms of 'genetic control of sensitivity to the environment' which seems to involve the assumption that the children of 'schizophrenic' mothers inherit a predisposition to respond in more extreme ways to their environments. The results have also been interpreted as supporting a genetic relationship between 'schizophrenia' and other diagnostic categories. Tienari *et al.* (1994), for example, claimed that 'the finding [of more serious psychiatric disturbance in index adoptees] hence supported the hypothesis that, as well as narrowly defined schizophrenia, a broader "spectrum" of other psychoses and some personality disorders are genetically related to schizophrenia' (22). The results certainly do suggest a relationship between adoptive environment and adoptees' psychological and behavioural problems, but it is not at all clear what other or more specific conclusions about genetics and schizophrenia could be drawn from the results.

The interpretation of these results is clearly made difficult by the methodological problems I described earlier and by the fact that we do not know about the direction of effects, a point made by the researchers themselves. There are, however, at least two additional major aspects of the study which raise serious questions about any interpretation which involves genetic transmission of 'schizophrenia' or 'genetic control of sensitivity to the environment'.

The first is that the reported analyses are dependent not only on the highly problematic 'schizophrenia spectrum' but also on the grouping together for statistical analysis of a wide range of adoptee diagnoses which have never been shown to be related in any important ways, such as schizophrenia, latent schizophrenia, pseudo-neurotic schizophrenia; paranoid personality disorder; ego-syntonic character disorders and narcissistic personality disorder. Similarly, and as we have seen, the index adoptees' biological mothers had been given a range of diagnoses. The reported analyses therefore do not allow *any* conclusions specifically about diagnoses of schizophrenia. In fact a crucial analysis, not reported by Tienari *et al.* but derived from their data, shows that there was no significant difference in the number of schizophrenia diagnoses between index and control adoptees either when the index adoptees were born to mothers with a diagnosis of schizophrenia or of schizophrenia spectrum ($\chi^2$ 2.36; 3.62; df 1 $p$ < 0.05). Unfortunately, this reliance on a vague spectrum concept, incorporating a wide range of social and psychological problems, is some-times played down in reports of the research by reference, for example, to 'schizophrenic mothers' when the mothers may have had a variety of diagnoses, or to a 'schizophrenic outcome' in the adoptees when the outcome actually refers to a wide range of diagnoses grouped together.

The second aspect of Tienari et al.'s study which makes interpretation diffi-cult is the lack of information on aspects of index adoptees' environment *before* adoption which might increase their risk of psychological or behavioural prob-lems later in life. This issue is crucial because a mother's diagnosis of schizophrenia, whether given before or after the adoption, may be associated with a wide range of factors which could affect foetal development, including medication taken by the mother, poor nutrition, misuse of legal and illegal drugs and poor antenatal care. Tienari et al. (1987) did discuss this problem but appear to have 'forgotten' it in later reports of the research. The problem is compounded by the fact that index adoptees could have been adopted up to the age of four years and eleven months. It is highly unlikely that living for several years with a mother with a serious psychiatric diagnosis, or who would be given one in the future, would have no effect on a child. It is also not clear whether children were adopted directly from their mothers or were in foster or state care for any length of time. Nor do we know why they were adopted. Tienari et al. (1985a) have reported on the proportion of children adopted at various ages, but this included only 108 of the 155 index adoptees eventually assessed and reported only on the numbers adopted at three age ranges: 0–6 months; 7–18 months and more than eighteen months (34 per cent of these 108 index adoptees were adopted when they were older than eighteen months). Tienari et al. reported on the mental health ratings of adoptees who were adopted at these three age ranges, but although the means for the three groups are similar no statistical analysis was reported. The ratings were also made rel-atively early in the research when one-third of the adoptees were younger than twenty. As the mental health ratings appear to worsen with age (Tienari et al., 1985a) these initial results may not reflect the final pattern.

The potentially important impact of the pre-adoption environment has been rendered virtually invisible in reports of the Finnish adoption study, not least by its authors persistently using the term 'genetic variable' to refer to the 'schizophrenic' status of the biological mother. The index children are also said to be 'at genetic risk'. Similarly, the phrase I quoted earlier – genetic sensitiv-ity to the environment – suggests that index adoptees' responses to their adoptive environment are mediated solely by their genetic endowment. Indeed, many reports of the research convey the strong impression that the bio-logical mother handed over for adoption a set of pure genes on which no other influence had ever acted.

These failures to appreciate the considerable problems of the spectrum con-cept, as well as the problems of writing about the index adoptees as if they were merely genetic carriers prior to their adoption, are well-illustrated by

Tienari *et al.*'s claim, quoted earlier, that the researchers' findings 'supported the hypothesis that . . . a broader "spectrum" of other psychoses and some personality disorders are genetically related to schizophrenia' (1994: 22). The researchers seem unable to imagine that some children who were potentially very disadvantaged before adoption might show a variety of serious social and psychological outcomes, related in subtle and complex ways, but which do not involve genetic explanations. Yet we would have no difficulty in imagining this conclusion if we were talking about physical illness:

> Imagine a group of children, born to mothers with a range of serious physical illnesses, possibly exposed to very adverse early environments such as mother's medication, birth complications, malnourishment, poor housing, mother's smoking, and so on. These children are then adopted up to the age of 59 months. In adulthood, they tend to show more serious physical illnesses (although none in particular, and not necessarily those shown by their mothers) than a group also adopted but born to healthy mothers and with possibly a less adverse early environment. Imagine also that a very strong relationship is found between the quality of the adoptive environment (nourishment, medical care, housing, etc.) and the general physical 'outcome' of the children.

It is unlikely that we would see these results as supporting the genetic transmission of any particular diagnosis, even in interaction with the environment, or as supporting the conclusion that a wide range of physical illnesses, say, cancer, heart disease and diabetes, were genetically related. Two reasons why Tienari *et al.* may have been less circumspect in their conclusions are that the unacknowledged conceptual incoherence of 'schizophrenia' allows its boundaries to shift and slide in any direction chosen by researchers and, second, that the genetic transmission of 'schizophrenia' is simply assumed before the research begins, so that genetic interpretations are ready to hand regardless of the ambiguities of the data.

## Genetic linkage studies

The data from twin and adoption studies have recently been supplemented by the results of what are known as genetic linkage studies. This research examines family patterns of genetic markers and of particular diagnoses. If the markers show a similar family pattern to the diagnoses, then it is assumed that there is 'linkage' between the marker(s) and a putative gene assumed to determine the diagnosis. A genetic marker is the biochemical product of a gene locus and it is assumed, as the name implies, to 'point to' the gene locus, although it may still, in genetic terms, be a considerable distance away. The data from these studies are usually expressed as lod, or logarithm of odds, scores. These are described by Watt *et al.* (1987) as 'an estimate of the relative likelihood that linkage at distance θ is occurring between the two loci against the alternative that linkage is not occurring' (365). Particular lod scores are associated with particular probabilities of linkage, although these may vary depending on the genetic model assumed to be operating for a given diagnosis.

Linkage studies of 'schizophrenia' have been of two main types. In the first, the inheritance pattern of a number of genetic markers, presumably from different chromosomes, have been examined and compared, in groups of families, to the pattern of schizophrenia and schizophrenia spectrum diagnoses. The data from these studies have been inconclusive (Turner, 1979) or negative (McGuffin et al., 1983; Watt et al., 1987). The second type of study is one which concentrates on a particular chromosome. The first major report of such a study claimed to have localised 'a susceptibility locus for schizophrenia on chromosome 5' and to have provided 'the first strong evidence for the involvement of a single gene in the causation of schizophrenia' (Sherrington et al., 1988: 164). This report, however, was accompanied in the same journal by the report of a study of a more extensive area of chromosome 5 and which claimed to find 'strong evidence against linkage between schizophrenia and . . . seven loci' (Kennedy et al., 1988: 167). These two studies used different populations, one Icelandic with a few English people, and one Swedish. Sherrington et al. also used three diagnostic groupings: schizophrenia, schizophrenia spectrum and a group with other, unspecified diagnoses. Kennedy et al. used only one group, probably similar to Sherrington et al.'s schizophrenia group. St. Clair et al. (1989), however, reported data from a Scottish sample, with similar diagnostic groupings to the Sherrington et al. study. They found 'no evidence for linkage, regardless of how broadly or narrowly the schizophrenia phenotype is defined' in the chromosome 5 area they studied and which included that studied by Sherrington et al. (St. Clair, 1989: 305).

This state of affairs, where a potentially controversial claim is accompanied in the same issue of a journal by a failure to replicate, and is quickly followed by a second failure to replicate, would normally lead others to report the first claim very cautiously and to make close critical analysis of the methods and data which led to it. It is testament to the public and professional popularity of claims about the genetic basis of 'schizophrenia' that this did not happen. Instead, the weight of negative evidence was subtly, or not so subtly, undermined, in four main ways. First, it was apparently assumed that a 'schizophrenia gene', or genes, exists and that it will one day be reliably detected, and that these conflicting results reflected the complexity of the search and the possible genetic heterogeneity of 'schizophrenia'. Perhaps not surprisingly, the twin and adoption studies reviewed earlier were uncritically cited in support of the belief that schizophrenia has a genetic basis (Watt et al., 1987; Lander, 1988; Nature Editorial, 10 November 1988; Lancet Editorial, 14 January 1989). Secondly, the specifics of Sherrington et al.'s results, and the considerable problems of interpretation which they present, were not always clearly reported. Sherrington et al. cited three maximum lod scores for their three diagnostic groups, the third of which, it will be recalled, had never been given schizophrenia or schizophrenia spectrum diagnoses. The lod score cited for the schizophrenia group was just below the acceptable level for 'good evidence of linkage' set by these authors; the scores for the other two groups were above it, with the 'fringe' group 3 achieving the highest score. This latter result suggests – to put it bluntly – that strong evidence for linkage of genetic markers and diagnoses can best be obtained when any old diagnoses are lumped together. Given the very weak theoretical foundations of the schizophrenia and schizophrenia spectrum diagnoses, and the lack of any theoretical justification for combining these with unspecified diagnoses, the result is a curious one. In fact, Sherrington et al. cautioned that it might have been obtained by chance. These details, however, were not clearly presented in secondary sources. On the contrary, there were indications of 'language slippage', with the diagnostically extremely heterogeneous sample studied by Sherrington et al. being transformed to 'schizophrenia' (Lander, 1988; Nature Editorial, 10 November 1988; Sherrington et al., 1988). The third method by which the negative results were undermined can perhaps best be dubbed the 'flight of ideas' around Sherrington et al.'s results. These included the ideas that the research offered the prospect of 'cloning and sequencing the chromosome 5 schizophrenia gene' (Gurling, 1989: 277); of 'a systematic route to an understanding of the mechanisms of schizophrenia'; of more effective drugs; of settling outright the 'contentious side issue' of the relativistic definition of madness; of discovering the familial advantages which must account for the fact that 'schizophrenia' remains extremely common in spite of the reproductive disadvantage to 'schizophrenics' (Nature Editorial, 10 November 1988: 95–96); of 'identifying non-penetrant carriers as well as fetuses at risk with a reasonably high level of probability' (Gurling, 1989: 277) and of considering 'genetic counselling in families where chromosome 5 linkage can be reliably established' (Sherrington et al., 1988: 167). To say the least, this does seem to be going beyond the data. Finally, perhaps the most popular way of reconciling these conflicting results was to see them as confirming the idea that schizophrenia has many causes, or that only some types of schizophrenia are genetically determined.

Since these first reports, genetic linkage studies have proliferated, though with less media attention, no doubt because of the lack of clearly positive results. There have, in fact, been many subsequent reports of negative results from a variety of chromosome regions apart from chromosome 5 (e.g. Crowe et al., 1991; Barr et al., 1994; Persico et al., 1995a, 1995b; Parsian et al., 1997; Neves-Pereira et al., 1998; Curtis et al., 1999; Antonarakis et al., 1999; Li et al., 1999; Hawi et al., 1999; Serretti et al., 1999). Other results are equivocal and inconclusive. DeLisi (1997), for example, notes that many 'weakly positive' linkages have been reported and that none has been consistently replicated. Hovatta et al. (1998) similarly point out that attempts to replicate potentially positive findings have rarely been successful, while Tsuang et al. (1999), in a considerable understatement, note that 'consistent results have been difficult to obtain' (185).

What is striking about genetic linkage studies, however, is how quickly they have assumed the characteristics of much other research on 'schizophrenia' in which an initial claim to have made an important discovery, particularly one which seems to prove that 'schizophrenia' has a biological basis, may be called into question but is speedily followed by a proliferation of research; the research, however, lacks a consistent guiding theoretical base (Ross and Pam, 1995) and instead adopts a 'scattergun' approach in which the research focus (in this case chromosome/chromosome region and genetic markers) quickly expands, with researchers in linkage studies choosing different chromosome foci for a variety of often unrelated reasons or even for no apparent reason. Some studies, for example, have looked at hundreds of genetic markers, while Gershon *et al.* (1998) hint at a project which would test every gene in the human genome for its association with major psychosis. This approach, in which technology appears to progress much faster than the theory or data which might guide its use, tends not only to produce very large amounts of conflicting and difficult to interpret data but can also lead to false 'positive' results.

As with other areas of 'schizophrenia' research, however, this mass of rapidly accumulating data has to be 'managed' and presented to researchers, professionals and the public in a way which creates an impression of, if not exactly coherence, then not incoherence, and which holds out promise for the future; that is, which averts the possible charge that researchers are wasting their time. I have already mentioned some of the ways this was achieved with the early linkage studies and the issue will be discussed more generally in the next chapter, but for the moment it is worth noting briefly some of the major ways in which genetic linkage research has recently been presented in order to maintain its credibility in the face of inconsistent and negative data.

A reasonable-sounding explanation first has to be offered for the failure to make significant progress. As with the failure to develop valid diagnostic criteria in DSM-IV, the idea of schizophrenia as a complex disease is brought into service, with the implication that setbacks are to be expected:

> Schizophrenia . . . is a complex and multi-factorial mental disorder . . . it perhaps represents several diseases . . . [its] pathophysiology is not localized to a single region of the brain . . . because of its complex pattern of inheritance genetic techniques are not readily applicable in identifying the genes responsible for the disorder.
>
> (Shastry, 1999: 149)

> It is highly likely that multiple genes and idiosyncratic environmental factors are involved.
>
> (Moldin and Gottesman, 1997: 547)

This impression of complexity, however, cannot be taken too far, otherwise it might seem that the task is hopeless and that researchers should turn their attention to a more soluble problem. The impression of complexity is therefore complemented by assurances that schizophrenia *does* have a genetic component and that this has been established by twin and adoption studies:

> Genetic factors make important contributions to the etiologies of schizophrenia.
>
> (Moldin and Gottesman, 1997: 547)

> Family, twin and adoption studies . . . provide strong but indirect support for genetic components in the etiology of schizophrenia.
>
> (Shastry, 1999: 149)

> [T]he advent of modern family, twin and adoption paradigms demonstrates the importance of genetic factors in understanding the familial basis of the disorder.
>
> (Tsuang *et al.*, 1999: 185)

> [A] genetic susceptibility for schizophrenia has been long established and even noted by Kraepelin . . .
>
> (DeLisi, 1997: 163)

Having established that 'schizophrenia' *does* have a genetic component, by uncritical reference to family studies, progress in genetic linkage research is then made to seem inevitable:

> [Reports of chromosomal linkages to diagnoses] have [not] *yet* been consistently replicated.
>
> (DeLisi, 1997: 163; my emphasis)

> [In this paper] we examine genetic linkage studies and our progress toward identifying the genes that cause schizophrenia.
>
> (Tsuang *et al.*, 1999: 185)

This impression of inevitable progress is reinforced by the promise of technological advances:

> As clinical molecular investigation methods advance, identification of disease susceptibility mutations and delineation of their pathophysiological roles may be expected.
>
> (Gershon *et al.*, 1998: 233)

> Rapidly evolving genetic technologies have been applied in the genetic analysis of schizophrenia . . .
>
> (Moldin and Gottesman, 1997: 547)

The idea of progress waiting to happen is reinforced even further by references to the new millennium and the twenty-first century, as well as by Gottesman and Moldin's claim that '[d]etermining the steps between the [chromosome] regions and the [schizophrenia] phenotype will challenge the next generation of scientists' (1997: 404). Finally, the title of Gershon *et al.*'s (1998) paper, 'Closing in on genes for manic-depressive illness and schizophrenia', conveys the impression so common in the 'schizophrenia' literature – of success not quite here but just round the corner.

## The social context and functions of genetic research

There is clearly a considerable gap between the original data from family studies of 'schizophrenia' and the claims made for them. Severe methodological and conceptual weaknesses have often been overlooked, while researchers in the twin and adoption studies have shown a dismaying tendency to omit important procedural details and analyses, to define variables in ways which support their hypotheses, to engage in strange statistical practices, and to gloss over non-significant results or to report them without comment in papers where they might well be overlooked. The obvious question arises as to why researchers should behave in this way. Although there is no clear answer to this question (which I will look at in more detail in the next chapter) we can consider it in terms of the functions which genetic theories of deviant behaviour have served since Kraepelin introduced the concept of dementia praecox. I mentioned earlier that both Kraepelin and Bleuler claimed that 'schizophrenia' was a genetic disorder. Although we have no way of knowing how they reached this conclusion, it could clearly have served to support the claim that many types of deviance were a medical matter; as we saw in Chapter 2, the credibility of the claim was by no means taken for granted at the end of the nineteenth century.

Later, however, one important function which could be served by genetic theories was to become apparent with the development of the Eugenics Movement in the US and Western Europe (see, e.g., Gould, 1981; Haller, 1963). Gottesman and Shields (1982) have described what they call an era of scientific genetics in psychiatry as beginning with the work of Ernst Rudin, and they discuss his work relatively uncritically. They did not mention the fact that Rudin, who was a committed supporter of Nazism and of Hitler, had founded a School of Racial Purity and Hygiene. He spoke of Hitler as enabling 'our more than 30-year dream [to] become reality and racial hygiene principles [to be] translated into action'. He went on to emphasise his 'deep gratitude' to his Führer (Marshall, 1985: 107). Rudin also served on the panel, chaired by Himmler, which drew up the 1933 sterilisation laws. It is perhaps not surprising that Rudin should have produced data in support of his belief in the genetic basis of dementia praecox. Kallmann's work has also been rather uncritically presented by Gottesman and Shields (who have on the contrary defended it) and by other commentators. While not showing Rudin's zeal for racial purity, Kallmann, by his own admission, was a supporter of eugenic policies (Kallmann, 1938). He expressed his strong belief in the genetic basis of schizophrenia before he started his own extensive studies, and then wrote of them in a rather exasperated way, as if they were a bothersome but necessary method of convincing sceptics.

There is no suggestion that most modern genetic researchers share Rudin's and Kallmann's ideas, although they are strangely reluctant to report the enthusiasm with which eugenic ideas were espoused by early genetic researchers and to consider the effect this might have had on their research practice. Nevertheless, it would be naive not to acknowledge the importance of genetic theory for the credibility of the modern concept of schizophrenia. Gottesman and Shields' comment still holds today and illustrates the point well: 'Our case for the role of genetic factors in the etiology of schizophrenia is built on clinical–population genetics data, *but it implies a biochemical and/or biophysical cause for the maladjustment of the brain that leads to the development of schizophrenia*' (1982: 235; my emphasis). In the continuing and predictable absence of consistent biochemical or neurological data in support of the assertion that schizophrenia is a brain disease, claims about the role of genetics in 'schizophrenia' assume considerable importance because they create the impression that the brain abnormality which causes bizarre behaviour is waiting to be discovered. It is also worth noting the suggestion that genetic linkage studies will benefit the psychiatric profession. The *Nature* Editorial which accompanied the report of Sherrington *et al.*'s study, for example, asserted that '[i]t goes without saying that psychiatry, for too long one of the Cinderella specialities of medicine, will profit enormously from the availability of objective tools for study' (95), while Lander (1988) declared that 'psychiatrists have now joined the ranks of experimental geneticists' (106). The subsequent proliferation of genetic linkage studies has also served to create the impression that psychiatry and 'schizophrenia' research are credible participants in the highly prestigious human genome project. Genetic theory and research thus bear the heavy burden of supporting or making credible the biological concept of schizophrenia in the absence of direct supporting evidence.

# Chapter 7

# Supporting and maintaining 'schizophrenia'

## Language, arguments and benefits

The concept of schizophrenia persists in the face of two major paradoxes. The first concerns its claim to scientific status, which ostensibly justifies the use of 'schizophrenia', as well as the search for its causes and cures. Yet as we have seen, the claim is clearly false. The second paradox is that it is not unusual for those who support the concept of schizophrenia to make statements which are, to put it bluntly, absurd but which are clearly intended or assumed to be sensible. For example, if we transferred to physics or chemistry DSM-IV's preoccupation with the 'user friendliness' of the criteria for inferring its concepts, it would be laughed to scorn, as would Andreasen and Carpenter's (1993) claim that DSM-IV's criteria for inferring schizophrenia are both 'arbitrary' and 'robustly valid' for some purposes. Similarly, Spitzer's introduction of the use of specific diagnostic criteria (the tying of concepts to observables) as 'a new approach to psychiatric diagnosis' (1975: 451) and DSM-IV's proclamation of this as a 'methodological innovation' (1994: xvii) are frankly embarrassing, referring to processes so basic in science that it is rather like a modern chef announcing a methodological innovation in cooking – that you switch the oven on first.

A major aim of this chapter is to make this state of affairs understandable; to discuss how and why 'schizophrenia' survives in spite of its exceptionally weak theoretical and empirical base; and how it comes to be surrounded by statements which often make little sense within the scientific framework said to underlie 'schizophrenia'. The starting point of the discussion is the idea that 'schizophrenia' has become part of our reality – a disorder or illness, once discovered and now to be diagnosed in individuals, to be treated and researched. The key question is how this version of reality has been achieved and maintained, how it is made to seem both reasonable and inevitable. This question assumes that maintaining 'schizophrenia' is an active process which requires work and effort, rather than something which simply happens because 'schizophrenia' is 'true'.

I shall examine these issues in four ways. The first is through an analysis of the particular forms of language which systematically construct 'schizophrenia'. Second, I shall examine some specific arguments frequently used to support 'schizophrenia' and thus make it look reasonable. Third, I shall discuss what might be called habits of thought – habitual ways in which all of us manage the complexity of the world – which have particular relevance in contributing to 'schizophrenia's' plausibility. These three sections will be concerned with the apparent reasonableness of 'schizophrenia'; the final section will address its *desirability* in terms of the benefits it confers on the public and professions and the role these play in encouraging its survival.

## Language and the 'realistic' construction of 'schizophrenia'

'Schizophrenia' is written and spoken about as if the language used simply reflected a reality already discovered or about to be discovered. Such a representational view of language has been strongly questioned in a range of theoretical ideas whose common assumption is that what we think of as reality or truth is not discovered or reported but is *constructed*, primarily through the strategic use of language (e.g. Foucault, 1976, 1979; Potter and Wetherell, 1987; Parker, 1992; Gergen, 1999). In this scheme, language is seen not as a mere 'carrier' of reality (Parker *et al.*, 1995) but as a means of actively constructing reality.

The idea of *discourse* is central to this approach (Foucault, 1976). 'Discourse' refers to patterns or regularities in the way we talk or write (and, by implication, think) about particular phenomena, which have certain important effects. Discourse is therefore not simply about words; to speak or write about an 'object' in a particular way is to 'produce' and make seem reasonable a particular version of reality (e.g. that there are mentally ill people and they are not responsible for their actions); it is also to invite or make seem reasonable particular kinds of actions or responses (e.g. that these people should not be punished) and to make other kinds of acts (sending them to prison) seem unreasonable or even unthinkable. Discourse is thus closely linked with social and institutional practices.

Of course, not all ways of speaking or all versions of reality have equal status. In Western society those versions of physical, mental and bodily events offered by what we think of as science and medicine are likely to be given greater credence, to take up more public space and to be challenged less than those offered by almost any other system of thought – for example, religious or astrological. It is unlikely to be accidental, then, that 'schizophrenia' is largely constructed within these two highly prestigious and overlapping systems; I will examine 'schizophrenia' in relation to each of them in turn, before looking at ways in which they may be mutually supportive in constructing 'schizophrenia' as reasonable.

### 'Schizophrenia' and the discourse of science

As Kirk and Kutchins (1992) have noted, science and images of science are used in the 'struggle for influence, position and advantage' and are used by professions 'to present themselves and their expertise to a wider public to gain legitimacy and prominence' (247). One way of doing this, of course, is simply to use the words 'science' and 'scientific' a great deal and to rely on shared cultural understandings of what these imply. As we have seen, the literature surrounding DSM-IV – and the manual itself – is characterised by frequent references to 'science' and to closely related terms such as 'research' and 'empirical evidence'. There are, however, a number of more subtle ways in which the literature on 'schizophrenia' draws on representations of science. The first of these is through what has been called the empiricist discourse or repertoire (Potter *et al.*, 1990; Gilbert and Mulkay, 1984), a systematic way of speaking and writing which allows researchers to present their preferred concepts and theories as neutral, objective decisions not involving any personal preferences or interests. In scientific writing, this impression is achieved, for example, by using the passive voice (the research was designed; the study was carried out), as well as by phrases which imply that research merely uncovers 'facts' (the results showed that . . .; the research found that . . .; it was discovered that . . ., and so on). It is, of course, much easier to maintain this apparently neutral stance when we are talking about things rather than people, particularly about things which involve complex and technical measures. It is significant, then, that so much of the literature on 'schizophrenia' is concerned with physical events such as brain chemistry, ventricular size and genetic markers. This focus not only fosters the impression that 'schizophrenia' is an organic disease, it also maintains the idea of an objectively described reality. And when physical events are not being studied, an impression of neutrality may still be fostered by the use of laboratory tasks or standard questionnaires with pre-set answer formats; in other words, by procedures which create distance between the researcher and the researched.

The process of *diagnosing* schizophrenia, however, presents a potential threat to the aura of neutrality, based as it is entirely on clinicians' judgements of behaviour and reports of private experiences. This problem was highlighted recently by a journalist questioning a doctor about the 'mental' assessment of a prominent politician: 'Can you observe [the mental state] accurately and scientifically *or* is it by observing and watching and talking to the person?' (BBC Radio 4, *World at One*, 17 February 2000; my emphasis). In this dichotomy the diagnosis of schizophrenia would clearly be considered 'not accurate' and 'not scientific'. It is not surprising, then, that so much effort has been expended on creating an impression of objectivity through the use of agreed diagnostic criteria, claimed to be derived from empirical research. Sabshin (1990), for example, claimed that the success of DSM-III was 'deeply influenced by the dire need for objectification in American psychiatry' (1272). In other words, the devisers of the DSM were well aware of the dichotomy inherent in the journalist's question and have strenuously sought to circumvent it. And we should not underestimate the importance of this effort: if 'schizophrenia' can be objectively 'found' in people through diagnosis then it must in some sense exist and be caused. Researchers' failure to find these causes can therefore be tolerated almost indefinitely. DSM-IV and its predecessors have also sought to create an impression of diagnosis as a neutral, objective activity by claiming that they do not categorise people (which might not be seen as neutral) but '[mental] disorders which people have' (1994: xxii). Mental disorders are thus represented as 'out there', as having a separate existence which can be objectively determined.

The use of an empiricist discourse to represent research and practice as objective, and thus reasonable, is closely related to a second way of speaking and writing which might be called a 'technical rational' repertoire[1] (Schon, 1983; Kirk and Kutchins, 1992). There are two main aspects of this repertoire. The first is the use of highly specialised language whose meaning will not be easily accessible to non-specialists. The second aspect is the presentation of a wide range of issues as technical problems responsive to the application of specialised, rational, problem-solving techniques. One of the most important aspects of this way of talking is its representation of problems as soluble by particular specialist groups. The paper I discussed in Chapter 5 which set out 'principles and approaches to guide the development of DSM-IV' in relation to 'schizophrenia' (Andreasen and Carpenter, 1993) provides an excellent example of the use of a technical–rational discourse to support 'schizophrenia' and to make the search for diagnostic criteria seem reasonable. The paper shows clearly the operation of the two aspects of technical–rational discourse: the use of a specialised technical language (e.g. modern biometric approaches; base rates, sensitivity and specificity of symptoms; discriminant function analysis) and the presentation of an issue (in this case the lack of a valid set of correspondence rules for 'schizophrenia') as a technical problem to be solved by quantifying the 'base-rate, sensitivity and specificity for each symptom included in . . . [draft] criteria sets [for schizophrenia]'. As I pointed out in Chapter 5, the ideas of base rates etc. were both misrepresented and entirely inappropriate for the conceptual problem faced by the devisers of DSM-IV; nevertheless, the rhetorical power of this technical language in making the search for valid correspondence rules for schizophrenia seem reasonable and likely to be successful, is clear.

I also showed in Chapter 5 that at precisely the time when it would have been called to account – on the publication of DSM-IV – this particular technical–rational discourse was replaced by a new version in which the problem of defining 'schizophrenia' would be addressed in the future through 'clinico-pathologic correlational validation using the new techniques of neuroscience' (Andreasen and Carpenter, 1993: 205). The importance of this process of change in technical language and in representation of problems and solutions is emphasised by Kirk and Kutchins' (1992) discussion of an earlier phase in

1 I am using the terms 'discourse' and 'repertoire' interchangeably here to refer to regularities in speech and writing about particular phenomena.

the development of the DSM in which the issue of reliability (rather than base rates etc.) was paramount. In a very detailed analysis of this issue in DSM-III, Kirk and Kutchins analysed the processes whereby diagnostic unreliability was transformed 'from a seriously threatening conceptual and practical problem into a technical problem, best left to experts who promised technical solutions' (13–14). As Kirk and Kutchins have pointed out, the power of this stance lay partly in the strong implication that if the problem of diagnostic unreliability were to be solved, then a solution to the even more threatening problem of validity could not be far away. This, of course, was nonsense but the overall effect is to make the continued use of 'schizophrenia' and other diagnostic concepts seem reasonable. Not only that, but the continual change in technical language over the years, to suit the needs of the moment – from reliability to base rates and symptom specificity to clinicopathologic correlational validation – may not be discerned or, worse, be mistaken for progress.

Empirical and technical–rational discourses are clearly related and both can function to create an air of reasonableness around a particular version of reality. They may achieve this effect, however, in different if complementary ways. Empiricist discourse can create an impression that a particular version of reality was objectively discovered, that it simply 'is'. Such accounts, as Kirk and Kutchins have put it, 'dull curiosity', making us less likely to question. Technical–rational accounts, however, tend to mystify; the highly specialised language and techniques of science are beyond the understanding of most non-specialists. This mystification is well illustrated by the response of a Nobel prize-winning physicist to a journalist's request that he describe the research which led to the prize: 'If I could describe it to you, I wouldn't have won the Nobel prize for it.' Technical–rational discourse, then, may not so much dull curiosity as make us reluctant to question; indeed, it may not be remotely obvious to us what would constitute an appropriate question. Not only that, but highly specialised language, used by those who claim the authority of science, may be accepted simply because we assume it must be true or meaningful (why would they talk like that otherwise?). This reluctance to question, however, allows one version of reality to become dominant and the less it is questioned, the less it seems to need to be questioned. Mystification, of course, may be an unintended by-product of scientific research; it is not intrinsically negative or sinister. But as Kirk and Kutchins have pointed out, speaking to non-specialist audiences also has its advantages:

> Listeners are not in a good position critically to assess scientific data, the methods used to gather them or the faithfulness of their interpretation. This provides scientists with some licence.
>
> (1992: 179)

And, as we have seen, this licence appears to have been used quite extensively in the case of 'schizophrenia'.

### 'Schizophrenia' and the discourse of medicine

The second major discursive framework which supports the idea of schizophrenia is that of medicine. As with the discourse of science, the question of interest here is how the discourse or repertoires of medicine function to support 'schizophrenia', to make it seem reasonable, to allow it to persist and to make its continued use understandable even in the face of its considerable conceptual and empirical problems. I shall look first at some general aspects of the medical language which surrounds and constructs 'schizophrenia' before discussing the joint role of scientific and medical discourse, and the additional advantages offered by the latter, in maintaining and protecting the concept of schizophrenia.

### 'Schizophrenia' and the everyday language of medicine

'Schizophrenia' is constructed within what might be called the everyday language of medicine. The behaviours and experiences from which it is inferred are called symptoms and signs; 'schizophrenia' is identified through 'diagnosis' and modified through 'treatment'. One of the most important effects of this language is to construct 'schizophrenia' both professionally and publicly as a taken-for-granted 'object' or phenomenon: if certain behaviours are symptoms or signs of schizophrenia, then schizophrenia must, in some sense, lie behind them; if schizophrenia can be identified through diagnosis, then it must, in some sense, however abstract, 'exist'; if it can be treated, then it must, in some sense, be capable of modification. Not only that, but the historical process whereby this kind of medical language came to be applied to disturbing behaviour is now obscure, so that the language may be seen as simply right and proper. But as I have shown, the language of symptoms, signs, diagnosis and treatment as used in medicine is capable of translation to the more general language of science, where signs and symptoms become patterns of regularities which serve as correspondence rules for concepts; where diagnosis becomes the recognition of patterns previously observed by researchers and the inferring of researchers' original concepts, and so on. The problem for 'schizophrenia', as we have seen, is that this translation cannot be done: from Kraepelin onwards, behaviours and experiences appear to have been interpreted as symptoms or signs of schizophrenia according to no clear set of rules or procedures; not only that, but the word 'sign' has been used in a very different way from its medical use, often as if it were interchangeable with 'symptom' or could be used to refer to any attribute which could be 'objectively' measured. Similarly, 'a diagnosis of schizophrenia' has to mean something different from the recognition of a previously identified pattern, as no pattern which would justify the concept has ever been observed.

But this translation problem can be difficult to see, not least because the translation from 'symptom', 'sign' and 'diagnosis' to the more general language of science is not often found in medical writings except in specialist theoretical or philosophical sources. The public and many professionals may therefore not readily understand what these terms refer to in medical contexts, far less that their meanings are quite different in psychiatry. Medical language therefore functions as an extraordinarily effective disguise which creates a spurious impression of similarity between medical concepts and the concept of schizophrenia, thus conferring on 'schizophrenia' an aura of reasonableness and respectability it would otherwise be difficult to sustain.

A further aspect of everyday medical discourse which has been particularly important in discussions of psychiatric diagnoses, including schizophrenia, is that of (mental) disease, disorder or illness. Indeed, the amount of attention which has been paid to these ideas in psychiatry – both defending and attacking them – is testament to their perceived importance. I shall discuss some specific arguments about 'mental illness' and 'mental disorder' in a later section, but simply say briefly here why the general concepts of mental illness or disorder are so central in supporting the specific concept of schizophrenia. First, if 'mental disorder' or 'mental illness' can be said to exist, or at the very least to be valid concepts, then it seems to make sense to talk about particular disorders or illnesses such as schizophrenia (and in many discussions, it seems to be taken for granted that if anything can be said to be a mental disorder, then it is surely schizophrenia). And the idea of specific illnesses, diseases or disorders is essential to the use of the language of symptoms, signs and diagnosis because designating behaviours as symptoms or signs carries with it the implicit question: symptoms or signs of what? As I pointed out in Chapter 1, the question is not appropriate – we are really asking for which concept are these observables the correspondence rules? – but it has become such a common way of talking that if psychiatrists wish to use terms like 'signs' and 'symptoms', then they had better have an answer to the 'of what' question in terms of specific diseases or disorders. A second reason why the general terms 'mental illness' and 'disorder' are so important is that if the validity of a specific 'disorder' is contested by critics, then it may look as if it simply needs to be adjusted or another specific mental disorder substituted, rather than the entire system of thought being re-examined. Finally, the terms 'mental illness' or 'disorder' keep alive the idea that such 'illnesses' have a physical or biological cause, even if present attempts to find it have not been successful.

### The linked discourses of science and medicine

The discourses of science and medicine through which 'schizophrenia' is constructed are closely related, not least because modern medicine has explicitly adopted the theoretical frameworks and research practices of the natural and biological sciences. Thus, although I have presented the two sets of discourses and their role in the maintenance of 'schizophrenia' separately, their effects can be seen as mutually reinforcing. In this section I shall look at two ways in which this process of mutual reinforcement might work in maintaining the idea of schizophrenia, in constructing it as part of a reasonable version of reality. The first is through the creation of what might be called narratives of progress; the second involves the special advantages conferred by adopting a medical framework over and above those conferred by the discourse of science.

## Schizophrenia and narratives of progress

As Kirk and Kutchins (1992) have pointed out, research data do not speak for themselves, but are given voice and purpose by researchers. One of the most consistent ways in which natural and medical scientists present their data is through narratives of progress in which each new set of data is presented as part of an incremental process, gradually moving us forward towards solving a particular problem. The narrative is often exciting with reports of 'discoveries' or 'innovations' or 'new research findings'. This type of narrative, however, presents considerable problems for 'schizophrenia' because there is so little progress to report. It is hardly exciting or progressive to report that the DSM-IV criteria for schizophrenia are arbitrary; or that schizophrenia has no biological markers; or that the genetic basis of schizophrenia has not been found; or that the claimed structural abnormalities in the brains of some 'schizophrenics' may be related to drugs or alcohol; or that clinicians cannot agree on the distinction between bizarre and non-bizarre delusions which is so important in the diagnosis of schizophrenia, and so on. Yet somehow a narrative of progress – a form of presentation which has become basic in the reporting of science and medicine – must be constructed. Indeed, the less progress there is to report, then the more effort must be expended in constructing a seemingly progressive narrative for both professionals and the public.

The literature on schizophrenia has constructed such a narrative in several ways. The first is through the creation of a linear history of 'schizophrenia'. This form of presentation is very familiar to us from medicine. It begins with the 'discovery' of a particular 'disease', through progressive research to reveal its causes and to discover its cure. The narrative is given credence thorough the existence of apparently completed stories such as the discovery of the infectious diseases, of vaccination and antibiotics. In the case of 'schizophrenia', this linear history is created through linking past and present by frequent references to the work of Kraepelin and Bleuler, with Kraepelin presented as the initial discoverer of 'schizophrenia' and Bleuler as building on his work. Andreasen and Carpenter (1993), for example, claimed that 'Kraepelin was the first clinician/scientist to develop a comprehensive definition of schizophrenia that gained wide acceptance . . . he identified a syndrome' (200–201) and that '[t]oday's construct is quite similar to that developed by Kraepelin and Bleuler' (210). As we saw in Chapter 3, this linear history is a myth; but if 'schizophrenia' is to be presented as a reasonable part of the present, then it must have been discovered or identified at some time in the past. And it is particularly important to remind us of this past when the present is so unpromising, in order to maintain the impression of a temporary problem, about to be overcome.

The second way in which a narrative of progress has been created for 'schizophrenia' is through a focus on the future, often using optimistic language which tells us more about researchers' hopes than about the quality of their data. In Chapter 5, I discussed Andreasen and Carpenter's (1993) paper on diagnostic criteria, in which far more space was devoted to the past and the future than to the unpromising present. Similarly, as I showed in Chapter 6, the negative and equivocal results from genetic linkage studies have been obscured by discussion of a highly promising future whose inevitability is signalled by the use of phrases such as 'has not *yet* been discovered' or 'researchers are making progress towards'.

A third means of creating a narrative of progress for 'schizophrenia is through the use of secondary sources. It is difficult to create a consistently progressive narrative in primary sources (although attempts may be made in the discussion sections, see Ross and Pam, 1995) because the often disappointing data and methodological details are there to be examined. In secondary sources, however, data may be presented in a simplified form or methodological problems may not be mentioned, or, if mentioned, their implications may not be made clear. Readers can thus be given a misleading impression of orderly progress which bears little resemblance to the actual results of research. As I showed in Chapter 6, these practices have been extensively applied to genetic research. Similarly, Andreasen and Carpenter's claim that today's concept of schizophrenia is quite similar to Kraepelin's and Bleuler's, is a travesty of primary sources. Although secondary sources use a variety of devices which create a misleading impression of progress in understanding 'schizophrenia' (and particularly progress in demonstrating its status as a 'biological disorder'), two are especially worth noting. First, detailed discussion of the many different ways in which research data may be interpreted is often avoided. Instead, readers' unfamiliarity with the implications of methodological problems, and our readiness to accept association as causation, are often exploited to imply biological causes of 'schizophrenia'. Second, *group* differences on an experimental task or measure – interpretable in many different ways – are transformed into attributes which are made to look as if they applied to every 'schizophrenic' and only to 'schizophrenics'. For example, it is often reported that 'schizophrenics have enlarged ventricles' or other structural brain abnormalities; the size of the effects (small), that they apply to only a minority of those diagnosed as schizophrenic as well as to people without the diagnosis; that they are associated with use and misuse of minor tranquillisers and alcohol and that they may apply far more to male than female 'schizophrenics', are often not reported in secondary sources (Lader *et al.*, 1984; Andreasen *et al.*, 1990b; Swayze *et al.*, 1990; Chua and McKenna, 1995; Harrop *et al.*, 1996;

Nopoulos *et al.*, 1997). More generally, the recently published text revision of DSM-IV (APA, 2000) provides a particularly striking example of the creation of a narrative of progress through secondary sources. The revision did not change diagnostic criteria or add new diagnostic categories; it simply drew attention to the long gap between DSM-IV and the planned DSM-V and 'updated' the text accompanying each diagnostic category; this text discusses 'associated features and disorders', 'prevalence', 'associated laboratory findings', 'course', 'familial pattern', and so on. It is not clear why the text is there at all; there is no equivalent in the ICD and such information is usually reserved for separate books and journals. What is notable, however, is that the DSM's claims, their expansion and 'updating', are entirely unreferenced; in effect, the DSM increasingly provides a secondary source of claims about 'schizophrenia' (and other 'disorders') which is completely separated from any primary source or from data which would allow readers to check the claims' validity. Given all of this, it is not surprising that McCulloch (1983) should have highlighted reliance on secondary sources as a major factor in the creation of scientific myths.

Finally, it is notable that much, if not most, of 'schizophrenia's' narrative of progress concerns implied progress in understanding 'schizophrenia' as a *biological* disorder. Given the difficulties in creating such a narrative within 'schizophrenia' research itself – at least if it is reported accurately – it is not surprising that perhaps more credibly progressive narratives in the biological sciences should have been spuriously linked to 'schizophrenia' research:

> As clinical molecular investigation methods advance, identification of [schizophrenia] susceptibility mutations . . . may be expected.
>
> (Gershon *et al.*, 1998: 233)

> The nature of the neurobiological lesions or the dysfunctions that cause schizophrenia remains elusive and will until our understanding of neuroscience advances considerably.
>
> (McGrath and Emmerson, 1999: 1045)

### The particular power of medical discourse

Although 'schizophrenia' is jointly constructed through the discourses of science and medicine, it can be argued that it receives special advantages, in terms of its seeming reasonableness, through its partial construction by medical discourse. The major reason for this lies in the fact that unlike natural or biological scientists, medical doctors are part of a *profession*, offering services directly to the public. Not only that, but the relationship between the medical profession and the public is very intimate: doctors have privileged and powerful access to our bodies and minds and see us at our most vulnerable, when our most basic concerns about life and death are to the fore.

This delicate situation is managed partly by an implicit exchange of privileges. On the one hand, the medical profession has been granted a status above that of technicians who use routinised knowledge and whom we might not wish to have such privileged and intimate access to us. Instead, as a number of writers have noted (e.g. Freidson, 1970; Lupton, 1994; Turner, 1995), medical practice is presented as based not only on facts and figures (i.e. on scientific discourse) but also as an intuitive process, based on 'clinical experience' or 'clinical judgement'. In return for this indeterminate knowledge base, for granting doctors the privilege of not having to justify every action by recourse to data, the public are offered a code of conduct, an undertaking about doctors' behaviour and trustworthiness, with severe sanctions for breaches of the code. These privileges are mutually dependent. Doctors provide assurances of absolute trustworthiness, of always acting in the patient's best interests; in return, we attribute to them qualities over and above the ordinary and the mechanised; we attribute to them a knowledge base which, as Turner has put it, has a 'distinctive mystique which suggests that there is a certain professional attitude and competence which cannot be reduced merely to systematic and routinised knowledge' (1995: 133). It is as if we require those who have such privileged access to us, such apparent control over our bodies, lives and deaths, to be above the ordinary and that this is 'proved' by their adherence to a code of conduct well beyond that which we expect in our ordinary interactions.

This is not to suggest that medical concepts and procedures are never justified by empirical evidence; on the contrary, many of them are (although it will be interesting to see how current demands for 'evidence-based practice' accommodate medicine's indeterminate knowledge base). In the case of 'schizophrenia', however, where empirical support is unavailable, then the assumption of an indeterminate knowledge base has worked greatly to the concept's advantage. For example, as I mentioned in Chapter 5, the introduction to DSM-IV cautions that 'The proper use of these criteria requires specialized clinical training that provides both a body of knowledge and clinical skills' (xxvii). Most readers are not to know that a search for this 'body of knowledge' or a request for the specifics of the 'clinical skills' would prove fruitless; the statement sounds reasonable not only because of the repeated use of 'clinical' – arguably the most important word in the language of the indeterminate knowledge base – but also because it fits our existing assumptions about a knowledge base which cannot easily be communicated and is not required to be communicated. Similarly, the fact that (unexplained) 'clinical utility' – a concept with no counterpart in science – was placed first in a list of 'domains considered in making decisions about diagnostic criteria' (xviii), demonstrates both the importance of this assumed esoteric knowledge and the way in which it is brought into service when more explicit scientific evidence is lacking.

Andreasen and Carpenter's (1993) claim that the DSM-IV criteria for schizophrenia are both 'arbitrary' and 'robustly valid' provides a further example of this process. Within a scientific framework, the claim is nonsense, unless we invoke a near miraculous level of coincidence, yet the claim was clearly neither intended nor accepted as such. The claim has an appearance of sense only if we accept that clinicians possess esoteric knowledge or skills which can transform arbitrary diagnostic criteria into something which is valid and useful in practice. Thus the assumption of an indeterminate knowledge base for medicine, with a 'distinctive mystique', arguably allows supporters of 'schizophrenia' considerable leeway in the claims which may be made and accepted as reasonable. I will argue in a later section that this leeway is further strengthened by the *desirability* of the idea of 'schizophrenia'.

## Arguing in defence of 'schizophrenia'

The previous sections have offered an analysis of some of the ways in which the language and representation of 'schizophrenia' may operate below our everyday level of awareness in constructing particular versions of reality as reasonable and plausible. But, as Billig (1990) has noted, talk about any issue – and certainly an issue as contentious as 'schizophrenia' – is also organised in *argument* in which speakers and writers explicitly try to persuade others of the reasonableness of their views by justifying their position and by countering criticism. In the next section, I will examine some specific arguments which draw on scientific or medical discourse and which have been used to defend 'schizophrenia'. As part of the success of these arguments in maintaining 'schizophrenia' lies in their seeming reasonableness, I shall highlight some of the factors which give the arguments their rhetorical power, and provide a critical evaluation of their status as arguments. The first three arguments draw mainly on scientific discourse and indirectly defend 'schizophrenia' by defending psychiatric classification; the final argument, about mental disorder, also offers an indirect defence of 'schizophrenia' and draws mainly on medical discourse.

### Schizophrenia and the defence of classification

The concept of schizophrenia has developed from psychiatrists' attempts to classify, or place into categories, 'abnormal' behaviours and experiences. One of the most important specific arguments which has been put forward within the language of science and used to defend 'schizophrenia' concerns the claimed reasonableness and necessity of psychiatric classification. Kendell's defence of psychiatric classification is worth quoting in detail:

> In any situation in which populations or groups of patients need to be considered . . . some form of classification or categorisation is unavoidable . . . Without diagnosis, or some comparable method of classification, epidemiological research would be impossible. We would have no way of

finding out whether mental illness was commoner in one culture than another . . . without a criterion for distinguishing between sickness and health . . . all scientific communication would be impossible and our professional journals would be restricted to individual case reports, anecdotes and statements of opinion . . . There is no point in defining a population unless its members possess something in common with one another which distinguish them from members of another population, and once this condition has been satisfied a classification has been created . . . I believe [this argument] to be irrefutable . . . it will be taken as proven that psychiatry cannot function at all without classifying its subject matter.

(1975b: 6–8)

Shepherd (1976) and Parsons and Armstrong (2000) have also bracketed classification, science and objectivity:

To discard classification . . . is to discard scientific thinking.

(Shepherd, 1976: 3)

The rise of science included the adoption of a scientific method which would become known as positivism. The central philosophy of positivistic classification was defined by Goldstein as 'The classification of data under clear and distinct rubrics'. In other words, the objective observation and classification of clusters of symptoms to hypothetical disorders which are then amenable to scientific investigation.

(Parsons and Armstrong, 2000: 205)

Put simply, these arguments say that scientists classify, therefore if psychiatrists wish to be scientific they too must classify and categorise. There are two major flaws in the arguments. The first is that while it is true that scientists classify, it is certainly not true that classifiers are therefore scientists. The arguments thus gain their plausibility by failing to make the crucial distinction between 'a classification system' and 'a classification system based on the observation of patterns and capable of predicting new observations'. In other words, the arguments imply that it is only scientists who classify when in fact all of us categorise objects and people in our day-to-day lives but, as I noted in Chapter 1, according to rather different procedures from those generally adopted by scientists. Kendell's and Shepherd's claims are thus rather misleading in that they fail to make clear that to *adopt* certain classification systems could be to discard scientific thinking and that to fill journals with papers based on such systems would be to fill them with anecdotes and statements of opinion. Parsons and Armstrong do acknowledge that we all classify, but perhaps hoped to evade the importance of this point by using the terms 'objective' and 'subject to scientific investigation' to reinforce their implication of affinity between psychiatric and scientific classification systems. In claiming that the devisers of psychiatric classification systems are simply doing what scientists have to do, these commentators seek to create an impression of naturalness or inevitability around the systems: there is nothing else we can do. The contents may be imperfect in terms of reliability and validity, but there is no other way to proceed if we wish to be scientific.

The second problem with these defences of psychiatric classification is that they misrepresent science. Scientists have certainly developed classification systems, but it is not all they have done, and they have not done so because they have followed a rule which says they must. The basic task of science is not to develop classification systems but to delineate patterns and regularities in its subject matter which are useful in making new observations; the classification systems developed by natural and biological scientists *are simply one (limited) type of pattern delineation* which happens to have proved useful for their subject matter. As Chalmers (1990) has noted – and the point can hardly be overemphasised – what has proved useful in understanding biological and physical phenomena will not necessarily prove useful in understanding psychological, behavioural and social phenomena. After all, the phenomena studied by natural and medical scientists have no language, emotions, social context or history; they do not form and break relationships with each other or reflect on their own existence or activities. There is thus no a priori reason to assume that, say, the relationships between language, behaviour and social context, will fall into the same kinds of groupings as the relationships between, say, infectious organisms and bodily responses. Defenders of psychiatric classification evade this crucial point by 'forgetting' that the subject matter of psychiatric classification systems *is* behaviour and experiences which occur in particular contexts and have particular meanings; instead, the subject matter is pre-packaged as an attribute of people (called mental disorders) or as clusters of symptoms which are simply assumed to form the same kind of patterns and be amenable to the same kind of theoretical analysis as bodily processes.

### But it's only a description . . .

I mentioned earlier that a particular way of speaking which has been called the empiricist discourse, or repertoire, could create the impression that scientists simply describe or discover reality. One argument which draws on empiricist discourse and which is used to defend psychiatric classification, is that it is 'atheoretical'; that it is simply descriptive. DSM-IV (1994), for example, claimed that its predecessor DSM-III introduced 'a descriptive approach which attempted to be neutral with respect to theories of etiology' (xvii) (see also Wakefield, 1999a and Parsons and Armstrong, 2000 for similar claims). This neutral, descriptive approach is also implied by claims that classification systems are simply agreements amongst professionals to talk in a particular shorthand way:

> The various diagnostic systems that are currently used in psychiatry rep-
> resent a provisional agreement to use the word 'schizophrenia' to refer to
> a group of patients in a consistent way.
>
> (Andreasen and Carpenter, 1993: 206)

> Because psychiatric diagnoses are sometimes misused to the detriment
> of patients does not seem to us an adequate reason for denying the pro-
> fession a classification system by which they can communicate with
> each other regarding the conditions for which they have professional
> responsibility.
>
> (Spitzer and Wilson, 1969: 422)

These arguments are extremely important because they create the impression
that psychiatric classification merely reflects the world as it is, that it makes no
particular assumptions or interpretations. At the very least, the impression is
given that psychiatric classification merely reflects ways of talking agreed by
psychiatrists which have no particular implications.

Psychiatric classification systems, however, are far from being merely
descriptive in the sense of involving as few theoretical inferences as possible.
On the contrary, they are laden with assumptions. They assume, for example, that their subject matter is 'mental disorders' and that people can be
said to 'have' these disorders (DSM-IV: xxii). The systems assume, further,
that these disorders manifest themselves in behaviours and experiences
which can be called symptoms and that these behaviours and experiences
can be understood using the conceptual frameworks which have been
applied to bodily processes. Finally, the classification systems assume that
these 'symptoms' *have already been shown* to cluster into particular patterns.
This last point is crucial because classification systems are systems of
assumed *relationships* and not simply lists of objects or physical features or
behaviours.

The claim that psychiatric classification and diagnostic systems are descriptive was in fact originally made in order to deflect some of the critics of
DSM-III. As Kirk and Kutchins (1992) have noted, many psychodynamic
clinicians objected to what they saw as the removal of implied psychodynamic
factors in 'mental disorders' (e.g. schizophrenic reaction) and the substitution
of a biomedical approach. The term 'descriptive' therefore served the useful
function of making it look as if no particular assumptions were being made, as
if no one theoretical orientation were being favoured over any other. The
'descriptive' claim, however, has since proved to have a wider utility in presenting diagnostic categories, including 'schizophrenia', as neutral, objective
givens over whose heads theoretical arguments might be conducted (is schizophrenia caused by biological or social factors?) but which themselves, simply
'are'.

## But they're only constructs . . .

In a paper published in the same year as DSM-IV, Alan Frances – Chair of the APA Task Force on DSM-IV – and his colleagues (Frances *et al.*, 1994) sought to defend psychiatric classification by claiming that DSM-IV was a 'heuristic and pragmatic classification' (they also suggested that it was a 'common sense nosology' which hardly fits with attempts to present the DSM as scientific or at least empirically based). The word pragmatic, however, is important here, suggesting that DSM-IV is a reasonable document, reflecting many views but giving preference to none; the term 'common sense', however ill-fitting in this context, also suggests a document with which no reasonable person could disagree. Such a stance was important in dealing with the hostility, from within and outside the APA, which surrounded DSM-IV. Frances *et al.* went on to argue that 'mental disorders are better conceived of as no more than (but also no less than) valuable heuristic constructs' (210). I have already criticised this kind of wording in relation to Kendell, in Chapter 4: it is not that mental disorders are constructs but that supporters of psychiatric classification insist on talking about diagnostic constructs as if they were synonymous with some separate and already identified phenomena called mental disorder. If however, we assume that Frances *et al.* are claiming that diagnostic labels or categories are constructs – a claim, incidentally, which contradicts DSM-IV's claim to take a 'descriptive approach' – then that is clearly the case; indeed, it is the entire basis of my arguments here that 'schizophrenia' is a construct which claims scientific status and must therefore be judged on that basis. What is interesting is that Frances *et al.* seem to see the claim that diagnostic labels are constructs as somehow offering a defence of diagnostic systems ('mental disorders are better conceived of as *no more than* . . . constructs'); but if we substitute 'diagnostic terms' for 'mental disorders', then the claim is not a defence of classification but a statement of the obvious (that diagnostic terms are constructs) and a necessary starting point for questions about the constructs' validity.

There is, however, a rhetorical value in this claim which could contribute to the impression of reasonableness which the devisers of psychiatric classifications clearly wish to create. The term 'constructs', unlike the idea of disease entities with which Frances *et al.* contrasts it, creates an impression of impermanence, of being subject to change and open to new evidence. This is, of course, exactly what constructs are meant to be, but, in the context of DSM-IV, claims about constructs could serve to ward off criticism (we're only using them provisionally, we'll change them when new evidence is available). The more fundamental issue, of whether the constructs should be used at all, is simply avoided.

The second part of Frances *et al.*'s claim, however – that diagnostic categories are valuable *heuristic* constructs – is also important in deflecting criticism by implying that these constructs have already proved their worth. The *OED* defines 'heuristic' as 'an aid to discovery'; in scientific terms, as I noted in Chapter 1, constructs are meant to predict new observations, unlikely to have been made without the construct. Frances *et al.* are thus claiming that DSM-IV's constructs, including schizophrenia, have enabled reliable observations of new phenomena unlikely to have been observed without these concepts. But what are these new observations? For want of better, Frances *et al.* are forced to fall back on the old and problematic ideas of course, family history and treatment response. As we have seen in the case of schizophrenia, this concept has never reliably predicted any of these. More generally, 'course', 'family history', etc. only make sense if the validity or usefulness of a construct has already been established or assumed, i.e. it must already have enabled the prediction of some other observations. Otherwise, we are left asking, course of what? Family history of what? In claiming that DSM-IV's categories are 'valuable heuristic constructs' Frances *et al.* are thus not only making a highly misleading claim, they are invoking prestigious scientific language while entirely avoiding the key issue of the constructs' validity.

### Defining and defending mental illness and disorder

The final specific set of arguments I shall discuss which are used to support 'schizophrenia' involve attempts to define 'disease', 'illness' or 'disorder'. Unlike the previous arguments which tried to compare psychiatric and scientific activities, these arguments try to compare psychiatric and medical activities. The arguments' common assumption seems to be that if we can find a 'proper' definition of 'disease' or 'disorder', which encompasses 'mental disease' or 'disorder', then it will be obvious which behaviours and experiences fall within the definition *and* that these should be understood using the language and theoretical frameworks of medicine. As I noted in Chapter 4, however, terms such as 'disease', 'illness' or 'disorder' are *lay* or social terms; they can no more have a proper or correct definition or tell us how to think about those to whom the terms are applied, than terms like 'courage' or 'sin'. Equally, trying to identify people who definitely have mental disorders makes no more sense than trying to identify people who are definitely courageous or sinful. This is not to suggest that there is no agreed usage of these terms, simply that no usage can be thought of as correct or definitive or tell us which theoretical frameworks to use in trying to understand whatever behaviours led us to apply the terms in the first place. It is not surprising, then, that most attempts to define 'disease', etc., proceed in a circular fashion by trying to identify common attributes of *what everyone already agrees are mental disorders* or by testing a definition against what everyone already agrees are mental disorders (and this, incidentally, always includes 'schizophrenia'). But in a culture which takes the existence of mental illness or disorder for granted, such fallacies are not always obvious and the arguments may be successful in maintaining the idea of schizophrenia by appearing to prove what is already assumed to be true. In the next sections I shall examine four attempts to define (and defend) 'mental illness' or 'disorder', and thus to support 'schizophrenia' as a medical concept.

Two early attempts to define 'disease' (including 'mental disease'), and to justify the application of medical theories to deviant behaviour, were made by Kendell (1975a) and Kräupl-Taylor (1971, 1976, 1979). Kendell suggested that the defining characteristics of 'disease' are that it represents a deviation from some normative standard *and* confers a biological disadvantage in the form of a reduction in fertility. Because those called 'schizophrenic' clearly deviate from normative standards of behaviour and have fewer than average children, Kendell concluded that schizophrenia is therefore 'justifiably regarded as illness' (314). Kräupl-Taylor's argument involved looking for the common attributes of those to whom the label 'patient' is applied and suggesting that they consisted of a statistically significant deviation of an attribute from a norm *and* therapeutic concern for a person felt by the person themselves and/or the social environment. Using set theory, he called the intension composed of these two attributes 'morbidity'. In turn, this set of 'morbid' attributes is seen as characterising all diseases.

Interestingly, Kendell (1975a, 1975b) and Kräupl-Taylor (1979) have provided critiques of the other's definitions, but unfortunately without acknowledging the futility of their attempts at definition. Kräupl-Taylor (1979) and Toon (1976) have pointed out that Kendell's definition encompasses phenomena such as voluntary sterilisation, celibacy via religious vocation or just by choice, and homosexuality (defined as not a disease by the American Psychiatric Association). Kendell, however, argued that Kräupl-Taylor's analysis would allow the medical profession and society free rein to label all deviants as ill and suggested that 'any definition of disease which boils down to "what people complain of" or "what doctors treat" or some combination of the two, is almost worse than no definition at all' (1975a: 307).

Clare (1976) took a rather different, but no less fallacious, approach to the task of defining mental illness. His major point was that critics of the term 'mental illness' have wrongly assumed that the term 'disease' is used in a straightforward and non-problematic way in medicine (to mean organic pathology), and that the term therefore cannot be used to describe behavioural or psychological phenomena. Clare's point may be valid in the sense that 'disease' is not used in a straightforward way in medicine, but his later conclusion is not. Clare has argued that the way in which the word 'disease' has been used in medicine has changed considerably over the last few centuries and that older usages which emphasised specific organ pathology, and assumed that psychic disease was brain disease, were based on a now outmoded dualistic view of the relationship between mind and body. Therefore, his argument implied, we can now apply the term 'disease' or 'disorder' to mental or behavioural phenomena where no bodily pathology can be found. A rather similar argument has been suggested by Roth and Kroll (1986) and by DSM-IV. The problem with these arguments is that they assume some logical connection between the widely accepted idea that the psychological may influence the physical, and the implied conclusion: that we are justified in adopting medicine's theoretical models and practices in dealing with certain deviant behaviour. We cannot, of course, assume any such connection, any more than we could argue the validity of specific gas laws merely by asserting that the physical and chemical interact. Arguments about dualism or about 'disease' being a social construct in medicine are simply a means of avoiding the crucial issue of the lack of empirical support for certain theories and concepts applied to disturbing behaviour.

A further attempt to define 'mental disorder' has been made more recently by Jerome Wakefield (e.g. Wakefield 1992a, 1992b, 1995, 1997a, 1997b, 1999a, 1999b). I will discuss this attempt in some detail because of the extensiveness of Wakefield's writings, his claim to have provided a scientific element for the definition of mental disorder, and because his discussion of the concept has received considerable attention in the literature.

Wakefield notes the 'vast literature' devoted to the concept of mental disorder which, he claims, has nevertheless failed to provide any widely accepted analysis 'that adequately explains even generally agreed upon and uncontroversial judgements about which constructions are disorders' (1992b: 374). He attempts to provide such an analysis and, rather ambitiously, to 'resolve the fact-value debate' (ibid.) in which the crucial argument has been whether terms like 'disease', 'illness' and 'disorder' are value-free scientific terms or social/political judgements.

The starting point of Wakefield's analysis is a critique of the definition of 'mental disorder' offered in DSM-IV and in earlier versions of the DSM. In a very detailed analysis (1992a, 1997a) Wakefield argues, for example, that DSM-IV's diagnostic criteria do not adhere to the goal implicit in the DSM definition of mental disorder of identifying dysfunction 'in the person'; that the contents of the manual are over-inclusive because the criteria encompass 'many conditions that are not true mental disorders in the relevant medical sense', and that the manual fails to distinguish disorders from non-disordered problems in living (1997a: 633). Wakefield also argues that there is a potential problem of *underinclusion* because of the DSM's requirement that 'symptoms' should not be an 'expectable response to a particular event'. As our knowledge changes, however, what was once unexpectable becomes expectable so that, to use Wakefield's examples, lung cancer becomes an entirely expectable response to smoking and post-traumatic stress becomes an expectable response to certain extreme situations.

Wakefield's aim is to provide an analysis and definition of 'mental disorder' which will avoid these problems and which will allow 'a coherent and valid distinction to be drawn between clear cases of mental disorder and non-disorder that is consistent with the use of disorder in the broader medical sciences' (1997a: 635). A crucial part of his argument, therefore, is that 'mental disorders are medical disorders' (1999b: 1007) or, to put it another way, mental disorders (as properly defined) 'legitimately fall within medicine's conceptual domain' (1995: 233).

Wakefield defines 'disorder' (the term is intended to encompass both physical and mental disorder) as 'harmful dysfunction' in which dysfunction 'is a scientific and factual term based in evolutionary biology that refers to the failure of an internal mechanism to perform a natural function for which it was designed, and *harmful* is a value term referring to the consequences that occur in the person because of the dysfunction and are deemed negative by sociocultural standards' (1992b: 374). In this definition, 'internal mechanism' is used to refer to both physical structures and organs and 'mental structures and dispositions' (ibid.), while 'natural function' is the 'function for which the mechanism was designed by natural selection' (1992a: 236).

Critics of Wakefield's attempt to define 'mental disorder' have contested his claim to have provided a factual definition of dysfunction; his presentation of evolutionary theory and the idea of natural function; his claim that the definition distinguishes what are thought of as disorders and non-disorders in medicine and the mentalistic assumptions underlying the analysis (e.g. Sadler and Agich, 1996; Lilienfeld and Marino, 1995; Houts and Follette, 1998). I will not repeat all of these criticisms here; instead, I will focus briefly on three of the more obviously problematic aspects of Wakefield's analysis, before looking at some of its more fundamental problems which call into question the whole enterprise of trying to define 'mental disorder'.

### Dysfunction as a failure in mental mechanisms

The idea of mental mechanisms or mental structures is simply taken as given in Wakefield's analysis. Indeed, in the face of criticism of his mentalistic assumptions he has simply asserted that '[m]ore or less everyone agrees that there are . . . functions [such as cognition, emotion and motivation] and that there are mental mechanisms designed to perform them' (1999b: 1013). Apart from the fact that appeals to what 'more or less everyone agrees' are entirely inadequate as a defence of a supposedly scientific and factual term (dysfunction), this assertion ignores the persistent and extensive controversy over the validity of the idea that 'what goes on in our heads' can be conceptualised as mental mechanisms or mental structures as well as the controversy over the relationship between 'what goes on in our heads' and our behaviour (e.g. Skinner, 1953, 1974; Coyne, 1982; Potter and Wetherell, 1987; Edwards, 1997; Gergen, 1999). The scale of the problem becomes apparent when we look at the mental mechanisms suggested or asserted by Wakefield, and implicated in various 'mental disorders'. These include: perception; language; learning; action; belief; thought; drive; hedonistic structures; internal reparative mechanisms; coping mechanisms; socialisation mechanisms; moral development and impulse control mechanisms; erectile mechanisms; loss-reaction regulating mechanisms; sadness generating mechanisms; anxiety regulating mechanisms; aggression inhibiting mechanisms; and exploitation inhibiting mechanisms. These supposed mechanisms, whose 'failure to function as designed' is necessary for mental disorder, appear to be generated *ad lib*, with little or no acknowledgement of the major validity problems they present. Not only that, but their existence is inferred in a circular fashion from the behaviour which the mechanism is then used to explain; there appears to be no independent means of inferring the mechanisms without reference to the supposed effects used to posit their existence in the first place. Wakefield has responded to this criticism (1999a) by claiming that it is reasonable to infer a cause from an effect, even if one does not know the nature of the causal mechanism. This may be so, but that does not mean it is reasonable to infer any specific cause. The problem here is that it is the existence of specific mental mechanisms and structures which is at issue, so that they cannot be inferred from their speculated effects in the absence of independent evidence of their 'existence'. It is because Wakefield takes their existence entirely for granted that he cannot 'see' the tautology.

### Establishing natural functions

Suppose for a moment that we do possess mental mechanisms or structures such as those generated by Wakefield; in order to identify a 'dysfunction' – the first stage of identifying a 'mental disorder' – we still have to establish the mechanism's 'natural function' *and* that the mechanism has failed to perform this function in a particular person. Wakefield has himself commented that 'discovering what in fact is natural or dysfunctional may be extraordinarily difficult' (1992a: 236); Lilienfeld and Marino (1995), however, have argued that it would be virtually impossible. Difficult or impossible, the fact remains that Wakefield has not provided any means whereby natural functions or dysfunctions could be directly established. Instead, he invokes his clinical experience, but has also suggested an indirect or 'circumstantial' route which involves judgements of, for example, whether the response (symptoms) is so extreme 'that nothing but the breakdown of internal mechanisms could be expected to cause them' (1992a: 243); or of whether the 'symptoms' are a 'natural response that is initiated and maintained directly by the ongoing stress' (1992a: 238), or of whether they are a 'normal response to problems in living' (1997a: 642), or a 'normal proportionate reaction to an unusual environmental stressor' (1997a: 646), or of whether the symptoms are caused by the 'right kind of triggering stimuli' (ibid.).

It is ironic that what Wakefield describes as a scientific and factual term (dysfunction) should have to be inferred from such highly evaluative criteria. Who is to decide what is a 'normal' or 'natural' or 'proportionate' reaction or what is the 'right' kind of triggering stimuli, and what standards are they to use? They cannot use statistical deviance, because Wakefield has already rejected that as a means of inferring dysfunction or disorder. We are left, it seems, with the personal views of those with the authority to judge. But given the extensive criticism of psychology's and psychiatry's tendency to see the world from the perspective of particular dominant groups (e.g. Sarason, 1981; Prilleltensky, 1989; Ussher and Nicolson, 1992; Fox and Prilleltensky, 1997), then it is difficult to share Wakefield's confidence in these judgements of 'dysfunction'.

### Disorder as harmful dysfunction

In Wakefield's argument, however, defining 'disorder' does not only involve establishing natural functions and dysfunctions. In order to be considered a disorder, '[a] dysfunction must also cause significant harm to the person under present environmental circumstances and according to present cultural standards . . . only dysfunctions that are socially disvalued are disorders' (1992b: 383–384). Thus the 'harmful' aspect of disorder, unlike the dysfunction aspect, is explicitly evaluative. It is therefore not appropriate to criticise this part of the definition simply because it involves value judgements; it can, however, be criticised on two grounds. First, Wakefield does not say exactly what he means by harm, possibly because he sees this as unnecessary if harm is explicitly acknowledged as a value judgement. But just as with judgements of 'dysfunction', this leaves the way open for systematic bias in these judgements. For example, socially dominant groups may be less likely to see *their* behaviour as harmful and to evaluate it negatively, particularly if it is behaviour they enjoy or which is important in maintaining existing power relationships. Thus the question of who decides what is harmful, and who decides whether this harm is caused by a mental dysfunction, is directly raised by Wakefield's analysis but is hardly addressed by his repeated reference to the 'common-sense' notion of harm.

The second point on which the 'harm' component of the definition of mental disorder can be criticised is that, having argued that it is necessary for inferring mental disorder, Wakefield subtly devalues it and implies that the supposedly scientific and factual idea of dysfunction is actually more important. For example, he implies that the concept of disorder exists 'over and above value judgements' (1999b: 1011). But since he himself has claimed that harm and dysfunction are equally necessary for judgements of mental disorder, then one element cannot be put 'over and above' the other. Nor does it make sense to suggest, as Wakefield appears to do, that the concept of mental disorder remains 'coherent' when the value element is removed. Wakefield also at times appears to forget that he *has* made 'harm' a necessary part of his definition of mental disorder, or at least he seems to take its application for granted. For example, he talks about 'mental functions fail[ing] to be performed, *yielding what we call disorder*' (1999a: 986; my emphasis) and claims that '[c]linical experience strongly suggests that . . . functions sometimes fail because of failures of underlying mechanisms to perform as designed, *warranting attribution of disorder*' (ibid.; my emphasis).

Both aspects of Wakefield's definition – dysfunction and harm – are therefore extremely problematic. And these problems are crucial, given Wakefield's claim that 'mental disorders' belong in the conceptual realm of medicine; in other words, having identified 'harmful dysfunctions' we are entitled to conceptualise and respond to them using a medical framework. This claim represents a fundamental problem of Wakefield's analysis; it will be considered, together with two equally fundamental problems, in the next section. And it is worth noting that the discussion applies to all attempts to define 'mental disorder'.

## Mental disorders as medical disorders

The claims that mental disorders are medical disorders and that they 'legitimately fall within medicine's conceptual realm' are made explicitly in Wakefield's analysis but are implicit in all attempts to define mental disorder. Wakefield, however, has also claimed that this does *not* necessitate physiological or organic accounts of 'mental disorders'. He argues instead that '[b]ecause the psychological systems with which the DSM and the mental health professions are concerned are biologically designed, DSM defined mental disorders are by definition a species of the general category of "medical disorder" . . . analogous to digestive disorders and circulatory disorders' (1999b: 1004–1005) and that '[d]isorders are failures of biologically designed functioning so in a trivial sense all disorders are biological. The judgement that "something has gone wrong" with psychological functioning must be made relative to some baseline of things "going right" and . . . evolution appears to be the only viable way to define the relevant baseline for how our minds are supposed to function. Evolution is part of biology so disorders are biological' (1999b: 1004–1005; 1007–1008).

The problem with this argument is that it involves many questionable assumptions which Wakefield simply takes for granted: that mental health professionals deal with psychological systems which are designed by evolution and which can fail to function as designed; that we have minds which are supposed to function in certain ways; that when 'something goes wrong' with psychological functioning, then we have a disorder in the medical sense. Not only that, but if all disorders are biological 'in a *trivial* sense', then in what *important* sense can 'mental disorders' be said to be 'medical disorders'? Wakefield does not discuss this, but what he and others assume is that the behaviours and experiences said to constitute 'mental disorders' will fall into the same kinds of patterns or regularities – symptoms and signs, syndromes, etc. – as do the bodily phenomena which constitute whatever we think of as physical disorders. But there is no reason to assume in advance that this will be the case, particularly as concepts and processes which appear to be very useful in understanding aspects of our behaviour – such as schedules of reinforcement, primacy and recency effects on memory or the regulatory effects of language – have no counterpart in the study of bodily processes. And even if we accept Wakefield's claims about evolution and mental mechanisms, we cannot assume in advance that when these mechanisms 'fail to perform as designed' the result will be conceptually identical to a 'failure' in a bodily mechanism. Wakefield evades this problem by frequently supporting his arguments about mental mechanisms with examples from physical medicine which simply assume that mental mechanisms are the same kind of phenomena as eyes or lungs or hearts, so that making a point about lungs is presented as if somehow the point also applies to, say, 'coping mechanisms'.

A second fundamental problem with Wakefield's and others' attempts to define mental disorder is that they assume the prior 'existence', or at least the validity, of 'mental disorders' and see their task as offering a definition or illuminating the nature of these pre-existing phenomena. In other words, they behave in exactly the same back-to-front manner as the devisers of the DSM by starting with an existing and very problematic concept and searching for a 'correct' set of correspondence rules for inferring it. Wakefield justifies this by arguing that we need to 'formulat[e] theories to explain a distinction [between disorder and non-disorder] we already use' (1999b: 1011), and that 'without the dysfunction analysis, I know of no way to explain the vast array of intuitions about disorder' (1995: 224). He also claims that such analyses 'do not stipulate how we *should* use mental disorder but attempt to capture how we *do* use it' (1999b: 1011; emphasis in original).

It is, of course, very reasonable to study how people use such socially important terms as 'mental disorder'. The problem with Wakefield's argument, however, is that in spite of his claims, he clearly sees himself as doing much more than 'capturing how we use the term'. It is difficult otherwise to account for his use of terms such as 'correct and incorrect' usages of 'mental disorder', or 'genuine disorders' or 'truly disordered'. Wakefield also claims that the question 'is there a failure of a strong function'? 'is good enough to be a scientific basis for the common sense distinction between mental disorders and other problematic behaviours' (1999b: 1017). But it is not the job of scientists to provide a scientific basis for common-sense distinctions between mental disorder and other problematic behaviours, any more than it is their task to provide a scientific basis for common-sense distinctions between sin and other forms of wrong-doing or between mild laziness and sloth. And the study of how people use terms like 'disorder' is no more capable of providing a scientific basis for the disorder/non-disorder distinction than the study of how people use the term 'sin' could provide a scientific basis for a sin/non-sin distinction. If this analogy seems strange, it is only because in the twentieth and twenty-first centuries mental disorder has assumed a reality in Western culture almost as unquestioned as the reality of sin in earlier times; it is this assumed reality which makes it look as if the task of finding a scientifically based definition of mental disorder is reasonable.

The third fundamental problem of Wakefield's and others' attempts to define mental disorder is that they assume the 'existence', if only in an abstract sense, of the specific 'disorders' named in the DSM. Wakefield, for example, claims that 'DSM obviously does classify *instances of disorder* into categories like schizophrenia' (1997b: 652; my emphasis). He acknowledges, however, that DSM's categories involve assumptions about 'the existence of co-varying symptoms' and about 'covariation derived from past observations' (1999a: 969, 989). Wakefield mentions this almost in passing, as if it were of no particular importance, when in fact it is a crucial and problematic assumption for anyone who wishes to talk about specific 'mental disorders'. As I have emphasised, the DSM does indeed involve assumptions that certain phenomena (its diagnostic criteria) cluster together in a meaningful way. Without this assumption, the DSM's categories do not even have the beginnings of a claim to scientific status. As I have shown, however, in the case of the most taken for granted of mental disorders, schizophrenia, the assumption is false: there is no evidence that the diagnostic criteria have ever represented, as Wakefield puts it, 'covariation derived from past observation'. As well as the arguments already presented here to demonstrate that lack of evidence, statistical studies of schizophrenia diagnoses have failed to find evidence of the statistical clusters assumed by the DSM (see Bentall, 1990b, for a review). Wakefield attempts to evade this crucial problem in a number of ways. He talks, for example, of the 'described pathological syndromes' in the DSM (1999a: 971) without considering what this claim requires in the way of evidence; he substitutes the vague term 'condition' for the specific medical term 'syndrome', thus again avoiding the need to examine exactly what is implied by 'syndrome' and whether the DSM meets the requirements; he claims that the DSM's categories represent an 'initial, purely descriptive phase' (ibid.: 973), thus making it look as if the categories can be taken for granted, when, as I noted earlier, far from being descriptive the categories are highly inferential and require close critical examination; Wakefield appeals to common sense by talking about 'known disorders', 'recognised disorders' and 'accepted disorders' (ibid.: 982); he implies that he is not really making any substantial claims about the DSM by claiming that it is more like a 'trouble-shooting guide to the human mind' than a theory or research programme, thus again avoiding having to confront the nature and problematic status of the assumptions made by the DSM. Yet these problems with DSM's categories present considerable obstacles for those who try to define mental disorder because they raise the question: what is a definition of mental disorder a definition of? Wakefield evades this question only by appeals to shared cultural beliefs: severe schizophrenia *is* a disorder; ignorance and greed are not; he also slides between the use of category names (schizophrenia, depression, anti-social personality disorder, etc.) and specific behaviours and experiences (hallucinations, extreme sadness, cruelty to animals) as the focus of his definition of mental disorder.

The result of all this is question-begging and conceptual confusion on a grand scale. It is not surprising, then, that no attempt to define 'mental disorder' should have escaped criticism, not least from those offering alternative definitions. I would emphasise again, however, that the entire enterprise of defining mental disorder is pointless, at least in so far as the goal is to allow us to recognise 'genuine' or 'true' disorders. Indeed, attempts to define 'mental illness/disease/disorder' can be seen as attempts to prove that we ought to respond to certain behaviours and experiences as if they were unwanted bodily phenomena *in the absence of evidence that this is a valid and useful way of proceeding*. I shall return to this issue in the discussion of the desirability of 'schizophrenia'.

## Habits of thought which support 'schizophrenia'

'Schizophrenia' may gain much of its plausibility through the strategic use of language and through specific arguments. There are, however, a number of habitual ways of thinking by which we manage the complexity of the world which also contribute to 'schizophrenia's' seeming reasonableness and therefore to its survival as an idea. Three of these will be discussed here: question-begging, reification and biases in pattern recognition.

### Question-begging and reification

In an analysis of popular forms of argument, Thouless (1974) identified a number of what he called 'dishonest tricks commonly used in arguments'. Most of them have been used in the 'schizophrenia' literature; indeed, one of the reasons for the concept's survival may be that no special form of argument is used to support it; instead, the arguments are in a form all of us use some of the time in good faith that we have a strong case, and are therefore less likely to be detected as false. (I should emphasise that Thouless was not suggesting that people who use these 'tricks' are conscious of doing so or are deliberately dishonest; part of their power is that they are not usually detected by either speaker or audience.)

Perhaps the most frequently used 'dishonest trick' in the 'schizophrenia' literature is that of begging the question, of taking for granted what is actually in dispute or of assuming to be true what has to be proved – in this case, the validity of the concept of schizophrenia. What is remarkable is the extent to which this device is used: the whole of Kraepelin's, Bleuler's and Schneider's writings are based on it, as is virtually the entire DSM literature on the search for an operational definition of schizophrenia. So too are defences of psychiatric classification which take for granted the existence of 'mental disorders', and the search for definitions of 'mental disorder'. As Thouless has pointed out, it is easier successfully to use this device, or indeed any false device, when the argument is stated in such a way that it is not apparent that it is being used.

It is easier to achieve this, to obscure the fact that important questions are being begged, when what is taken for granted is strongly and widely believed. In the case of 'schizophrenia', its validity seems self-evident (if a little difficult to demonstrate at the moment) when we believe in mental disorders or mental illnesses; mental illnesses seem self-evident when we believe that bizarre behaviour is caused by brain disorder; that, in turn, seems self-evident because we cannot think of any other way to explain such bizarreness. Above all, the self-evidence of these ideas increases with their use, to the point where even imagining an alternative becomes difficult.

Question-begging may also be accomplished more easily in the presence of the habit of reification, of talking about ideas or concepts as if they were things. This habit has been well described (see, e.g., Ryle, 1949; Young, 1951); Szasz's (1987) observation that the *Dictionary of the History of Ideas* has no entry for 'mental illness' is a good example of it. Crookshank (1956), in a sharply critical paper condemning the widespread use of reification in medicine (actually written in 1923), talked of the 'tyranny of names' and claimed that 'few now comprehend the distinctions between Words, Thoughts and Things, or the relations engaged between them when statements are communicated' (340). Emmet (1968) expressed the hope that reification was now less prevalent in medicine but this seems not to be the case. The 8th edition of the ICD still talked of constructs as being 'the names of diseases' and DSM-IV talks of psychiatrists diagnosing 'disorders which people have'.

It is not difficult to see why we might reify ideas. It is, after all, much more difficult to juggle with abstract concepts and symbols than with material entities. Ogden and Richards (1956) have suggested another reason: that 'if we are ever to finish making any general remark, [we must] contract and condense our language' (133). But as Ogden and Richards were well aware, it is precisely these contractions which allow reification, *if they are used without acknowledgement of what is being done.* Examples of this kind of contraction are easy to find in medicine: 'You have diabetes' (or multiple sclerosis, rheumatoid arthritis, etc.) instead of 'Your body shows a cluster of phenomena which previous research suggests is a pattern which justifies inferring a hypothetical construct which in this case we call diabetes.' 'Doctors find new treatment for multiple sclerosis' instead of 'Researchers have identified a biochemical agent which changes (or abolishes) some parts of the pattern from which they infer the construct of multiple sclerosis.' The problem is that these semantic devices are often used without acknowledgement that the contractions do not mean what they seem to mean; that is, acknowledgement that they are, to use Ogden and Richards' phrase, conveniences in description and not necessities in the structure of things. This means that when psychiatrists employ the same contractions, it is not at all obvious that the expansion statement has a quite different meaning from that which it would have in medicine. Thus, when a psychiatrist says, 'You have schizophrenia', the medical expansion is false, because no pattern which would justify inferring the concept has ever been observed. And, because the true expansion is rarely made, the concept is protected.

This habit of reification may encourage question-begging because it is, after all, easier to take for granted the existence of a thing than of an idea. Conversely, it is much more difficult for critics to convince an audience that a thing does not exist than that an idea might be wrong or a concept be invalid. It is perhaps, then, easier to understand why the search for diagnostic criteria for schizophrenia should have proceeded back to front, if the search is seen as based on both reification and question-begging. Instead of treating 'schizophrenia' as a concept whose lack of an original empirical base meant that it could not constructively be used, those seeking diagnostic criteria treated the term as if it referred, say, to a car which did not work very well, which had to have some bits removed and new bits added and which might very well improve even more in the future but which was always indisputably a car.

## The problem of pattern recognition

The question of the validity of 'schizophrenia' centres on the demonstration that it is derived from a reliably observed pattern, an above chance co-occurrence of phenomena. Many of those who use the concept clearly believe that it is derived from a pattern, but it is equally clear, from the literature reviewed in earlier chapters, that this is not and never has been the case. Why, then, does this belief persist? One reason may lie in the human tendency to 'see' patterns which are not there. It is well demonstrated, for example, that we tend to assume that unusual or distinctive phenomena are related when they are shown by the same person or group (Hamilton, 1981). The behaviours from which schizophrenia is inferred are both unusual and distinctive and this may encourage the belief not only that, for example, delusions and hallucinations are related but that both are related to other unusual and distinctive acts such as murder or arson (Leudar and Thomas, 2000). This process is not dissimilar to that suggested by Slade and Cooper (1979) – that a spurious impression of co-occurrence of 'schizophrenic symptoms' might be fostered simply by the fact that several odd behaviours, even if they co-occur by chance, are more noticeable than only one. Thus, the psychiatric population who are, after all, those who have been noticed and brought to psychiatric attention, will by definition contain more cases of co-occurrence than of single disturbing behaviours. Although this process is likely to create a strong subjective impression of a pattern of co-occurrence where none exists, it might also be responsible for the creation of apparently significant statistical patterns. Indeed, Slade and Cooper reported that the correlation amongst 'symptoms' for those diagnosed as schizophrenic was no greater than the correlation found in a group of 'artificial' cases whose symptoms had been assigned randomly by the researchers. And if those brought to psychiatric attention already contain an excess of 'co-occurrences', then this impression is likely to be further

strengthened by diagnostic practices. If psychiatrists regularly apply an official definition of 'schizophrenia', then inevitably a population will be created
who seem to show a similar cluster of behaviours.

Further examples of our general tendency to 'see' illusory patterns have
been provided by Chapman and Chapman (1967, 1982) and Shweder (1977).
Using random pairings of symptom statements and test results, Chapman
and Chapman showed that lay people 'found' relationships between the two
which apparently reflected cultural beliefs about how people with various
characteristics would respond to projective tests. Chapman and Chapman were
also able to show that the effect, which they called the 'illusory correlation',
was remarkably resistant to their attempts to abolish it. Shweder, in an ingenious reanalysis of Newcomb's 1929 study of co-operation and competition in
a boys' camp, showed that camp staff using rating forms, reported highly significant co-occurrences between various behaviours which observation of the
boys had shown not to co-occur at all. Shweder was able to demonstrate that
the *reported* (i.e. false) co-occurrences reflected commonly held beliefs that certain behaviours 'were like each other'. Although this research has used lay
people as participants, there is no reason to suppose that the same effect does
not hold for 'specialist' beliefs. Bennett (1983), for example, presented psychiatrists and lay people with 'cases' showing psychiatric symptoms. Half the
participants were also told that the cases had a diagnosis, either schizophrenia
or manic depressive psychosis. One week later, participants were asked to
recognise, from a long list of 'symptoms', those which had been shown by
'their' cases. For those participants whose cases had been given a diagnosis, psychiatrists were significantly more likely than lay people mistakenly to choose
symptoms which their cases had not shown, but which were consistent with
the diagnosis they had been given.

It is not surprising, then, that a number of writers have commented on –
and provided strong evidence for – the considerable difficulties we seem to
have in making accurate judgements of correlations or covariation (Shweder,
1977; Nisbett and Ross, 1980; Crocker, 1981; Kahneman *et al.*, 1982).
Indeed, we might argue that the whole scientific enterprise – whose task,
after all, is to identify meaningful rather than illusory covariation – seeks to
reduce these biases as much as possible. This is reflected partly in the demand
that concepts inferred from putative patterns should have predictive power
and, similarly, in medicine's demand that the criteria for inferring diagnostic
concepts should include reliably observable 'signs'. It is therefore rather disturbing to find an apparently total lack of awareness of these effects in the
'schizophrenia' literature; on the contrary, there is open acceptance of processes
which give considerable scope for the operation of biases – Kraepelin's and
Bleuler's method of introducing concepts on the basis of personal beliefs completely unsupported by data; the defence of 'schizophrenia' merely by offering
shared beliefs; the practice of allowing committee judgement to determine
diagnostic criteria; the failure to appreciate the profound effects on research

results of using strongly pre-selected 'psychiatric' samples, and so on. It is difficult to avoid the conclusion that when the subject matter is ourselves, we are inclined to overestimate the veracity of our beliefs.

## The desirability of 'schizophrenia'

I have focused so far on the construction of 'schizophrenia' as a reasonable version of reality, and therefore one which seemingly ought to be maintained. But particular ways of speaking and writing are used purposefully, to achieve particular ends, to bring about certain effects; as Gergen (1999) has put it, 'structures of language are used to build *favored* realities' (64; my emphasis). Given this, we need to ask not only why the version of reality represented by 'schizophrenia' seems so reasonable, but also why and to whom it should be so desirable? In posing this question, I am not assuming a direct relationship between the outcomes people desire, the ways they write and talk and the effects of that talk. On the contrary, as Foucault emphasised, people do not deliberately think up discourse and disseminate it in order to achieve desired outcomes. Rather, changing economic, social, scientific and political conditions may facilitate the development of certain ways of talking which in turn make particular social, economic or scientific developments more likely. I discussed some aspects of this process in relation to 'madness' in Chapter 2. Eventually, one discourse may become so dominant that many people may not know of any other way to talk about a particular topic. As Potter and Wetherell (1987) have pointed out, when people talk in particular ways they may simply be doing what seems natural or appropriate in that context. It is important to emphasise, however, that once certain ways of talking or writing become culturally available, they may be appropriated by dominant groups to further their interests. In the case of 'schizophrenia', then, the relationship between reasonableness and desirability is not likely to be straightforward. It may be that 'schizophrenia' is desirable because it seems so reasonable, and what are taken to be reasonable versions of reality are prized in Western society. Or, it may be that so much work and effort must be expended in making 'schizophrenia' seem reasonable precisely because it is so desirable, but that the issue of its desirability or its social benefits is too threatening or contentious to be openly and directly discussed. In practice, both of these processes are likely to be operating simultaneously and their joint action serves as a reminder that no person or group has *planned* the maintenance of 'schizophrenia'. Rather, it is a dynamic process in which all of us participate and which involves understandable fears and anxieties as well as the construction of a version of reality which draws on widely available and prestigious ways of speaking and thinking. But although I am not assuming a planned or conscious process of maintaining 'schizophrenia', I am assuming that talking about 'schizophrenia' in certain ways, or, more accurately, talking about behaviour *as* schizophrenia, does have important social and psychological effects, and that we are entitled to ask what and whose interests these appear to serve.

One final point needs emphasis. The idea of schizophrenia is so closely intertwined with the idea of behaviour as illness or mental disorder that it is virtually impossible to discuss the desirability of schizophrenia without discussing the desirability of the idea of mental illness or disorder. This point is particularly important in view of the status of 'schizophrenia' as *the* taken-for-granted mental disorder: to maintain the idea of schizophrenia is simultaneously to maintain 'mental illness/disorder', while to maintain the idea of mental disorder is almost automatically to maintain 'schizophrenia'.

## The desirability of 'schizophrenia' – for psychiatry

One of the most important aspects of the desirability of 'schizophrenia' for psychiatry relates to psychiatry's ambiguous professional position. Just as it is difficult to imagine a branch of the legal profession whose activities have nothing whatsoever in common with solicitors or barristers or judges, it is difficult to imagine a branch of the medical profession whose activities bear no relationship to the practice of medicine. That this is indeed the case is emphasised by the remarks of a US Professor of Psychiatry:

> Now, it is in the tradition of such experts [medical specialists] that they are masters of knowledge about an organ system. What is the organ system of psychiatrists? If the domain of the cardiologist is the heart and circulatory system, then surely the domain of the psychiatrist is the brain and its system therein. To qualify and *survive* as physician specialists, we must become better brain specialists.
>
> (Hanley, 1985; cited in Szasz, 1987: 69; my emphasis)

Psychiatrists, however, are in the potentially embarrassing position of being brain specialists who for the most part rely on judgements about behaviour, not brain functioning, to make their diagnoses, and who have failed to demonstrate reliable links between these behaviours and brain functioning. We might argue that the *language*, or the *idea*, of behaviour as illness and of 'schizophrenia' as a particular and serious form of illness is important in maintaining the impression of similarity between psychiatry and the various medical specialities, in the absence of important actual similarities in their activities. The crucial differences between medicine and psychiatry can perhaps best be summarised by saying that whereas medical scientists study bodily functioning and describe patterns in it, psychiatrists behave *as if* they were studying bodily functioning and *as if* they had described patterns there, when in fact they are studying behaviour and have assumed – but not demonstrated – that certain types of pattern *will be* found there. We could argue that it is this 'as if' or metaphorical quality of psychiatry which makes the concept of mental illness or disorder, and attempts at definition, so important to it as a discipline. It is not accidental that so much more effort should have been expended on these attempts in psychiatry than in medicine *and* that the discipline which has expended less effort should be the more successful. It is precisely the lack of direct evidence that the concepts and theories of medicine can usefully be applied to behaviour which makes the idea of mental disorder – which implies that they can – so important. Equally, it is because medicine does not need continually to defend its concepts and theories in relation to the study of bodies that the idea of disease, illness or disorder is far less important to its status as a profession or scientific discipline. The idea of mental illness or disorder, then, serves as a crucial substitute for research evidence. And if the concept of mental disease or disorder is indispensable to psychiatry, then it is equally important to identify specific mental diseases, otherwise we might begin to suspect that they did not exist. The very bizarreness of behaviours and reported experience used to infer 'schizophrenia', and the difficulties we have in empathising with them, certainly provide more scope than in other diagnostic categories for making apparently credible links between psychiatry, medicine and the biological sciences; Lander's rather premature remark following the now discredited early genetic linkage studies, that 'psychiatrists have now joined the ranks of experimental geneticists' (1988: 106), illustrates just how keenly, if inappropriately, such links will be made.

There is a second, and related, benefit to psychiatry in maintaining the idea of schizophrenia as illness, and that is in deflecting criticism that psychiatrists act as agents of social control. Indeed, it is notable that this has repeatedly been given as a reason for finding a definition of 'mental disorder' which would 'correctly' identify sufferers and justify the claim that psychiatry simply diagnoses and treats specific forms of illness. Wakefield (1995), for example, has claimed that '[w]ithout an adequate analysis of "mental disorder" . . . one cannot correctly judge when human interests are covertly influencing diagnostic judgements versus when there is only overt adherence to the correct standard of judgement' (245). I have argued (Boyle, 1996a) that this fear of being seen as agents of social control is one reason why so little attention has been paid to the specific *content* of psychotic experiences, in case this should be interpreted as selectively suppressing particular beliefs or utterances, rather than simply treating general 'symptoms' such as delusions and hallucinations.

But although the idea of schizophrenia as illness is very important for the status of psychiatry, it is equally important that the concept of schizophrenia should remain vague and non-specific – a complex disorder whose diagnostic 'signs and symptoms' may change; whose biological causes and cures will be discovered at some unspecified point in the future. This uncertainty has the triple advantage of retaining within psychiatry a 'disorder' which would have to be given over to neurology were it a *literal* brain disease; of creating an impression of important and progressive research whose future prospects are always bright and of ensuring that it is never quite clear what does and does not serve as evidence for or against the concept.

The problem remains of why professional groups which have no obvious vested interest in maintaining concepts of illness and schizophrenia, should still do so. One answer may lie in the fact that, as Kirk and Kutchins (1992) have pointed out, all 'mental health' professions aspire to use science to help people, and the process of diagnosing 'mental disorder' does '[provide] a powerful framework for mental health professionals to demonstrate the connection between science and practice' (23). In defending the idea of mental disorder, Wakefield (1992a: 232) has also argued that it is 'the glue that holds together the mental health field' and that there is a 'critical need for the mental health professions to continue to be seen as genuinely medical disciplines' (1997a: 643). The idea of mental illness/disorder, and of specific disorders such as 'schizophrenia', may therefore provide a sense of identity for people who might otherwise wonder about the nature of their job. As well as this, all 'mental health' professionals are protected from accusations of being agents of social control by the use of diagnostic concepts with a claimed scientific base. It may also be that the use of the concept of schizophrenia in the face of incomprehensible behaviour gives the impression of knowledge so important in maintaining the credibility of any group who claims expertise. This is not to suggest that professionals who use 'schizophrenia' are deliberately pretending knowledge; an understandable reliance on secondary sources, together with the processes which construct 'schizophrenia' as reasonable, may have convinced them of the concept's validity.

## The desirability of 'schizophrenia' – for the public

Although the psychiatric and related professions clearly have much to gain by retaining the concept of schizophrenia, the idea of schizophrenia as a brain disease is arguably equally desirable to the general public. Indeed, this joint desirability may be necessary for the maintenance of schizophrenia: if the idea only benefited the public, then professionals could override it with their 'expert' knowledge. On the other hand, if 'schizophrenia' were only of benefit to professionals, the public might be more critical and questioning.

One possible function which 'schizophrenia' might serve for the public was unwittingly suggested by Jablensky, interviewed about research which supposedly showed 'schizophrenia' to have a biological basis: 'Those who take comfort from the evidence that schizophrenia has a biological basis should be further reassured' (*The Times*, 3 March 1986). It is not immediately obvious why we should be comforted by the fact that at least one in every hundred people in the population is suffering from an incurable brain disease. There has certainly never been the slightest suggestion in any neurology text that people should be comforted by the idea that their relatives have a brain disease; on the contrary, this news is usually seen as meriting sympathy and pity. In the case of 'schizophrenia', however, the answer is apparently that the idea of brain disease somehow absolves the 'victim', their relatives or society in general, from responsibility for having caused the person's disturbing behaviour:

> Even though [the genetic evidence] exonerates parents from having caused their child's schizophrenia by their methods of rearing . . .
>
> (Gottesman and Shields, 1982: 200)

> The study should relieve any feelings of guilt. Families cannot be blamed . . .
>
> (Jablensky, *The Times*, 3 March 1986)

> We, as a parent support group (People Acting Together in Hope) are extremely grateful for your series on schizophrenia . . . Recognition has long been overdue that this terrible brain disease is the fault of neither the victim nor their families, but is of neurobiological or genetic origin . . . We need the understanding and help of all society to see this disease as it truly is – a disabling brain disease.
>
> (Rose, 1986; cited in Szasz, 1987: 76)

> The recognition that schizophrenia is an organic brain disease means that families can be relieved of the burden of guilt that the illness is a consequence of bad parenting.
>
> (Iverson, *The Guardian*, 4 September 1997)

It appears, then, that if the concept of schizophrenia as brain disease were to be abandoned, the blame for disturbing behaviour might be placed squarely on either the person or their family. Given the potency of the ideas of guilt and blame in our society, it is hardly surprising that we should wish to evade them. But the idea of people being comforted or exonerated by particular ideas recalls not scientific but lay theories (that there is life after death; that education will harm women's brains; that black people are inferior to white people) – ideas which are expressly designed to comfort particular groups and may be used to justify actions which could otherwise be called into question.

To claim that we should not be concerned with how comforting our theories of disturbing behaviour might be, and, indeed, that we should be suspicious of theories with no direct support but which are said to comfort or exonerate, is not to downgrade the plight of those diagnosed schizophrenic or their relatives. It is, however, to emphasise that when people are faced with incomprehensible, disturbing and aversive phenomena for which they might be blamed, then they are likely to grasp at explanations which not only appear to exonerate them but which also remove the disturbance. In the case of behaviours which lead to a diagnosis of schizophrenia, the disease or illness idea is used to justify removing the person to 'a place of safety' and 'treating' them without their consent. The concept and the assumptions which surround it thus have the threefold advantage of exonerating disturbing people and their relatives, of removing and apparently helping 'the sufferer', and of apparently achieving this not only with humanity but also with the support of science.

The ways in which this issue of blame and exoneration may be of joint concern to, and be jointly managed by, professionals and the public is strikingly illustrated by research on family interaction and 'schizophrenia'. In the 1970s and 1980s, a number of researchers studied the relationship between patterns of family interaction and what was called relapse in 'schizophrenia' (e.g. Vaughn and Leff, 1976; Leff and Vaughn, 1981; Leff *et al.*, 1982; Falloon *et al.*, 1984). It was reported that certain types of behaviour from relatives (e.g. criticism, hostile statements, disregard for privacy, interrupting, and so on – called 'high expressed emotion') appeared to be associated with high rates of 'relapse' and readmission in the 'schizophrenic' family member. Perhaps inevitably, families felt they were being blamed for the negative behaviour of the 'schizophrenic' to the point where the research was said to be a 'public relations disaster' (Strachan, 1986; Hatfield, 1987). Obviously, serious and complex issues are raised here. For example: What is the relationship between the content of theories of madness and public sensibilities? How are researchers to proceed when their attempts to describe have become so intertwined with perceived accusations of blame? But rather than addressing these issues, research on family interaction quickly moved to protect relatives from accusations of blame by claiming or implying that relatives' behaviour could only influence 'relapse' and not the development of 'schizophrenia'; that is, relatives could only influence 'schizophrenic' behaviour *after* the diagnosis had been given and not before. (There is, incidentally, no clear evidence for this position and some evidence that certain 'affective styles', very similar to negative 'expressed emotion', precede the development of 'schizophrenia'; see, e.g., Doane *et al.*, 1981; Goldstein, 1987). In line with the idea of relatives only influencing 'relapse', it has also been claimed that the aim of 'family management' is to help relatives 'cope better' with the 'sick' person suffering from a 'defined disease' (Kuipers *et al.*, 1992). More recently, and more subtly, the difficulties raised for theory construction by our propensity to blame and exonerate have been entirely avoided by presenting expressed emotion research as part of more general research on 'health care' (by both relatives and professionals) or 'care burden' (e.g. Kuipers, 1998; Wearden *et al.*, 2000). Relatives are positioned as 'carers' of an 'ill' person, while the integrated discussion in research papers of relatives and professionals as 'carers' can obscure important differences in the relationship of these two groups to the person diagnosed as 'schizophrenic'. I am not suggesting that these research developments have been planned or that we should not sympathise with or try to relieve the impact on relatives of living with someone whose behaviour is bizarre and possibly frightening. But the joint benefits of the approach adopted by 'family research' are obvious: professionals avoid what may be very public criticism from relatives and maintain the idea of behaviour as illness; in turn, relatives avoid implications of blame and receive the socially valued role of 'carer'.

The idea of schizophrenia as brain disorder might offer further comfort by distancing 'normal' from disturbing people. It may do this by placing disturbing people in a separate category and by suggesting uncommon processes to account for their behaviour, processes which by definition do not operate for ordinary people. Lerner (1980) has emphasised our apparent need to believe in a stable and orderly world and our tendency to use 'internal' and pejorative labels to characterise those who in some way challenge this belief. This not only achieves distance between 'them' and 'us' but also fosters the belief that 'we' can avoid a similar fate.

Another way of looking at this process of separation between the mad and the sane is through Foucault's (1971) analysis of the modern links between madness and irrationality. Foucault highlighted the historical connection between the growing importance of the idea of rationality in Western culture from the Enlightenment, and the parallel construction of madness as irrationality. These two developments are closely related, if not inseparable. Human attributes are often valued to the extent that they are unequally distributed. Rationality, then, is hierarchical and linked to social status, with white men (who invented the idea) given more than women, adults more than children, white people more than black people and the mad least of all. It can be argued that this process has allowed the mad (and, to a lesser extent, women, children and black people), to become the repositories of society's irrationality and has thus fostered the comforting belief in the intrinsic rationality of the rest of us. This point was tellingly illustrated by a judge's comments during the trial of a man who had been diagnosed as schizophrenic and who had attacked a group of children with a machete:

> In some ways it is a relief to know that it was a profoundly sick and deluded individual who committed these offences. To believe such an attack could be carried out by a sane person would shake belief in humanity.
>
> (*The Guardian*, 8 March 1997)

But the idea of madness as irrationality is jointly beneficial to psychiatry and the public. In the absence of direct evidence for the major claim made about 'schizophrenia' – that it is a brain disease – then the idea of madness as irrationality, as not understandable in relation to the person's context or culture, becomes crucial in implying that the behaviour must therefore be caused by brain pathology even if this pathology has not yet been found.

The desirability of 'schizophrenia' (and other diagnostic categories) for the public is further fostered by the persistent creation of a dichotomy which implies that the only alternative to an illness model of 'abnormal' behaviour is a return to primitive and pre-scientific thinking which may also involve guilt and blame:

[Schizophrenia] is not mystical; it has physical causes . . .

(*New Scientist* Editorial, 1970)

[Schizophrenia] is not caused by devils or difficult mothers or tyrannical fathers or latent homosexuality or stress . . . Schizophrenia is a physical *disease* . . .

(Hoffer and Osmond, 1965; cited in Szasz, 1976: 113; emphasis in original)

Fifty per cent of prisoners have committed offences not because they are evil but because they are sick.

(BBC2, *Out of Court*, February 1987)

Schizophrenia is not a punishment from God. It is not a product of faulty upbringing. It is a disease of the brain and mind.

(Blakemore, BBC2, *The Mind Machine*, 18 October 1988)

Violence is biochemically caused. To say otherwise is to turn people into baddies.

(BBC Radio 4, *Does He Take Sugar*, 4 April 1994)

Is there any lingering worry that [post-traumatic stress disorder] is moral weakness or just malingering?

(BBC Radio 4, *Face the Facts*, 29 September 1998)

These dichotomies are reminiscent of the nineteenth-century debates I discussed in Chapter 2, where medical explanations of lunacy were presented as the only alternative to spiritual or religious accounts. But the credibility or reasonableness of the dichotomies is fostered by the behavioural and social sciences' lack of success in providing the public with alternative accounts, so that the idea that unwanted, distressing and disturbing behaviour can be explained only by scientific biology *or* by moral failure remains extremely powerful.

It is, finally, worth noting again the importance of the apparent ability of 'schizophrenia' to provide an explanation of unwanted, distressing and disturbing behaviour. Of course, it does nothing of the sort, but by providing a name, a label, professionals convey the powerful and comforting message that they are familiar with these behaviours and experiences, that they have seen them before and (it is implied) have some understanding of them. 'Schizophrenia' is therefore a highly seductive label, for professionals, for relatives, for the public and for those whose behaviour has given cause for concern.

## Reasonableness, desirability and alternatives to 'schizophrenia'

Lakatos (1978) has argued that it is the presence of a plausible alternative, rather than the weight of negative evidence, which mainly determines whether a concept or theory will persist. But he was talking about theories in the natural sciences whose proponents, as Kuhn (1970: 164) has noted, have experienced an 'unparalleled separation from the demands of the laity and everyday life' (and see Boyle, 1994). 'Schizophrenia' and its surrounding theories could hardly be in a more contrasting position. Theories of madness are of profound concern both to the public and to professionals who provide services to that public. Not surprisingly, then, in spite of the weight of negative evidence, schizophrenia appears to be maintained through a powerful web of apparently reasonable argument and through its ability to provide important professional, social and psychological benefits. But I shall argue in the final chapter that plausible alternatives to the concept of schizophrenia (to describing and interpreting 'schizophrenic' behaviours and experiences) do exist. As we might expect, however, the formidable structures and processes which support 'schizophrenia' mean that the development and dissemination of alternatives is a far from straightforward process.

# Chapter 8

# Living without 'schizophrenia'
## Issues and some alternatives

A few years ago, I attended a conference on 'Alternatives to Schizophrenia' where speaker after speaker discussed alternative diagnostic criteria for schizophrenia or whether 'schizophrenia' and 'schizoaffective disorder' really were separate 'illnesses'. It was rather like a conference on 'Alternatives to Religion' where speakers suggested different deities we might worship if we abandoned the idea of God. But perhaps I should not have been surprised. I knew, after all, about the social and professional forces which hold 'schizophrenia' in place, and which make it difficult even to imagine a world which contains neither schizophrenia nor the assumption that certain behaviours and experiences should be understood as symptoms of disease or pathology. The same problem is evident in remarks I have heard which acknowledge that 'schizophrenia' is problematic but claim that 'there is nothing else'. If we expect to identify symptoms, to diagnose and treat disorder in terms of what is wrong with an individual, then, no, there is little else except debates about classificatory boundaries and diagnostic criteria. But if we acknowledge that the 'symptoms of schizophrenia' are actually behaviours carried out by people in a social context, statements they make about their experiences, about themselves and about the world, then there is no reason to assume that alternatives to 'schizophrenia' will look anything like the present medical system of understanding, a system which was, after all, developed for phenomena quite different from those used to infer 'schizophrenia'. The subject matter of this chapter, then, will be the behaviours and experiences from which schizophrenia is inferred. The focus will be on voice-hearing (verbal hallucinations) and 'delusions' (reports of highly implausible beliefs not shared by others). This is partly for reasons of space but also because these phenomena have been and remain central to the diagnosis of madness or schizophrenia. They are the first mentioned 'symptoms' in DSM-IV's diagnostic criteria for schizophrenia, and, under some circumstances, either of them may be the only 'characteristic symptom' needed to make the diagnosis (APA, 1994). My aim is not to provide an alternative to 'schizophrenia' which can be easily substituted for it – that would be to ignore the problems of the theoretical model which supports the concept – but to discuss alternative ways of understanding and ameliorating some of the behaviours and experiences from which 'schizophrenia' is inferred. The emphasis here is on 'discuss': this area has suffered badly from premature theorising and prescription, when what is needed is more open debate. What is offered, then, is a critical analysis of possibilities which will draw on a range of theoretical ideas but with the assumption that hallucinations and 'delusions' can be understood within the same theoretical frameworks as any other behaviour or experience. This is not to suggest that our present frameworks for understanding behaviour are adequate, simply that there is no reason to assume in advance that the 'symptoms of schizophrenia' require different frameworks from other behaviours and experiences. In other words, developing alternatives to 'schizophrenia', like all research and theorising, involves looking for relationships and regularities amongst the phenomena of interest; but the starting point is not an assumed disorder called 'schizophrenia' (i.e. an assumed relationship amongst 'symptoms') and the types of regularities which might be identified are not assumed to be like those found in the study of unwanted bodily phenomena.

With this in mind, several points should be emphasised:

1   The study of 'delusions' and hallucinations as phenomena in their own right emphatically does not entail adopting a 'single symptom' model (cf. Costello, 1992; Marshall and Halligan, 1996; Garety and Freeman, 1999). This is for two reasons. First, 'symptom' is a medical term which reflects potentially problematic assumptions and raises questions about any behaviour it is applied to, not least the popular question: symptom of what? Seeing 'symptoms' as synonymous with 'complaints' is no solution, because it still leaves the problem of how we can know which of the many behavioural or psychological complaints we make, or have made about us, should be called 'symptoms'. The use of 'symptom' also makes it much more difficult to abandon the additional assumptions of a medical framework, particularly that symptoms cluster together, that they have an underlying pathological cause which lies within the person, and that they should be removed. Second, within medicine, a 'single symptom' approach would be seen as a seriously backward step: we should hardly consider it a sign of progress if medical researchers announced that they were abandoning the study of, say, tuberculosis, to concentrate instead on the separate study of coughing or weight loss. But if we step outside a medical framework (which some of those advocating a single symptom approach do not) then the study of 'delusions' and hallucinations as phenomena in their own right is potentially progressive, not least because it allows questions which may make little sense within a medical framework, questions about context, about content and function, and about social and personal meanings (Boyle, 1996a; Leudar and Thomas, 2000).

2    If studying hallucinations and 'delusions' as phenomena in their own right definitely does not entail a single symptom model, then it does not necessarily entail a 'continuum model'. Claridge (1994) has discussed two approaches to continuity: the 'quasi-dimensional', which sees continuity in terms of degrees of expression of signs and symptoms of an abnormal state, and the 'fully dimensional' in which 'psychotic symptoms' are the manifestations of a widely distributed and assumed personality trait (schizotypy) whose expression may represent healthy diversity in personality as well as 'illness'. Both of these models have the advantage of drawing attention to the lack of qualitative difference between psychiatric and non-psychiatric groups. Both models, however, appear to accept at least some behaviours as illness; they are also highly individualistic and could convey the impression (more so for the quasi-dimensional model) that the difference between those who do and do not receive a psychiatric diagnosis is the possession of more of a trait or the expression of more 'signs and symptoms'. Thus, the contribution of interpersonal or social factors to the designation of 'patient' may be obscured.

3    To seek alternatives to 'schizophrenia' outside of a medical framework is not to deny the distress and difficulties which may be experienced by those diagnosed as schizophrenic or by their families. This should hardly need to be said, but those who have been critical of 'schizophrenia' have so often been accused of indifference to the plight of 'the mentally ill' that the point needs to be made with some force. The issue is not one of acknowledging distress but of how we conceptualise and respond to it. The problem is compounded by statements such as Jones's (1999) that 'to say to those who may be subject [to misdiagnosis of schizophrenia] that there is nothing wrong does not help them' (281). This dichotomy ('you have schizophrenia' versus 'there is nothing wrong') remains firmly within a medical framework and appears to deny the possibility of constructive help without diagnosis.

4    This discussion of alternatives will focus on social and psychological aspects of hallucinations and 'delusions', not least to redress the balance in an area which has given such primacy to supposed biological causes of 'schizophrenia'. This is not to deny the potential contribution of biological factors to hallucinations or 'delusions', but their contribution is likely to be far more complex than is implied by research seeking the 'biological basis' of 'schizophrenia' or, indeed, of hallucinations or 'delusions'. In thinking about this issue, four points are worth bearing in mind. First, biology is involved in *everything* we do and experience, from supporting a political party to feeling bored; obviously, then, it must be involved in hearing voices and expressing beliefs; the issue is how we conceptualise that involvement and how useful it might be in accounts of particular behaviours or experiences. Second, the idea that the relationship between biology and behaviour is one-way (the biological *basis* of behaviour) is

highly misleading: behaviour and experience may influence biology as much as the other way round (see Harrop *et al.*, 1996, for a discussion of this issue in relation to psychosis); third, there is a dismaying tendency to treat any association between biological events or processes and diagnoses of schizophrenia as if it directly indicated something about a biological or neurodevelopmental substrate of schizophrenia when in fact the relationship between biological events and psychotic experiences is likely to be highly variable and indirect. For example, birth complications, which show a weak relationship with a range of psychiatric diagnoses, may lead to brain dysfunction, which may lead to difficulties with school work or lack of skill at sports, which may lead to bullying and social isolation, which may lead to poor employment prospects, stressful life events and more social isolation, which may facilitate psychotic experiences, and so on; when we consider that birth complications are themselves linked to familial and social disadvantage, then the potential complexities and indirectness of the relationships between biology and psychosis become apparent. Finally, if we remove the problematic concept of schizophrenia, then we are left with the complex question of what exactly is to be explained biologically: is it holding highly implausible beliefs which have no evidence in support? Or disagreeing with cultural norms? Or not being able to persuade others about one's beliefs? Or being indifferent to others' opinions about one's beliefs? Or hearing voices which comfort and direct in times of crises? Or hearing voices which insult and abuse? Or hearing voices which bring social status and public acclaim? Or not being able to cope with voices? Or not carrying out valued social roles? Put like this, then it is clear that simply replacing a search for the biological basis of schizophrenia with a search for the biological basis of 'delusions' and hallucinations is as unlikely to be successful.

5   The term 'psychosis' is increasingly used, particularly in Britain, in preference to the more problematic-seeming 'schizophrenia'. I will use the term rather reluctantly here because of the danger, already evident in the literature, that it will simply become a substitute for 'schizophrenia' with the latter's assumptions intact. We could thus find ourselves searching for the biological or neurodevelopmental basis of psychosis or trying to 'treat' the 'symptoms' of psychosis. In other words, 'psychosis' may simply become a way of assimilating criticisms of 'schizophrenia' without making any fundamental changes to the systems of thought which support the concept.

6   Abandoning the concept of schizophrenia raises the issue of how the wide range of phenomena subsumed by the term ought to be responded to by professionals and society. The complexity of this issue will be evident in the discussion which follows; but although I will discuss some psychological interventions, discussion of the wider issues of social and professional responses and service structure, and the relationship of these

to research, is beyond the scope of a chapter which is mainly concerned with alternatives to the concept of schizophrenia. It should be emphasised, however, that the issues involved are moral and political as well as scientific and professional (see Boyle, 1997; Newnes *et al.*, 1999 and Johnstone, 2000 for further discussion of research–policy relationships and of services which do not depend on a medical framework).

7   As earlier chapters have shown, theories of madness are deeply embedded in particular social and professional contexts and are informed by often unarticulated assumptions about people and their behaviour. It would therefore be naive to expect the development of alternatives to 'schizophrenia' to be exempt from this process, to develop by the neutral accretion of disinterested knowledge. I shall therefore comment quite extensively on these issues in discussing alternatives to 'schizophrenia'.

Finally, a word about language. The negative and assumption-laden language which surrounds 'schizophrenia' is so woven into our thought that it is extremely difficult to find an alternative that is not either cumbersome or obscure. With this in mind, I will use some of this language as neutrally as possible. *Bizarre* will be used to mean behaviour or experiences which disturb observers and are incomprehensible to them; *hallucinations* to mean experiences which would seem to require the presence of an external stimulus or non-self source, but where none is obviously present, and *psychosis* to mean behaviour and experiences which seem to lie beyond what is regarded as consensual reality. Other terms, such as 'symptoms' and 'delusions' will remain within quotation marks to reflect their exceptionally problematic status in this context.

## Verbal hallucinations or hearing voices

Hallucinations have been defined in a number of ways. Behrendt (1998), for example, calls them 'perceptions that are underconstrained by sensory stimulation' (247); Honig *et al.* (1998) have suggested that they are 'perceptions experienced in the absence of a corresponding sensory stimulus with an immediate vivid character, independent of will and felt to be real' (646). This definition is similar to that offered by Slade and Bentall (1988: 23): that hallucinations are any precept-like experience that occurs in the absence of an appropriate stimulus, have the full impact of the corresponding actual stimulus and are not amenable to direct voluntary control by the experiencer. Sarbin (1967) has suggested that different usages of the term 'hallucination' have in common the idea of reported imaginings or, more specifically, reporting imaginings as real.[1] Verbal hallucinations or hearing voices will be considered here

1   These definitions share the assumption that hallucinations are not the result of 'real' spirit or divine voices, although this interpretation may be made by some voice-hearers. The discussion here will also be based on that assumption.

in relation to two major questions. First, what factors are associated with or facilitate reports of voice-hearing and, second, what factors are associated with or facilitate the labelling of some of these reports as pathological.

## Reports of hearing voices

We cannot think about reports of hearing voices (or seeing visions) independently of their social context or of social reactions to them. There is general agreement (see, e.g., Wallace, 1959; Holt, 1964; Al-Issa, 1977) that while reactions differ across social groups, modern Western societies are particularly hostile to such reports:

> In a factually oriented, skepical [sic], anti-intraceptive, brass-tacks culture like ours, where the para-normal is scoffed at and myth and religion are in decline, the capacity for vivid imagery has little survival value and even less social acceptability. We live in an age of literalism, an era that distrusts the imagination, while at the same time it develops its beat fringe of avid seekers after drugs that may artificially restore the capacity for poetic vision. It is little wonder that adults are made uneasy by the admission that they can experience things that are not factually present.
>
> (Holt, 1964: 262)

> Rational cultures that make a rigid distinction between reality and fantasy tend to consider hallucinations negatively, as they are expected to interfere with daily activities and interaction with the physical environment. Individuals are thus actively discouraged from assigning credibility to certain imaginings. They even learn to ignore these experiences and to remain unaware of their existence. These cultures would generally be conducive to a high threshold in the observation of hallucinations and to a negative attitude towards these experiences.
>
> (Al-Issa, 1977: 576)

Both Al-Issa and Wallace have emphasised that reports of hallucinations are often accompanied by anxiety in Western groups. By contrast, in some non-Western groups the experience may not only be accepted but actively sought (under certain socially approved conditions), using, for example, sleep deprivation, fasting, intense pain or social isolation. Al-Issa has linked the strict social control over the initiation, content and duration of such hallucinatory experiences with the fact that they are generally short-lived and distress-free.

Jaynes (1976) has developed a rather more elaborate theory of the suppression of hallucinatory experiences which, he suggests, paralleled the development of what we think of as consciousness and the ability to reflect on our own behaviour and mental processes. Jaynes's thesis (which even he admits sounds preposterous) is that this habit of self-reflection, the awareness of an 'I', is relatively recent – Jaynes dates it at after 2,000–1,000 BCE. Before this, Jaynes suggests, the place of 'consciousness' was taken by auditory hallucinations which were reported as the voices of gods. These were heard when plans had to be made, or decisions taken, whenever behaviour might depart from clear, habitual (and unconscious) paths. Jaynes suggests that the hallucinated voices reflected right hemispheric activity channelled via cerebral commissures to the left or speech hemisphere and interpreted as linguistic utterances. One of Jaynes's major sources of support is the *Iliad*, the early part of which (in so far as it can be accurately dated) apparently contains no reference to consciousness, to mental acts, to free-will or to self-reflection (cf. Leudar and Thomas, 2000). Instead, Jaynes has argued, action was to a large extent initiated by the hallucinated voices (of gods), which directed, commented and advised. Jaynes implicates increases in population and social complexity, and the development of writing, in the 'breakdown' of what he calls the bicameral mind. Direct communication with the gods, via their hallucinated voices, was, he claims, replaced by indirect communications, via prophets, oracles and divination. It is interesting to note Jones's (1974) suggestion (cited in Witelson, 1986) that the Greek word *phronĕsis*, representing inwardly conscious awareness or introspection, was introduced by the philosopher Heraclitus during the sixth century BCE. He was, Jones suggests, seeking a new word which would denote a mental process that he, but not many of his contemporaries, believed was going on in the mind.

It must be said that it is exceptionally difficult to offer direct support for Jaynes's theory, based as it is on a particular interpretation of generally accepted events. Certainly critics (see, e.g. Miller, 1986) are able to offer only alternative interpretations with no obvious criteria for choosing amongst them. It is not disputed that reports of hearing the voices of gods were a 'normal' part of Ancient Greek culture. Similarly, the importance of hearing voices and seeing 'visions' as part of religious or spiritual experience has long been noted (van Marrelo and van der Stap, 1993; Jackson and Fulford, 1997a). Indeed, so common are hallucinatory experiences that Wallace (1959) has called them 'one of the most ancient and most widely distributed modes of human experience' (58). It is perhaps ironic that an experience which formed the basis of the modern world's major organised religions should so often now be seen as a symptom of major mental illness, as an indication of pathology within the person. This negative interpretation presents particular problems for the study of reported imaginings in Western groups, but at the very least the importance of hallucinatory experiences in the development of Western culture should alert us to the need to adopt a much broader approach to their study than would be suggested by a framework which emphasises pathology.

The need for a broader approach is also emphasised by studies of non-psychiatric groups which suggest that hallucinatory experiences are relatively common, and that between 10 and 40 per cent of people have experienced auditory or visual hallucinations (McKellar, 1968; Posey and Losch, 1983;

Bentall and Slade, 1985; Tien, 1991; Barrett and Etherbridge, 1992). Most of these experiences are not distressing and are not reported to medical professionals (Tien, 1991).

Detailed study of the characteristics of auditory hallucinations, in both psychiatric and non-psychiatric groups, shows that voices may be experienced as internal or external to the person; that they are frequently, though not always, identified as specific people known to the hearer; that the hearer is almost always the 'target' of voices' comments and that the voices' common feature is one of regulating activity through commands, questions, comments, propositions, criticism and evaluations (Romme and Escher, 1993; Nayani and David, 1996; Leudar et al., 1997; Honig et al., 1998). What is particularly interesting about this descriptive research are the *similarities* it suggests between the hallucinatory experiences of psychiatric and non-psychiatric groups. The groups' experiences do differ in potentially important ways which will be considered in a later section; the differences, however, are not those which would be expected from diagnostic criteria, including Schneider's postulated list of first-rank symptoms of schizophrenia.

## Psychological theories of verbal hallucinations

It is important to emphasise that there is no one theory of hallucinatory experiences which clearly accounts for our observations about them or which can provide strong evidence in support of all its theoretical tenets. Nevertheless, there is some provisional agreement, or, at least, shared assumptions, about two aspects of hallucinatory experiences. First, at least some auditory hallucinations appear to be associated with inner, sub-vocal speech (Gould, 1949, 1950; Inouye and Shimizu, 1970) which may correspond to the content of 'voices'; second, hallucinatory experiences involve the attribution of internal or mental events to an external source or, at least, a non-self source. In other words, hallucinations are seen as self-generated mental events which are experienced as alien to the self and may be interpreted as of external origin (Hoffman, 1986; Bentall, 1990a). We might add to this McGuire et al.'s (1993) 'cautious interpretation' that the generation of auditory hallucinations is associated with increased activity in a network of cortical language areas and in particular in an area implicated in the production of inner speech. It could be argued, of course, that the idea of auditory hallucinations involving the attribution of self-generated internal events to an external or non-self source is almost true by definition (Bentall, 1990a), at least if we put aside the idea of non-visible spirits; certainly, Sarbin and Juhasz's (1967) definition 'reporting imaginings as real' seems to include this idea. The framework, however, has important advantages over one which simply sees hallucinations as a symptom of mental illness in that it raises questions which would otherwise be obscured or not thought important within an illness model. These include questions of how distinctions between the 'real' and the 'imaginary' are made by all of us on a moment-to-moment basis (Bentall, 1990a); of how only certain imaginary material is reported as real; of how particular contexts or personal experiences might facilitate reporting imaginings as real or, indeed, reporting the 'real' as imaginary. Questions like these allow us to approach the analysis of hallucinations while bearing in mind two important factors. First, that reporting imaginings as real is a ubiquitous human feature which must be studied as such in both non-psychiatric and psychiatric groups; and, second, that what we think of as hallucinations involve something a person *does*, rather than something they *have* and are therefore subject to the same questions we might ask about any human activity.

A number of theorists have suggested that auditory hallucinations are the result of defects, deficits or disorders in brain or cognitive systems concerned with processing linguistic information. Frith (1992), for example, has argued that auditory hallucinations reflect a deficit in a neurological system responsible for the internal monitoring of willed action, so that self-generated speech is attributed to an external source. David (1994) has suggested that auditory hallucinations result from defects in language input and output systems, while Hoffman (1986) and Hoffman and Rapaport (1994) have posited a disorder of discourse planning in which certain linguistic information stored in long-term memory is brought into consciousness in unplanned and unexpected ways, is experienced as alien and unintended, and attributed to an external source. The evidence for these deficit accounts, however, is weak (Bentall and Slade, 1986; Bentall, 1990a; Bentall *et al.*, 1994; Boyle, 1996b; Morrison and Haddock, 1997). The theories also present additional problems which will be discussed later.

As an alternative to deficit theories of hallucinations, Bentall (1990a) has argued that hallucinations reflect a bias, an error of judgement in discriminating the origins of mental events, or a failure of the meta-cognitive skill of reality testing, rather than a global neuropsychological deficit. Several kinds of evidence have been proposed in support of this theory. First, Young *et al.* (1987) found that psychiatric patients who experienced hallucinations were more likely to report auditory hallucinations in line with researchers' suggestions than patients who did not; second, Bentall and Slade (1985) and Rankin and O'Carroll (1995) found significant differences in a measure of bias in a signal detection task (i.e. reporting the signal present when absent) between non-psychiatric groups who had scored highly on the Launay–Slade Hallucinations Scale, but no significant differences in a measure of perceptual sensitivity. Bentall and Slade reported the same pattern of results in two groups of people diagnosed as schizophrenic who did and did not experience hallucinations. Finally, Morrison and Haddock (1997) compared the performance of three groups on a source-monitoring task. One group met DSM-IV criteria for schizophrenia and experienced hallucinations; a second group also met the DSM criteria but did not experience hallucinations, while a third group were not in contact with psychiatric services and did not experience hallucinations, although it is not clear how this was checked. The source-monitoring task consisted of presenting words to participants with the request that they 'Think of the first word that comes to mind when I say . . .' Participants were then asked to rate how much the word that came to mind was their own (immediate source monitoring) and, after another series of tasks, to indicate whether words then read out by the researcher (original stimulus words plus the participant's associative responses) had been generated by themselves or the researcher (delayed source monitoring). Morrison and Haddock reported significant differences between the group experiencing auditory hallucinations and the two other groups on immediate source monitoring but no significant difference on delayed source monitoring. Across the three groups, however, more errors were made on the delayed source-monitoring task for words with an emotional content (e.g. 'frightened' versus 'bookcase'). Morrison and Haddock suggested that their data were consistent with an immediate, moment to moment, bias in perception among the group who experienced auditory hallucinations rather than a global deficit in production processes.

Although deficit and bias theories seem to suggest different mechanisms or processes in relation to auditory hallucinations, the theories share important similarities which are very problematic. For example, both types of theory are characterised by the search for a general underlying feature, trait or attribute (e.g. defective internal monitoring; abnormal perceptual bias; deficient or biased reality testing) which is 'possessed' by those who experience hallucinations. This 'feature' may also be presented as if it were always present, as when Morrison and Haddock (1997) talk of 'a hallucinator's tendency to misattribute internally generated events to external sources' and when McGuire *et al.* (1993: 703) describe psychological theories of auditory hallucinations as hypothesising that 'schizophrenic subjects are unable to monitor the generation of their own thoughts'. These global individualistic accounts have the potential to direct our attention away from the *variability* in hallucinatory experiences: for example, why is *this* thought and not *that* thought attributed to an external source? Why do many people who hear voices have no difficulty in discriminating the origins of most of their thoughts? What accounts for the intensely self-referential nature of voices? Why should the defect or bias assumed to underlie hallucinatory experiences apparently be more pronounced among Afro-Caribbean men living in Britain (Jarvis, 1998) or among women in the general population (Tien, 1991)? This variability is much more of a problem for defect than for bias theories; for both theories, however, there is a tendency to lose sight of the fact that we are talking about something a person does in relation to some mental events on some occasions, not something they have or are.

A second problem with defect and bias theories is their apparent assumption that these defects or biases *cause* someone to experience auditory hallucinations, as is clear from phrases such as 'the fundamental cognitive disorder implicated in hallucinations'; 'evidence that hallucinations result from a failure in reality testing'; 'data consistent with the account that auditory hallucinations result from a bias in normal information processing'; 'underlying pathophysiology of auditory hallucinations'; 'biases that determine their interpretation of inner speech' (Bentall, 1990a; McGuire *et al.*, 1993; Bentall *et al.*, 1994; Rankin and O'Carroll, 1995; Haddock *et al.*, 1998b). The research designs used to generate and test these models, however, cannot support such conclusions because they involve people who have already experienced auditory hallucinations. We do not know whether the experience of hallucinations changes the way people judge auditory information, particularly under the kinds of conditions of uncertainty induced in this research. There is, too, the problem of confounding variables which could affect performance on cognitive tasks. For example, in Morrison and Haddock's (1997) study, the group diagnosed as schizophrenic who were experiencing hallucinations scored significantly higher than the non-psychiatric group on an anxiety scale and also higher, though not significantly so, than the group diagnosed as schizophrenic who did not experience hallucinations. We therefore need to be cautious in assuming that performance on these cognitive tasks tells us something specific about auditory hallucinations, far less that it tells us about their causes.

The need for caution is further underlined by two factors. First, tasks purporting to measure source monitoring which have been used in much 'bias' research may show little agreement in their results (Johnson *et al.*, 1993; Morrison and Haddock, 1997), thus emphasising the problems of knowing what such tasks are actually measuring. Second, research on biases and defects said to be associated with auditory hallucinations produces *group* data; regrettably, this data may later be inappropriately reported as if whatever (usually negative) attribute is inferred from it applied equally to everyone in the hallucinators' group or to everyone who experiences auditory hallucinations, and not to non-hallucinators. This kind of reporting, together with the tendency to assume that the attribute is general and always present, is particularly powerful in supporting individualistic models which assume that the underlying causes of hallucinations are to be sought in the heads of 'hallucinators'. As statisticians have frequently pointed out, however, it is possible to obtain significant differences between groups on a measure even when there is a great deal of overlap between the groups and where the 'attribute' in question applies only to a minority of group members.

A final problem of deficit and bias accounts of hallucinations is their use of extremely negative evaluative language. People who experience hallucinations are, for example, hypothesised to have defective judgement; abnormal perceptual biases; deficits in speech-processing mechanisms; defective reality testing; parasitic memories; impairments in reality testing; pathologically stored linguistic information; deficits in internal monitoring systems; they make errors of judgement; are deficient in reality testing; are hasty, over-confident and suggestible. As well as this, McGuire *et al.* (1993)

talk of the 'pathophysiology' of auditory hallucinations and Nayani and David (1996) of their 'pathogenesis'. Indeed, Nayani and David also talk of people 'admitting' to auditory hallucinations as if they were some form of wrongdoing. It is not only that this negative and evaluative language – which is quite unnecessary for conveying the results of research – constructs a devalued and demeaning identity for those who experience hallucinations; it also, again, reinforces a narrow, individualistic and abnormal framework in which it seems reasonable – following the traditions of psychology and psychiatry – to search inside the heads of those who hear voices in order to find out what is 'wrong' with them. Such an approach obscures the sheer commonness of auditory hallucinations, the rich and varied roles they have played for both individuals and cultures and, if Jaynes's account is taken seriously, their normality as part of human development.

Clearly, then, broader accounts of hallucinations are needed than those offered by the ideas of bias or deficit. As we shall see, such accounts have actually been offered as part of bias theory. Unfortunately, psychology and psychiatry's habit – one might say, bias – of assuming that a negatively judged behaviour or experience can best be explained by positing a general abnormal feature 'possessed' by the person, is extremely strong; it has tended to elevate the potentially tautological idea of bias at the expense of other aspects of this theoretical model.

## Hearing voices in context

Slade (1972, 1974), Slade and Bentall (1988) and Bentall (1990a) have suggested three major factors, apart from an assumed bias or predisposition, which might influence hallucinatory experiences: stress, environmental stimulation and reinforcement. These will be considered in turn, followed by a discussion of particular forms of aversive experiences, especially sexual abuse, which may be linked to auditory hallucinations.

### STRESS AND ANXIETY

I am not using these terms as if they referred to definite psychological states; on the contrary, both terms are problematic when thought of in this way (Sarbin, 1968; Hallam, 1985a, 1985b). I will, however, adopt Slade's working definition of stress as referring to aversive events associated with reports of negative mood states.

It has often been noted that hallucinatory experiences are associated with reports of major stresses such as bereavement, military activity, torture and other traumatic events (Slade and Bentall, 1988). Studies of psychiatric groups also suggest a relationship between hearing voices and negative mood states. Slade (1972), for example, noted that hallucinations seemed more likely to happen during periods of reported anxiety and stress. Nayani and David (1996) reported a variety of negative states, dominated by sadness and 'stomach churning', associated with the onset of auditory hallucinations. It is perhaps also worth noting Morrison and Haddock's (1997) study in which the psychiatric group reporting auditory hallucinations also had the highest mean score on an anxiety scale. We must be careful here, of course, not to confuse cause and effect: the experience of hallucinations may itself produce very negative states particularly if, as is often the case, their content is also negative or is interpreted as malevolent (Chadwick and Birchwood, 1994). Nevertheless, there is some evidence that aversive events and negative moods do precede hallucinatory experiences. Slade (1972), for example, was able to show an apparently systematic relationship between reports of anxiety and reports of auditory hallucinations such that 'anxiety' seemed to precede hearing voices. Perhaps more important, he also reported that training in relaxation and imaginal desensitisation to stressful events produced a significant decrease in reports of auditory hallucinations. Personal accounts of voice-hearers also suggest strongly that hallucinations are often preceded by intense stress or personal or social crises and that the content of voices relates directly to this (Romme and Escher, 1993; Jackson and Fulford, 1997a).

Bentall (1990a) has suggested that it is in this state of high arousal that information processing and discrimination between what is 'real' and what imaginary, which thoughts are intended and which unintended, may be disrupted or at least be different from when someone is in a more relaxed state. Similarly, Morrison and Haddock (1997) reported that their research participants – both psychiatric and non-psychiatric groups – made significantly more errors in a source-monitoring task when the content of the material was emotional rather than neutral. More specifically, Behrendt (1998) has suggested that some kinds of persistent social or interpersonal stress may result in increasing attention being paid to events which communicate a social message; that the person might intensely observe their environment for hints that help them make inferences about their social value and acceptance and might thus pay close attention to how others think or talk about them. Behrendt argues that an intense preoccupation with one's own hopes, wishes and fears could lead to 'underconstrained perceptions' in which external stimulation sets fewer restrictions than usual on what is perceived. In turn, this *social* anxiety is related to the fact that voices so often comment on, criticise and evaluate the person. But before we assume that such voices must be caused by a problem in the person, it is worth noting Romme's (1993) suggestion that when voices are triggered by intolerable circumstances their content tends to reflect how the hearer is actually treated by others. Birchwood *et al.* (2000) have similarly reported that the characteristics of voices (e.g. how powerful or dominant they are perceived to be) is related to the voice-hearer's perception of their own power, or lack of it, in relationships.

## ENVIRONMENTAL STIMULATION

A number of writers have noted a possible relationship between hallucinations, structured external stimuli and the extent to which these stimuli engage a person's attention (Schultz, 1965; Slade, 1974; Margo *et al.*, 1981). Auditory hallucinations seem to be more likely in the absence of meaningful auditory stimulation or in the absence of a requirement to respond. Slade (1974), for example, manipulated the reported frequency of auditory hallucinations in a psychiatric group by asking them to process auditory information. Margo *et al.* (1981) found that ratings of intensity and duration of auditory hallucinations were lowest in an experimental condition in which (psychiatric) participants read aloud a prose passage whose content they knew they would later be asked to describe, and highest in a white noise condition. Bentall (1990a) has suggested that having to process external auditory information may reduce hallucinatory experiences because it inhibits normal inner speech, while Antrobus *et al.* (1966) noted that 'stimulus independent thoughts', which may be seen as unintended and alien, tend to increase when our attention is not engaged by external stimuli.

Of course, environmental stimulation and processing and responding to auditory stimulation are closely related to the extent of someone's social isolation. It is not surprising, then, that 80 per cent of Nayani and David's (1996) psychiatric sample reported that being alone worsened their hallucinations. These authors also noted that sadness – the most common 'state' reported to encourage hallucinations – was often associated with being alone or lonely. Extended periods of social isolation also allow people to re-live earlier interactions, to 'mull over' how others have talked about or evaluated them, with little opportunity for alternative external feedback. This isolation also produces opportunities for what Morrison *et al.* (2000) have called 'cognitive self-consciousness': they reported a significant correlation between positive responses to questions such as 'I think a lot about how my mind works'; 'I pay close attention to my thoughts' and scores on a revised Launay–Slade Hallucinations Scale.

But social isolation is obviously not the same as the absence of auditory stimulation. The possible importance of social *inter*action or being required to respond meaningfully, in reducing auditory hallucinations, is suggested by Nayani and David's (1996) report that watching TV and listening to the radio were more likely than any other activity mentioned to increase the frequency of auditory hallucinations. By contrast, talking, more than any other activity mentioned, was reported to reduce their frequency.

## REINFORCEMENT

The inclusion of reinforcement as a factor in both Slade's (1976) and Bentall's (1990a) model of hallucinations serves as a reminder of the point I made earlier:

that hallucinations are not something a person *has* but something they *do* – an experience in which they actively participate, and which, like any other activity, is shaped by its consequences.

There are numerous examples in the literature of auditory hallucinations having positive consequences. Posey and Losch (1983), for example, reported that many of their (non-psychiatric) sample claimed to find their voices comforting or that they provided positive guidance. Similarly, over 50 per cent of Miller *et al.*'s (1993) psychiatric sample reported positive effects such as relaxation and companionship, while both psychiatric and non-psychiatric participants from Jackson's (1991) study reported positive effects from hallucinations which some of the psychiatric group saw as outweighing the negative consequences. Heery (1993) has highlighted one particular positive effect of auditory hallucinations: when they are interpreted as part of a spiritual experience, as 'channels towards and beyond a higher self' (92). Jackson and Fulford (1997a) have also emphasised the spiritual dimension of hallucinations for some voice-hearers. This aspect is not surprising, given the centrality of hallucinatory experiences to the development of the major organised religions. As might be expected from this evidence of hallucinations serving directly positive functions, Chadwick and Birchwood (1994) reported that, in their psychiatric sample, when a voice was interpreted as benevolent, then 'without fail', the person willingly engaged with it. Nayani and David (1996) similarly found that 38 per cent of their participants could start at least some of their voices by concentrating on the voice or asking it questions, thus implying that the voice was being actively sought. Morrison *et al.*'s (2000) study also implies positive consequences for some hallucinations: they reported a significant correlation between scores on a revised Launay–Slade Hallucinations Scale and scores on a scale of positive beliefs about unusual experiences.

Although there is good evidence that auditory hallucinations can serve straightforwardly positive functions for the voice-hearer, hallucinatory experiences may more usually be influenced by a complex mix of positive and negative reinforcement; that is, by creating directly positive effects *and* by warding off or ameliorating aversive or negative events; for many voice-hearers, negative reinforcement seems to predominate. Three possible aspects of these mixed functions of voices will be considered: the role of voices in regulating behaviour and solving problems; their role in allowing fantasy control of difficult situations and their role in allowing projection or externalisation of intolerable thoughts or feelings.

In their descriptive study of voice-hearing, Leudar *et al.* (1997) concluded that the most common function of voices was to regulate ongoing activity, often quite mundane activity, through comments, questions, directives and evaluations. Nayani and David (1996) similarly found that some voice-hearers relied on voices to guide them when they were confronted by dilemmas. This regulatory aspect of voices is, of course, exactly what was highlighted by

Jaynes's analysis of the *Iliad*. Guidance or regulation by voices may be seen as positive, as in the woman who described her voices as helping her to 'think things through a bit. It is like people doing your reasoning for you in your head' (cited in Romme and Escher, 1993: 127). In other cases, regulation by voices could be seen as more of an avoidance of the stress of making independent decisions, as in the young man who reported, 'I mean it [voice] finished the relationship, which was the appropriate and healthy thing to do at the same time. I . . . didn't know how to do that so the voice took over' (Heery, 1993: 91).

What conditions might foster the regulation of some behaviour by externalised rather than internalised 'mental processes'? One possibility is that external control is more likely when people are suddenly deprived of important sources of discussion, advice and guidance at the same time as they are exposed to new situations requiring 'new' decisions, as in bereavement or when young people leave home for the first time. In these cases, we might expect voice-hearing to lessen as the new situation becomes more familiar and new sources of discussion and guidance are found. More seriously, the persistent regulation of behaviour by voices may be fostered by circumstances where the person's behaviour and emotions are intensely and extensively controlled by dominant others, often parents. The result may be a person for whom independent thought or decisions are not only very difficult but also very threatening, so that externalised voices can both reproduce the way the person is treated in relationships *and* reduce anxiety engendered by having to make independent decisions. In line with this, Nayani and David (1996) emphasised the critical, admonitory nature of many hallucinated voices in people diagnosed as schizophrenic and that for many voice-hearers, voices had seemingly come to replace the inner 'voice of conscience'. These ideas are particularly interesting in relation to the research on 'expressed emotion' which I discussed in the previous chapter. It is notable that the characteristics of many of the voices of those diagnosed as schizophrenic – hostile, judgemental, critical, intrusive – are very similar to the characteristics which would lead a family to be described as 'high in expressed emotion'.

Jackson and Fulford (1997a) have suggested a possibly more constructive role for voices in guiding and regulating behaviour, but one which still involves negative reinforcement. Based on detailed accounts of voice-hearing and 'delusional' beliefs in psychiatric and non-psychiatric groups, they have argued that these phenomena can be considered to be 'an intrinsic feature of an essentially adaptive problem solving process' (Jackson and Fulford, 1997a: 57). This process, they suggest, is triggered by intense stress in the context of existential crises – for example, severe threats to health, livelihood or identity. The content of voices or 'delusional' beliefs 'acts directly to resolve the triggering stress by producing a paradigm shift for the individual' (ibid.). Thus voices (or beliefs) might predict a secure future, provide a radically different interpretation of the present, or provide guidance or approval for particular actions. The immediate effect is to lessen very negative moods and to provide negative reinforcement for voice-hearing or for 'delusional' beliefs.

A further important way in which hallucinated voices might reduce negative mood states, and thus be maintained through negative reinforcement, is through allowing unacceptable or threatening thoughts and feelings to be separated from the self and attributed to a non-self source. Bentall (1990a), for example, has noted that people who hear voices often become very anxious when asked to reattribute their voices to themselves. Haddock *et al.* (1996) have provided a striking example of this process in the case of a woman whose voices increased following rows with her husband. While she gradually became aware that the content of the voices reflected what she thought and felt about her husband but was unable to express, she did not accept that the voices were self-generated but attributed them instead to the devil. The woman was, presumably, unwilling or unable to confront the implications of accepting that she herself might be capable of such negative thoughts about her husband. Davey (1993) has also suggested that intense regulation by others may result in what are seen as unacceptable thoughts and feelings being perceived as alien (and very threatening) to the self and lead to their being attributed to a non-self source. This idea again recalls the relationship between 'high expressed emotion' and 'schizophrenic' experiences.

A rather different way of looking at possible functions of auditory hallucinations is in terms of their role in allowing fantasy control over difficult, threatening or otherwise uncontrollable situations or simply allowing the fantasy creation of a more acceptable 'reality' (Mednick, 1958; Sarbin, 1970; Sarbin and Juhasz, 1978; Behrendt, 1998). Behrendt, for example, links intense social anxiety to voice-hearing in which the person 'more and more withdraws into a world of interactions with people who are present only through their voices' (245). In turn, social isolation is seen as fostering perceptions underconstrained by external stimuli in which the person's self-image 'can be controlled in a short-cut manner without application of social behaviour' (ibid.).

It is, finally, important to note that hallucinations do not serve important functions only for individuals; I have already emphasised the centrality of hallucinatory experiences in the development of organised religions. One social function particularly emphasised by anthropologists (e.g. Wallace, 1959; Murphy, 1978) is that of fostering the belief that it is possible to communicate with the dead and with spirits, to control them and to convey messages from them. This power may allow the occupation of a valued social role as prophet, shaman or medium. The English medium Doris Stokes, for example, published books with titles such as *Voices in My Ear*, *A Host of Voices* and *Whispering Voices* and was able to fill Sydney Opera House and many other venues with people anxious to benefit from her voice-hearing. Her social standing is illustrated by the fact that her death merited obituaries in the 'quality' press, where she was lauded for her 'great gift'.

## VOICE-HEARING AND ABUSE

There is now general agreement that traumatic experiences, including severe physical and sexual abuse, can be associated with a variety of behaviours and experiences which would be called psychiatric symptoms (Sakheim and Devine, 1995). The possible scale of this association is suggested by Jacobson and Richardson's (1987) study of one hundred psychiatric in-patients: 81 per cent had experienced major physical or sexual assaults, many of which were not known to staff. Bryer et al. (1987) also reported a high rate of childhood sexual and physical abuse in a sample of sixty-six adult female psychiatric in-patients. More specific links between psychosis and abuse are suggested by several studies. Forty-six per cent of a group of in-patients who remained 'actively psychotic', despite medication and other therapy, reported histories of severe childhood sexual abuse (Beck and van der Kolk, 1987); similarly, Greenfield et al. (1994) reported histories of childhood abuse in 52 per cent of 'psychotic' adults admitted to hospital for the first time.

In line with this, Stampfer (1990) has highlighted the striking similarity between what are said to be symptoms or features of chronic post-traumatic stress disorder – assumed by definition to be the result of trauma – and what are called negative symptoms of schizophrenia, such as severe loss of pleasure and social withdrawal (see also Harrop et al., 1996). As Stampfer points out, 'trauma' need not be sudden and discrete; instead, he suggests, '[n]egative symptoms would emerge only when the accumulation of trauma or conflict began to overwhelm the individual and hence threaten his or her functional integrity, hold on life or whatever else one chooses to call such a feature' (521). Startup (1999) has also drawn attention to the overlap between 'pathological dissociative experiences' – said to be linked theoretically and empirically with histories of trauma and maltreatment – and 'schizotypy', a constellation of experiences and behaviours assumed to be on a continuum with 'schizophrenia'. In a general population study, Startup found significant correlations between scores on a Dissociative Experiences Scale and on two Schizotypy Scales assessing unusual perceptual experiences and 'cognitive disorganisation', even when overlapping items were removed.

Honig et al. (1998) investigated the more specific relationship between abuse and auditory hallucinations. In a study of three groups of voice-hearers diagnosed as schizophrenic, dissociative disorder or with no diagnosis, only a minority reported *not* having suffered some form of abuse or severe maltreatment as a child: 17, 14 and 27 per cent, respectively. Ensink's (1993) study began with a group of one hundred women who had been sexually abused in childhood for four years or more, mostly by their father or stepfather. Almost 30 per cent of the women reported hearing voices and 43 per cent reported visual hallucinations. Moreover, the reports of the large majority of women who experienced auditory hallucinations (85 per cent), met Schneider's criteria for schizophrenic hallucinations.

Given the possible relationship between abuse and psychotic experiences, it is interesting to note Nayani and David's study of the content of auditory hallucinations in a sample of one hundred people with a diagnosis of psychosis. The authors commented that:

> [T]he most commonly encountered hallucinated utterances, occurring in 60% of the whole sample, were simple terms of abuse. Female subjects described words of abuse conventionally directed at women (e.g. slut) and 32 male subjects similarly described 'male' insults such as those imputing homosexuality.

> (1996: 182)

Of course, this does not mean that abuse or maltreatment has happened, but psychological theories of voice-hearing still have to provide an account of why abusive voices are so frequent, particularly in psychiatric groups. It is also perhaps worth noting that in Tien's (1991) general population study of hallucinatory experiences, the prevalence rates for females (reportedly the majority victims of sexual abuse) were 40–50 per cent higher than those for males; Tien suggested 'false positive reports in histrionic women' as a possible explanation (291). He later rejected this hypothesis (not because it might be insulting to women, but because his data did not fit with what was known about 'histrionic personality'); he did not, however, suggest any alternative. Again, these figures do not necessarily implicate sexual abuse, but they do merit further attention.

If there *is* a relationship between abuse, trauma and auditory hallucinations, then what mechanisms might account for it? Ensink (1993) has suggested that sexual abuse could make it difficult to learn or sustain a distinction between 'reality' and fantasy; for example, the abuser may insist that the child enjoys the abuse or deny that certain events happened. Indeed, as Ensink points out, in this situation it might be advantageous *not* to learn a distinction: imagination, possibly peopled with protective voices, could provide the only bearable 'reality'.

A second possible mechanism, prominent in psychoanalytic theory, involves 'splitting', a process in which, it is suggested, people react to very traumatic events by isolating those memories and associated thoughts and emotions from conscious awareness. The events may 'return', however, in the form of flashbacks, images or voices; they may also return in a fragmented and distorted form which, together with their separateness from the stream of consciousness designated as 'me', makes them more likely to be experienced as external and alien to the self (Ensink, 1993; Heery, 1993). Some hallucinatory injunctions to violence might also be understandable in this framework. Aggressive thoughts and feelings towards an abuser, or those who did not protect the child, may be so threatening as to be experienced only as hallucinated injunctions from an external source.

The fact that two relatively common events – abuse and hearing voices – often happen together, does not mean that they are meaningfully related. Three factors, however, suggest that the relationship is likely to be meaningful. First, the figures for hallucinatory experiences in those with a history of abuse, and the figures for abuse experiences in those diagnosed as psychotic, are consistently higher than the reported rates of either experience in the general population and much higher than the expected rate of co-occurrence if the two events are unrelated. The figures raise problems of sampling and definitions of abuse, but clearly need further study. There is, second, the very negative and abusive content of many voices, particularly in psychiatric groups. Finally, there are at least plausible psychological mechanisms posited across a range of traumatic situations which provide a starting point for understanding the possible relationship between trauma/abuse and hallucinatory experiences.

## Labelling reported imaginings as pathological

I emphasised earlier that not all reports of hearing voices result in a psychiatric diagnosis. This section is concerned with some of the factors which might contribute to the selective labelling of some hallucinatory experiences as pathological. It is important, however, to clarify two points in relation to the now well-acknowledged experience of auditory hallucinations or voice-hearing among the general population. The first is that, by itself, the relatively common reporting of auditory hallucinations by non-psychiatric groups cannot be used to criticise the concept of schizophrenia. This is because symptoms or complaints which form part of the cluster from which medical concepts are inferred are often widely distributed in the general population: we would obviously not consider the frequent experiences of nausea or thirst as evidence against the concepts of cancer or diabetes. And, certainly, users of 'schizophrenia' have never suggested that hearing voices is always a symptom of schizophrenia. The reason why the general population data are so problematic for the concept of schizophrenia is that, unlike concepts such as cancer and diabetes, 'schizophrenia' is inferred only from its widely distributed and supposed symptoms, so that there is no valid and independent way of designating any instance of voice-hearing as (or as not) a symptom of schizophrenia. Not only that, but descriptive studies of voice-hearers have shown that it is not possible clearly to discriminate psychiatric and non-psychiatric groups by the very criteria suggested in the psychiatric literature for designating any instance of voice-hearing as a symptom of schizophrenia (e.g. Leudar *et al.*, 1997; Jackson and Fulford, 1997a; Honig *et al.*, 1998). For example, what would be called first-rank symptoms of schizophrenia, such as voices conversing or keeping a running commentary on the person's behaviour, can be found in both psychiatric and non-psychiatric groups. Of course, this is not surprising as all suggested criteria for discriminating symptoms of schizophrenia from other experiences are inevitably arbitrary. It is this combination of the relatively frequent occurrence of auditory hallucinations in the general population, the failure to discriminate psychiatric and non-psychiatric groups by traditional diagnostic rules *and* the lack of any independent criteria for discriminating 'schizophrenic' from 'non-schizophrenic' voice-hearing, which makes the general population data so problematic for 'schizophrenia'.

The second issue which arises in relation to the general population data is this: there has always been concern to distinguish 'good' (or neutral) and 'bad' hallucinations – those calling for action from authority and those not. Sarbin (1967) and Sarbin and Juhasz (1978) have noted that in the West this concern can be traced (at least) to the preoccupations of medieval theologians, anxious to distinguish potential sainthood from heresy, or spirit possession from witchcraft. This concern to distinguish good from bad hallucinations is still very much with us and it is rather dismaying to find that even some of those who have provided important descriptive data showing the lack of distinction in form or structure, between the hallucinatory experiences of psychiatric and non-psychiatric groups, are nevertheless still preoccupied with the need to distinguish 'pathological' from 'non-pathological' hallucinations. For example, after providing an extremely thoughtful discussion of the difficulties in distinguishing what they called pathological from benign spiritual psychotic experiences, Jackson and Fulford (1997b) still concluded not only that the distinction was meaningful but also that it needed to be 'correctly drawn' (87). As I pointed out in relation to 'mental illness', however, there is no possible way in which we can 'correctly' distinguish two lay concepts, in this case pathology and benign spiritual experience (and see also Littlewood, 1997). Jackson and Fulford (1997a) also appear to adopt two opposing positions: they seem to define pathological psychotic experiences as 'symptoms of illness' but at the same time argue that it is 'unlikely that a psychopathology which is capable of accommodating the distinction [between pathological and spiritual psychotic experience] will be developed within the restrictions of the traditional medical model' (60). But if we step outside the medical model, the identification of pathological forms of psychotic experience becomes meaningless, in the same way that distinguishing sin from states of grace is meaningless outside of a Christian model. The point here is that even when we try to move away from a medical framework, the continued use of medical language – which seems not to be recognised as only making sense within the model – inevitably draws us back in. The result is the persistent belief that some forms of voice-hearing must be intrinsically pathological; it is a short step from that to the search for something pathological about some people who hear voices. This tendency is also apparent when psychological researchers emphasise that 'circumstances' could cause any of us to experience auditory hallucinations, yet assume that these are best accounted for by cognitive abnormalities in those diagnosed as schizophrenic. At best, these ways of thinking are misleading; at worst, they excuse us from spelling out the full range of factors which influence our response to bizarre and incomprehensible behaviour and from explaining clearly why some instances and not others should call for action by authority.

None of this alters the facts that some instances of auditory hallucinations *are* labelled as pathological and that, for some people, the experience of voice-hearing is extremely negative and disruptive. But there is no reason to assume that this calls for a 'correct' distinction between pathological and non-pathological, or schizophrenic and non-schizophrenic experiences; instead, we can argue that the important questions concern the process by which professionals come to label some voice-hearers as pathological, as ill, *and* the processes by which some experiences of voice-hearing become so negative and disruptive that the person comes to psychiatric attention, possibly to be called schizophrenic.

## Professional judgements of pathology

There is very little research on how professionals come to decide that any instance of voice-hearing is pathological or a symptom of illness. Sarbin and Juhasz (1978), however, have suggested that observers, in this case psychiatrists, are more likely to judge reported imaginings as pathological when the report is made by someone who has already been devalued in some way – who is of low social status, poor education, who is less powerful, who has 'failed' in the performance of certain social roles, etc. Sarbin and Juhasz suggest, with Szasz and Goffman, that diagnostic labels, or the claim that certain behaviours are symptoms, occur *after* the person has violated other social norms. Several sources suggest that these ideas are at least worthy of further consideration.

The first is the relationship of diagnoses to judgements of 'social competence'. Phillips *et al.* (1966) rated over 500 psychiatric patients, on occupation, IQ and education, and also computed a global 'social maturity' score for each person. The group who reported hallucinations had the second lowest mean social maturity score. The authors also grouped 'symptoms' according to their 'social maturity level' and showed that diagnoses of schizophrenia were in general associated with lower-level (in terms of their scale) symptoms than were diagnoses of, for example, manic depressive psychosis or character disorder. Phillips *et al.* concluded that 'a patient's level of social maturity finds expression in his symptomatology and this combination of maturity and symptom expression is an important factor in the diagnosis he receives' (213). The hypothesis might have been better put that when someone judged to be of low social maturity also reports imaginings as real, then he or she is more likely to be said to be hallucinating and more likely to be called schizophrenic. But Phillips *et al.* only studied people who had come to the attention of psychiatrists. We have no way of knowing how these psychiatrists would have reacted to the imaginings of those who reported hallucinations in general population surveys. Interestingly, however, Honig *et al.* (1998) reported that amongst a group of voice-hearers, those diagnosed as schizophrenic had, overall, a lower educational level than either a non-psychiatric group or a group diagnosed as dissociative disorder, although this could have been a function of sample selection. Posey and Losch (1983) also asked clinicians to examine psychiatric questionnaires completed by their hallucinating students – all were pronounced 'completely normal'.

A second source of support for the idea that voice-hearing is likely to lead to a diagnostic label for those whose social functioning has already been devalued comes from the DSM itself. I pointed out in Chapter 5 that one of the criteria for inferring schizophrenia is deterioration from a previous level of functioning in areas such as work, social relations and self-care. I discussed the problems of the deterioration criterion in Chapter 5, but the criterion does suggest that reports of bizarre behaviour or experience are by definition more likely to be labelled as 'schizophrenic' when they are made by or about people whose social functioning is otherwise deemed inadequate.

Further, albeit very indirect, support for the importance of social behaviour is provided by Falloon *et al.* (1984). They pointed out that when relatives were asked to comment on the behaviour of the 'schizophrenic' in the family, by far the most frequent cause for complaint was not the so-called symptoms but failure to perform valued social behaviours – to talk to family members or visitors; get up in the morning; make friends; obtain employment; take up hobbies, etc. It seems reasonable to suggest that relatives are more likely to complain to the psychiatric services when bizarre behaviour is accompanied by 'social failure'. This 'failure', in turn, can provide justification for the application of a diagnosis of schizophrenia.

A more specific factor which might influence professional judgements of voice-hearing is that of language. Al-Issa has argued that:

> the linguistic sophistication of the suspected hallucinator seems to play a dominant part in influencing the decision of the diagnostician. His public report is, for example, unlikely to be declared false or considered hallucinatory if he includes in his statements such qualifiers as 'it is *as if* I hear . . ., I *thought* I saw.'
>
> (1977: 574)

Sarbin has made a similar point:

> In reporting his construction [that he saw the Virgin Mary] *literally* the speaker might show ignorance of current norms regarding language constraints to be used when talking about [the world of imaginings]; in interpreting such a report *literally* the hearer might mistake the metaphoric intent of the speaker. These confusions, which may lead to tragic or comic outcomes, are not just signs of ignorance or lack of knowledge but a predictable result of the metaphorical language when employed to communicate about imaginings.
>
> (1970: 66–67)

Although there are virtually no data available which would clarify this suggested role of language in determining responses to reported imaginings, it is interesting to note that Miller *et al.* (1965), using a descriptive language task, found that the performance of hallucinating 'schizophrenics' was inferior to that of non-hallucinating 'schizophrenics'. Their vocabulary was also described as more restricted (using a different test). In addition, their performance on a 'metaphor selection test' deviated more from normative standards than did that of the non-hallucinating 'schizophrenics'. Miller *et al.* concluded that '[t]he deviant language observed in hallucinating schizophrenics may not only reflect an attempt to describe inner experiences which are vague, strange and frightening, but may also reflect a lack of sufficient language skills to formulate metaphors which meaningfully convey these inner experiences' (51). Unfortunately, Miller *et al.* did not study voice-hearers who had not been diagnosed as schizophrenic. Obviously, no strong conclusions can be drawn from so few data, but they do suggest that the issue is worth pursuing. Language skills may, of course, interact with the kind of variable used by Phillips *et al.* to rate 'social maturity'.

Finally, the context in which voice-hearing is experienced is likely to influence judgements of its pathology. Littlewood and Lipsedge (1982), for example, suggested that it is not necessarily the performance of certain behaviours *per se* which invites pathological labels, but their performance outside a prescribed social context. Although the frequent use of terms like 'mental illness' in Western society gives the impression that pathological labels are attached to pathological people, there is little reason not to suppose that it is performance outside accepted social contexts which attracts 'illness' or 'symptom' labels. In modern Western societies, there are few contexts where reporting imaginings as real is acceptable. One is when reported imaginings have a religious content, but this may be more acceptable in European countries with a strong Catholic tradition than in northern European Protestant culture. It is also increasingly being suggested (see Littlewood and Lipsedge, 1982, 1997) that reports of hearing voices should not be called symptoms if they are made by certain immigrant groups and are understandable within the person's cultural context. Reporting hearing voices is also acceptable in the context of the Spiritualist Church when the claim is made by a recognised or aspiring medium. A key factor in all of these cases may be the extent to which others outside the psychiatric services can be persuaded to accept the reported imaginings as non-pathological.

## Becoming 'pathological': negative experiences of voices

As with the closely related issue of professional judgements of pathology, there is little research which addresses the issue of how the experience of voice-hearing – interpretable in many different ways – may be so negative or disruptive for someone that they come to psychiatric attention and receive a diagnosis. One reason for this lack of research is that if certain types of voice-hearing are called symptoms of schizophrenia, then there is no apparent need to ask how the person came to psychiatric attention and how they received a diagnosis of schizophrenia. The answer is obvious: they came to psychiatric attention because they were displaying symptoms of psychiatric illness and they received the diagnosis of schizophrenia because that is the illness they were suffering from. If, however, voice-hearing is seen differently – as a human characteristic, more or less suppressed by cultural influences; as an experience which can be positive, neutral or negative – then the question of how only some voice-hearers come to psychiatric attention becomes crucial. A small number of recent descriptive studies of the experiences of psychiatric and non-psychiatric groups of voice-hearers has provided a valuable starting point for thinking about this issue. Indeed, the unanimous conclusion of these studies that the voice-hearing of psychiatric and non-psychiatric groups cannot easily be distinguished by classical psychiatric criteria, makes the question of how only some of them become 'patients' even more important. Three factors which might influence this process will be considered: the content and characteristics of voices; the response of the person themselves and of those around them and, finally, the ways in which voice-hearing might lead to other behaviours which would be labelled as symptoms of schizophrenia.

## VOICE CONTENT

Two studies which compared voice-hearing experiences of psychiatric and non-psychiatric groups suggest potentially important differences in the *content* of voices. In Leudar *et al.*'s (1997) study, significantly more of the psychiatric ('schizophrenic') group reported voices which abused them, while Honig *et al.* (1998) reported significant differences between 'schizophrenic' and non-patient groups in the experiences of critical voices or voices which restricted activities. As well as this, all of Leudar *et al.*'s 'schizophrenic' group, but only 60 per cent of the non-patient group, reported that voices which directed action were persistent, often becoming aggressive if not obeyed. These authors also noted that of seven voices which instigated violence, six were reported by the 'schizophrenic' group. Similarly, significantly more of Honig *et al.*'s patient groups ('schizophrenic' and 'dissociative disorder') reported hearing voices daily and continuously and that their voices disturbed their life. Intensely negative experiences of voices were also 'unanimously' reported by Jackson's (1991) psychiatric group, in contrast to more positive and mixed experiences of the non-psychiatric group.

Research which has looked only at voice-hearing in psychiatric groups, usually with a diagnosis of schizophrenia, supports this very negative picture of their experience. Nayani and David (1996), for example, concluded that the most frequent function of voice-hearing in this group was negative evaluations, including criticism and abuse. Only 23 per cent of Chadwick and Birchwood's

(1994) psychiatric group reported voices perceived as benevolent, while 65 per cent reported malevolent voices. It is not difficult to see how the negative, at times very abusive, content of voices reported by psychiatric groups could prove very distressing and disruptive and increase the likelihood of the person's coming to psychiatric attention. It is also not difficult to see how experiencing voices daily and persistently – voices, moreover, which may demand to be obeyed – could also have this outcome. But not all psychiatric patients experience very negative voices, while some non-patients do. This suggests that other factors also influence the process of becoming a psychiatric patient.

## RESPONSES TO VOICE-HEARING

Honig *et al.* (1998) reported a highly significant difference between psychiatric and non-psychiatric groups of voice-hearers in the extent to which they were afraid of their voices; the groups also differed in how far they felt in control of their voices. The potential importance of the perceived power of voices is emphasised by Chadwick and Birchwood's (1994) study of a psychiatric group of voice-hearers, all of whom perceived their voices as extraordinarily powerful. Not surprisingly, voices which were also perceived as malevolent or at least as not benevolent – the large majority – elicited very negative responses such as anger, fear or depression. Romme *et al.* (1992) and Romme and Escher (1993) reached rather similar conclusions about the importance of voices' perceived power. A study of people who believed they coped either well or badly with their voices suggested that one important factor was how far the person felt themselves to be stronger than their voices, how far they felt able to say 'no' to them.

We are reminded here again of the suggested links between voice-hearing and abuse, of the links between 'schizophrenic' symptoms in general and 'expressed emotion', *and* of Romme *et al.*'s and Birchwood *et al.*'s suggestion that voice content may reflect the way people are treated in relationships. People who have experienced intense control by others, whether through sexual or physical abuse, or intrusive 'over-protection', are likely to experience themselves as less powerful than others. Some voice-hearing, with its critical, abusive or simply regulatory characteristics, may replicate aspects of these relationships, including their hierarchies of power. The result may be an extremely distressing, even overwhelming, experience to which the person is unable to respond constructively.

But it is not simply the response of the person themselves which determines whether they will 'cope' with the experience of voice-hearing or whether they come to psychiatric attention. Romme and Escher (1993) and Jackson and Fulford (1997a) have emphasised the importance of others' responses in influencing the outcome of the experience. Romme and Escher (1993) noted that, initially at least, most voice-hearers believe their experience is unique, feel ashamed and fear 'going mad'. Participants in their study of 'copers' and 'non-copers' emphasised the importance of a supportive friend, relative or partner who 'listened to them, accepted them and with whom they felt secure' (34). Jackson and Fulford (1997a) have argued that whether someone's psychotic experience becomes 'pathological' is crucially influenced by whether they can constructively use the 'insight' provided by the psychotic experience. This might be more easily achieved for some experiences than others (e.g. 'hearing' that you are under God's protection rather than that you are a fat cow); nevertheless, as Jackson and Fulford have shown, the reactions of those with whom the person first discusses the experience may be crucial in determining how the experience is interpreted and whether it leads to a psychiatric outcome.

These two factors – the content and persistence of voices and people's responses to them – could in a general way lead to such distress and disruption to someone's life that they seek or are brought to psychiatric attention. In the next section I will discuss three more specific ways in which voice-hearing might lead directly to other behaviours or reported beliefs which would be seen as symptoms of illness and thus as justifying or reinforcing a psychiatric diagnosis.

The first is through the relationship of voice-hearing to the development of 'delusional' beliefs. Leudar *et al.* (1997), for example, reported a significant difference in the proportion of 'schizophrenic' and non-psychiatric voice-hearers whose voices had told them something they did not know. Such an experience could be interpreted as evidence of special status, of being 'chosen', particularly if the voice is thought to belong to a public figure. (Alternatively, it could simply reinforce the belief in the 'otherness' of voices.) Behrendt (1998) has suggested that the belief that one's thoughts are being broadcast to others (said to be a first-rank symptom of schizophrenia) could arise from voices appearing to know about and react to the voice-hearer's thoughts. Similarly, if voices are thought to come from real people, and if the voices can be partly controlled, then 'delusions of influence' might be an understandable response. So too would the belief that others can read the voice-hearer's mind, in the face of any correspondence between the person's thoughts and the content of voices.

A second way in which voice-hearing might lead to or reinforce a psychiatric diagnosis is through its effects on social behaviour. I noted earlier that the diagnostic criteria for schizophrenia require a deterioration, or deficit, in the person's social behaviour or self-care. It is easy to see in a general way how the distress and preoccupation produced by some voice-hearing could have this effect; Behrendt (1998), however, has argued more specifically that social behaviour degrades when it is no longer needed for controlling the perception of social stimuli. In other words, if voice-hearing functions to provide imaginal control of interpersonal situations, and if it involves social isolation, then 'normative' social behaviour becomes less important and less necessary.

Finally, Behrendt has suggested that so-called negative symptoms of schizophrenia might persist or worsen through the avoidance of social contact which may be both the antecedent and consequence of auditory hallucinations. Behrendt links social avoidance both to fears of social failure or of endangering a compensatory grandiose self-image; in either case, it is not difficult to see how the resulting isolation could foster or reinforce 'negative symptoms' such as 'affective flattening', 'lack of will' and so on.

### Auditory hallucinations: an overview

I have argued here that if we see voice-hearing not as a symptom of schizophrenia but as a widely distributed human experience, then we are led to a set of questions, involving social and personal antecedents, content, function and meaning, entirely different from those traditionally posed in the psychiatric literature. We are also, crucially, led to the question of why only some voice-hearers receive psychiatric diagnoses. It is important to emphasise, however, that research in these areas is still at a preliminary stage and that much of the discussion here is necessarily speculative. It is also important to emphasise how easily psychological research on hallucinations can simply replicate traditional psychiatric models, by positing and searching for something abnormal 'in the person' which causes them to hear voices. Yet this replication is achieved not only at the expense of most of the factors actually posited in psychological models of auditory hallucinations, it can also obscure the important question of how only some instances of voice-hearing come to be labelled pathological. A fuller understanding of voice-hearing will involve acknowledging that voice-hearing is a *social* phenomenon, involving those immediately around the voice-hearer as well as social authorities and wider cultural practices.

## Bizarre beliefs or 'delusions'[2]

Traditional attempts to define 'delusion' have focused on a number of factors, including the claimed falsity or absurdity of the belief; that it is held with absolute conviction; is based on incorrect inferences about reality; is not amenable to reason, evidence or persuasion; is preoccupying and is not culturally shared (APA, 1987, 1994; Oltmanns, 1988; Butler and Braff, 1991). When they are not explicable by known organic factors, such beliefs are claimed to be important indicators of mental disorder, including schizophrenia. In other words, theories which deal with 'ordinary' false or highly implausible beliefs will not do for 'delusions'.

It is not difficult to show that these attempts to distinguish 'normal' from 'abnormal' false or implausible beliefs are based, to say the least, on weak foundations. For example, there is no evidence that delusional beliefs said to be symptoms of mental disorder are held with any greater conviction than equally improbable beliefs which would not be called symptoms; indeed there is evidence that some religious beliefs are held with just as much conviction as

2 I am using the term 'belief' here simply to mean 'a persistent claim that such and such is the case'.

beliefs labelled pathological (e.g. Jackson and Fulford, 1997a; Jones and Watson, 1997; Peters *et al.*, 1999a), although the latter may be more preoccupying, a point I will return to later. Nor is there evidence that 'delusional' beliefs are impervious to evidence or persuasion. Again, there is good evidence to the contrary (Watts *et al.*, 1973; Milton *et al.*, 1978; Johnson *et al.*, 1977; Chadwick and Lowe, 1990). But even if this were not the case, a distinction based on being amenable to reason remains problematic because it involves the highly questionable assumption that 'ordinary' beliefs *are* routinely changed by rational means (see, e.g., Anderson *et al.*, 1980). The criterion of falsity or improbability is equally problematic. To someone from outside the culture it is surely difficult to choose, on that criterion, between the ideas that an invisible being can 'hear' and respond to certain thought patterns called 'prayers' and that the BBC send coded personal messages through the radio. Indeed, as Harper (1999) has pointed out, 'deluded' people may be judged by and expected to adopt a standard of rationality that most 'normal' people do not reach most of the time (and see Gaines, 1995 and Harper, 1999, for discussion of some of the implausible beliefs widely held in the general population).

But if these criteria for 'delusions' are problematic, then we are left with the idea that a delusion is an odd belief which is idiosyncratic and not culturally shared; in other words, it supposedly cannot be explained by cultural learning. It is this criterion which is increasingly being emphasised in the face of Western psychiatry's dealings with minority ethnic groups (e.g. Mercer, 1986; Littlewood and Lipsedge, 1997); it is explicitly used by DSM-IV to define bizarre delusions: 'Delusions are decreed bizarre if they are clearly implausible and not understandable and do not derive from ordinary life experiences' (1994: 275).

There are two major problems with this emphasis on cultural sharing or understanding of beliefs. First, it is apparently based on the assumption that the number of people in a particular social group who make certain belief claims should influence the judgement as to whether the claim is a symptom of mental illness. This implies that it is a priori impossible for someone to construct and defend a radically different belief system, seen by the majority culture as highly improbable, except under the influence of pathological processes. And if we accept this criterion, then we must also accept that, for example, Christians (judged not to be ill) are in fact victims of a *folie à millions* because they subscribe to the (now) culturally acceptable but, some would say, highly implausible or false claim (that he was the Son of God) put forward with great conviction by one apparently preoccupied man, against what was culturally acceptable at the time. Littlewood and Lipsedge (1982) provided a tautological escape route from this paradox by claiming that psychotics are rarely able to convince others of the validity of their beliefs. The opposite is just as likely: that when someone, for whatever reasons, cannot convince others of the validity of their odd beliefs, then they are more likely to be called psychotic or deluded.

The second and much more serious problem with the cultural under-standability criterion for identifying delusions is that it implies that an observer's ability or willingness to understand how a belief system could have come about in terms of someone's life experiences or cultural back-ground should serve as a criterion of whether the belief is a symptom of mental illness. The arrogance, absurdity and dangers of such a criterion can hardly be overstated. It implies, first, that psychiatrists (who are the defining observers in this context) could be omniscient, that they know or could know everything that could ever possibly be known about how environmental and personal factors interact to produce certain beliefs and are thus in a position to pronounce on when a belief falls outside this process; the criterion implies, second, that psychiatrists systematically and comprehensively assess the pres-ence or absence of each of these factors and, third, having concluded that none is present, they are then entitled to infer mental illness or even brain disor-der, even in the absence of any direct evidence of such abnormality. None of these, of course, is true and Wing's (1978b) comment that a psychiatric examination must be grounded in a thorough familiarity with the subjective experience of human beings (intended to offer reassurance about how some behaviours are labelled 'symptoms'), shows a dismaying lack of appreciation of these problems. So too do Sims' (1997) claims about using the 'method of empathy' in order to 'feel oneself into the situation of the other person', so as to distinguish pathological from non-pathological beliefs and experiences (80). In practice, psychiatry and psychology have shown and continue to show a dismaying lack of understanding of possible links between cultural context and disturbing behaviour and experience (e.g. Ussher and Nicolson, 1992; Fernando, 1993; Stoppard, 2000), so that even if understandability *were* a valid criterion for identifying 'delusions' we would be very far from being able to apply it.

What is obscured by attempts to identify the essence of 'delusions', and to define them objectively, is that the judgement is always social and relational; it involves an interaction between a speaker and hearer, 'a comparison of minds, in which one is treated as authoritative and the other as deficient . . . A belief becomes a delusion when the psychiatrist judges that no-one wants to hear it and that the patient does not care to adjust the belief in the direction of social value' (Heise, 1988: 267, 270). Clearly, how far someone can convince others of the value of their beliefs will vary with time and place, as well as with other characteristics of the 'believer'. Given this, and the problematic nature of the criteria for defining 'delusion', we should not be surprised that in a study of psychiatrists' accounts of how they came to decide that certain people had paranoid delusions, Harper (1999) should have found little evidence that this was achieved through the systematic application of objective criteria. Instead, Harper argued that professionals drew on a number of rhetorical resources to construct the beliefs as implausible. These varied both within and between patients, and included references to people's physical characteristics, social status, gender and emotional state. It could be argued, of course, that this illustrates the application of the understandability criterion. But we are then simply returned to the problems of that criterion; in any case, and in line with Maher's (1992) claim, the clinicians' studies by Harper appeared to draw more on common-sense notions of what certain people ought to believe under certain circumstances, rather than on a detailed assessment of the links between belief and life experiences.

## The development and maintenance of 'delusions'

Perhaps because it has traditionally been assumed that certain belief systems are simply symptoms of schizophrenia or mental disorder – as Berrios (1991) put it, 'empty speech acts' – the literature on the development and maintenance of beliefs called 'delusions' has until recently been sparse. Ironically, this is in spite of a large psychological literature on 'normal' beliefs, but as I noted earlier it has been assumed that theories which apply to ordinary beliefs do not necessary apply to their 'pathological' counterparts. Unfortunately, much recent research on 'delusions' has implicitly adopted a rather essentialising approach, rather than regarding 'delusion' as a construction rising from an interaction between a speaker and a hearer. I shall return to this point later, but for the moment simply describe briefly some of the ideas which have been put forward to explain what are thought of as delusions.

Scheibe and Sarbin (1965) drew on a range of ideas from anthropology, from Skinner's (1948) observations on 'superstitious' behaviour in animals and on Rotter's (1954) theory of generalised expectancy, to suggest that individual and social belief systems, whether bizarre or not, develop in response to gaps about cause–effect relationships in important areas of knowledge and as part of a general human habit of constructing explanations – with little regard for their validity – which can be used to justify and support behaviour. One important setting condition for the development of personal and cultural belief systems is uncertainty about a valued outcome. Falling in love, for example, and especially unrequited love, is notorious for fostering odd beliefs.

Maher and Ross (1984) and Maher (1988) have put forward a framework rather similar to that of Scheibe and Sarbin in its emphasis on our constant search for explanations and on the continuity between ordinary and 'delusional' beliefs. Their model, however, gives prominence to the role of anomalous personal experiences in the development of 'delusional' beliefs. Maher (1988) reviewed some of the research which emphasises the apparent ease with which 'irrational' beliefs can be provoked in ordinary people under anomalous environmental conditions. He also discussed the work of Southward, early in this century, in which post-mortem findings for patients said to have been deluded suggested that many of their beliefs served an explanatory function for symptoms of pathology undiagnosed in life but obvious at post-mortem. It is interesting to recall here the plight of Kraepelin's and Bleuler's patients, probably suffering from post-encephalitic Parkinsonism, many of whom experienced anomalous physical and cognitive changes which were as bewildering to their doctors as to themselves. Not surprisingly, some of their beliefs appear to be attempts to explain the inexplicable: their inability to carry out 'willed' acts; impulsive acts they had not 'willed'; chronic constipation, and so on. One anomalous experience now said to be characteristic of schizophrenia is, of course, hearing voices. Chadwick and Birchwood (1994) and Birchwood and Chadwick (1997) have emphasised the importance of focusing on how people make sense of this experience – often in ways which would be called delusional. Maher's emphasis on anomalous experiences could, however, be rather problematic for the model if only because there may be no clear means of determining in advance what constitutes such an experience; rather, it is defined by the person themselves. Maher talks also of 'puzzles', of 'discrepancies between what we expect to observe and what we do observe', but, as Maher is well aware, this still leaves us with the problem of knowing why people react to the same 'puzzle' in such different ways or why what is self-evident or trivial to one person should be puzzling or significant to another. It is difficult to see how this can be understood without reference to other aspects of people's belief systems and life experiences.

More recently, a number of cognitive theories have been suggested which link 'delusions' to social and probabilistic reasoning and to the ability to infer others' intentions. These ideas can only be described briefly here (but see Garety and Freeman, 1999, for a detailed review). The theories do, however, raise important issues for the study of 'delusions' which will be discussed in a later section.

Bentall and colleagues (e.g. Bentall et al., 1991, 1994; Lyon et al., 1994; Kinderman and Bentall, 1996, 1997; Bentall, 1999) have focused mainly on persecutory 'delusions' and have suggested that these function as a defence against an underlying and not explicitly acknowledged negative view of the self. These researchers have drawn on similar earlier ideas from a number of sources including psychoanalytic theory (see, e.g., Zigler and Glick, 1988; Hingley, 1997a), but have framed their research within a cognitive-attribution model. It is suggested that people who hold persecutory 'delusions' are more likely than others to make external attributions for negative events, thus avoiding having to confront potentially threatening discrepancies between perceptions of actual and ideal self. This tendency is not assumed to be absolute; as Lyon et al. (1994) have pointed out, it is widely observed in non-psychiatric groups. It is, however, presumed to operate to a greater extent in 'paranoid' groups. More specifically, it is suggested that people said to have persecutory delusions will be more likely to attribute the causes of negative events to other people (i.e. external personal attributions) rather than to external circumstances. These researchers have also made a number of complex predictions about the relationships of overt and covert views of the self and about the relationship amongst different 'versions' of the self, such as actual and ideal selves, reflecting their view of persecutory 'delusions' as functioning to defend against low self-esteem.

A second set of theories – not necessarily incompatible with those just described – implicates probabilistic reasoning as one factor in the development and maintenance of 'delusions' (e.g. Huq et al., 1988; Garety, 1991; Garety and Hemsley, 1994; Dudley et al., 1997a; Fear and Healy, 1997). It is suggested that people who are 'deluded' may reach conclusions from evidence, or gather information, or test hypotheses, in ways that are different from 'normal' groups. It is particularly suggested that 'deluded' people may 'jump to conclusions'; that is, draw conclusions on the basis of inadequate evidence. These theories have been tested mainly using reasoning tasks unconnected with the content of delusions.

Finally, Frith (1992) and Corcoran et al. (1995) have noted that 'delusions' of persecution and reference, almost by definition, involve misinterpretation of another person's behaviour or intentions. They have argued, rather more contentiously, that these 'symptoms' arise 'as a result of a deficit in a system which enables us to infer what is in the minds of other people' (Corcoran et al., 1995: 6). Tests of the theory involve tasks – often called theory of mind tasks – but again unconnected with 'delusional' content, which ask people about a story character's beliefs or intentions; in more complex tasks, participants are asked about a story character's beliefs about the beliefs or intentions of someone else.

The results of attempts to test these psychological theories of 'delusions' are very mixed. There is some evidence that people said to have persecutory delusions are more likely than non-psychiatric groups to attribute negative events, imagined as happening to the self, to external causes. These results, however, have been obtained using a questionnaire (The Attributional Style Questionnaire) whose reliability is unsatisfactory. There is also no widely agreed method of measuring this 'external bias' and results may depend on the method of measurement. Using a questionnaire with more satisfactory reliability (The Internal Personal and Situational Attributions Questionnaire), Kinderman and Bentall (1997) were unable to replicate the finding that 'paranoid' psychiatric groups had a general 'external bias'; they did, however, report that people said to have persecutory delusions were more likely than non-psychiatric groups to make attributions to other people for negative events, imagined as happening to the self, rather than to circumstances or situations. It is also not clear whether any 'external bias' is specific to persecutory 'delusions'; again the results are mixed (Fear et al., 1996; Sharp et al., 1997). As to whether persecutory 'delusions' serve a defensive function in protecting self-esteem, Garety and Freeman (1999) have provided a very fair assessment of the evidence, highlighting not only inconsistent results but also the considerable difficulties of testing this hypothesis within an experimental framework. Their conclusion that the defensive function may apply to some people said to have persecutory 'delusion' may be the best that can be said at the moment.

It is easier to present the results of studies of probabilistic reasoning and 'delusions' if I first briefly describe the tasks typically used in this research. Participants are usually presented with two sources of information (e.g. two jars with coloured beads; two lists of names of pupils at two schools, etc.). For each source, participants are told the ratio of contents (e.g. jar 1 = 60:40 red to green beads; jar 2 = 40:60 red to green; school 1 = 80:20 girls to boys; school 2 = 20:80 girls to boys). The researcher then removes the source from view and presents, one at a time, a pre-set sequence of beads, names, etc. from one of the sources only. The participant's task is to decide from which of the two sources the sequence of beads, names, etc. is being drawn. The task ends when the decision is made and the researcher records both the number of trials ('draws to decision') and whether the decision was correct. In a variant of this task, participants may be given a fixed number of trials in which a sequence is built up, again from one source only, and asked at each stage in the sequence to estimate the probability that the beads/names are from, for example, the 20:80 source or the 80:20 one (see, e.g., Dudley *et al.*, 1997a; Young and Bentall, 1997a; Linney *et al.*, 1998 for examples of these and other reasoning tasks).

The results of this research are fairly consistent. Studies using 'draws to decision' – that is, the number of trials before someone decides which source the beads, names, etc. are being drawn from – report that the group said to have delusions (usually diagnosed as schizophrenia or delusional disorder) makes the decision after significantly fewer trials than non-psychiatric and, usually, other psychiatric groups. (It is the group scores which differ here, not the scores of every individual.) The results of studies using other reasoning tasks, however, are much less consistent. For example, when participants are given a fixed number of trials and asked at each stage in the sequence to estimate the probability of the bead/name etc. being drawn from a particular source, then the performance of groups of people said to be deluded is not consistently different from that of non-psychiatric groups. Similarly, Bentall and Young (1996) found no evidence of what they called abnormal hypothesis testing strategies in people said to be deluded. As Garety and Freeman (1999) have pointed out, there is no evidence that 'deluded' people have an absolute deficit in reasoning; their performance, or, more accurately, the performance of some of them, on some reasoning tasks does appear to differ from that of non-psychiatric and some psychiatric groups, but the interpretation of these data is still open to question.

The final psychological theory suggested that 'delusions' of persecution and reference arose from a deficit in a system which enables us to infer what is in the minds of other people. This theory, however, has received little support. Instead, performance on tasks said to measure this deficit appears to be related to a range of factors, including diagnoses of depression and anxiety, a diagnosis of schizophrenia, especially with 'negative symptoms' and general cognitive functioning (e.g. Corcoran *et al.*, 1997; Langdon *et al.*, 1997; Mitchley *et al.*, 1998).

Several writers have commented on the problems and limitations of research designed to test these cognitive theories of 'delusions' (e.g. Bentall, 1999; Garety and Freeman, 1999; Birchwood, 1999). Five major problems have been highlighted. There are, first, many potentially important variables in these studies whose contribution to task performance is not clear. For example, there is a marked bias to male participants in the 'deluded' groups, while performance on some probabilistic reasoning and 'theory of mind' tasks may vary with IQ. Scores on depression inventories, when reported, also tend to be higher in groups said to be deluded than in non-psychiatric control groups. Interestingly, scores on anxiety scales are almost never reported, nor are people with a diagnosis of anxiety disorder usually used as controls, in spite of Garety *et al.*'s (1991) report that the performance of an anxious control group on a probabilistic reasoning task was not significantly different from that of a group said to have delusional disorder. Similarly, the possible effects of medication on these tasks has not been systematically studied.

A second, and closely related, problem concerns the resulting heterogeneity within experimental and control groups, as well as possible overlap between them. Groups said to be deluded (the experimental group) may have a variety of psychiatric diagnoses, but other 'symptoms' they may have which could influence performance on cognitive tasks are rarely reported. Of particular concern is the lack of control groups of people diagnosed as schizophrenic who are not judged to be deluded. Allocation to the experimental group may also be based on psychiatric judgements of unknown reliability, while different studies may focus on different types of 'delusion'. The psychometric properties of the tasks and measures used in the research present a third problem. I have already mentioned this in relation to some attribution questionnaires, but, as Bentall (1999) has pointed out, the psychometric properties of many reasoning and 'theory of mind' tasks have hardly been investigated.

There is, fourth, the problem of what has become known as the multidimensional nature of 'delusions'. Rather than being static beliefs, either present or absent, 'delusions' are now said to vary along several (possibly independent) dimensions such as conviction, preoccupation and distress. Inevitably, this would lead to even greater (uninvestigated) heterogeneity in research groups said to be deluded. Finally, the research uses cross-sectional designs which study associations amongst variables and not antecedent–consequent relationships. As Garety and Freeman (1999) point out, the processes examined may act as antecedents, maintaining factors or consequences, or, they might have added, as all three; there is no easy way of clarifying this point within a cross-sectional design. The issue is highlighted by the fact that when 'deluded' groups are said to be in remission, their performance on some of the tasks used in this research may be similar to non-psychiatric groups (Birchwood, 1999; Garety and Freeman, 1999).

Several solutions to these problems or, at least, ways forward, have been suggested. These include more precise specification of sample characteristics, including delusional content and position on delusional dimensions; further investigation of psychometric properties of tasks and of the constructs they claim to measure; systematic study of the contribution of variables such as IQ, depression and medication; clarification of the aetiological status of the processes studied, possibly through the use of longitudinal studies and non-clinical groups said to be high on delusional ideation; attempts to specify more precisely the relationships amongst the variables and processes studied, possibly through the use of mathematical models (Bentall, 1999; Garety and Freeman, 1999). The aim is to develop a multifactorial account of 'delusions' which can specify with more precision 'which processes are likely to be active in which people with delusions' (Garety and Freeman, 1999: 148).

These suggestions for progress make very good sense within what might be called the assumptive framework which underlies most psychological research on 'delusions'. But they leave the framework itself unexamined or even unarticulated; instead, research procedures and proposed solutions to research problems appear simply as taken for granted rather than as being derived from a set of implicit assumptions about people, their behaviour, and how they should be studied.

### Investigating 'delusions' – some assumptions, problems and alternatives

Much of the recent psychological research on 'delusions' is informed by the same implicit framework as the research I discussed earlier on hallucinations. Such research is characterised by the search for a general, underlying defect, trait or attribute which is posed by or is characteristic of 'deluded' people and is implicated in the development of their 'delusions'. Research participants are thus given tasks unrelated to their beliefs, which are assumed to measure particular intra-psychic attributes, with the aim of demonstrating significant differences in the 'amount' of the attribute possessed by 'deluded' and non-deluded groups. This framework is borrowed directly from medicine, and, as in medicine, involves the implicit assumption that researchers are studying the *antecedents* of 'delusions'. It is interesting that researchers occasionally comment that their experimental designs do not necessarily allow conclusions about causes of 'delusions'. What is notable, however, is that the caution has to be given at all. The fact that it has, clearly highlights the default assumption, very apparent in the literature, that researchers are actually studying the antecedents of 'delusions'.

The following sections will focus on some of the restrictions this framework potentially places on the study and understanding of 'delusions' and will suggest some ways of broadening the research. It is important to emphasise that it is not a matter of dismissing research which is based on a medically derived model. On the contrary, the research has highlighted processes, such as how people account for positive and negative events, how they interpret others' intentions, how they gather evidence for particular conclusions likely to be extremely important in the development and maintenance of belief claims. I would argue, however, that it is the unarticulated assumptions of the model on which the research is based that are problematic in this context, and which seriously restrict both the conduct of research and the interpretation of its results.

## MEASURING VARIABLES MORE PRECISELY

I noted earlier that some researchers had commented on the unsatisfactory psychometric qualities of tests and measures used in psychological research on 'delusions'. The answer is usually assumed to be the development of more precise and reliable measures of inferred internal processes or attributes assumed to be implicated in 'delusions' such as attribution style or self-esteem. The problem, however, is arguably more fundamental than this and arises from the assumption, which I queried in Chapter 7, that we 'possess' specific intrapsychic attributes or processes which manifest themselves through performance on tests, questionnaires and experimental procedures and which can be precisely quantified and measured through these means in much the same way as we might measure heart rhythm or blood glucose. Inevitably, because the assumption is problematic, measurement of these assumed attributes and processes is also problematic. But this assumption about intra-psychic attributes and their potential for precise measurement means that, for example, when two forms of a questionnaire purporting to measure 'attribution style' turn out to have very little shared variance (see Lyon *et al.*, 1994), or when researchers disagree on how to measure 'external bias', it seems to suggest a need to find the most reliable and accurate measure of these characteristics, rather than suggesting a need to re-examine our assumptions about intra-psychic processes. More naturalistic studies of people's attempts to account for particular events (which is what attribution questionnaires ask them to do) suggest, however, that people use a variety of rhetorical strategies which cannot easily be accommodated within the idea of a stable attribution style, and which cannot easily be 'measured' via closed questionnaires (e.g. Potter and Reicher, 1987; Gill, 1993). Similarly, 'self-esteem', which persecutory 'delusions' are hypothesised to protect, turns out to be a problematic concept when viewed from constructionist perspectives on the self (e.g. Sampson, 1989; Davies and Harré, 1990) and not one whose problems can be dealt with by seeking a more accurate or reliable measure. It is precisely because concepts like these are so problematic, and because they have been inferred on inadequate conceptual and empirical grounds, that researchers seem unable to find the 'right' measure or at least one which would meet the standards we impose on measures of physical or biological attributes. In other words, the psychometric problems which attend psychological research on 'delusions' are not a temporary blip, a sign that researchers need to increase their efforts at precise measurement, but an inevitable and permanent result of the unarticulated conceptual foundations of the research. If we add to this the perceived need to control for a host of variables which might influence scores in any test or questionnaire, and which themselves may be conceptually problematic (e.g. IQ, depression, anxiety), then we face not the gradual accumulation of knowledge through increased precision but increasing diversity, inconsistency and fragmentation.

## ESSENTIALISING 'DELUSIONS'

The starting point of most psychological research on 'delusions' is a group of people within psychiatric services identified as 'deluded'. Indeed, this group is frequently referred to, without qualification or comment, as 'the deluded group'. Such language and research practices create the impression of 'delusions' or 'the deluded' as natural categories, forms of what Harper (1999) has called pure pathology, capable of separate, objective study. Frith (1999) presents an extreme form of this essentialising tendency when he talks of 'acquiring clues for the brain systems underlying true and false beliefs' (320). But if we return to Heise's (1988) point, then we are reminded that 'delusion' is *always* a social and relational judgement: a 'delusion' only 'officially' comes into being when a speaker and a more powerful hearer disagree about a belief claim; to study one side of this interaction or to reify its result as a characteristic of one participant is like trying to understand a marriage by studying only one of the partners. We cannot get round this problem by saying that the speaker is obviously expressing an absurd or false belief which others do not share; this simply returns us to the problems I discussed earlier and, indeed, by that standard most of us would qualify at one time or another as participants in a 'deluded' research group. Nor do we necessarily avoid essentialising 'delusions' by adopting a 'multidimensional' approach. It has been suggested (see Strauss, 1969; Chadwick and Lowe, 1990; Garety and Hemsley, 1994; Garety and Freeman, 1999) that 'delusions' are not static, unitary beliefs but may vary along a number of important dimensions, such as conviction, preoccupation and distress, which will vary both within and between those said to be deluded. These ideas have the potential to broaden our understanding of 'delusions' in a very constructive way. The problem, however, has been the tendency to essentialise and reify the dimensions, to see them as attributes of the belief or the person, capable of objective measurement through questions such as 'How strongly do you believe this to be true?' or 'How much do you think about it?', with the answers measured on five- or seven-point scales. But as Gergen (1999) has pointed out, we do not consult an internal scale and read off a score in pre-set units when asked questions like these about what we believe.

Responses to such questions must therefore be produced in a more complex and obscure way. Georgaca (2000), for example, has argued that 'conviction' is not an attribute of a belief, nor an internal state of certainty concerning the truth of a statement, but is a rhetorical effect of the actions of defending and negotiating the belief claim with others. We might, alternatively, see statements about 'conviction' as related to the threat presented by the 'loss' of the belief, which in turn is related to the circumstances of people's lives (Roberts, 1991). Similarly, statements about 'preoccupation' may be a function of how far a belief claim is shared and integrated into relationships and action. The more someone's belief is shared by others, the more it is integrated into day-to-day life, the fewer threats are presented to it, then the less the person may judge themselves to think about or be preoccupied by it. Finally, statements about distress may be related to the content of beliefs – for example, believing you are being threatened by others – but many 'delusions' have a positive content and distress may then be related to difficulties in persuading others to accept that the belief is true, or to other negative reactions.

What we think of as belief dimensions, then, may be seen as constructed through interaction, rather than being inherent, measurable qualities of beliefs or of those who express them. It is not that they are unimportant in understanding belief claims which come to be called 'delusions' – far from it – but they may benefit from being conceptualised differently.

It is also worth noting here research which has failed to find any significant difference in ratings of belief conviction (and other belief dimensions) between psychiatric and non-psychiatric groups. Peters *et al.* (1999b), for example, found no significant difference in 'delusional ideation' scores on the Peters *et al.* Delusions Inventory (PDI[3]), between a psychiatric group said to be deluded and a group of adherents to several religious movements outside the mainstream. The groups also did not differ in how true they thought their endorsed beliefs to be. The groups did differ, however, in distress associated with their beliefs and in how much they reported thinking about them. Similarly, Jones and Watson (1997) found no significant differences on nine of twelve 'belief dimensions', including conviction, impact on thinking, impact on behaviour, strength of feeling evoked, and importance to the person, between a group of 'schizophrenics' said to be deluded and a group who held mainstream Christian beliefs and attended church regularly. Peters *et al.* (1999a) also reported considerable overlap between a psychiatric group with 'delusions' and a non-psychiatric group, in the range of overall scores on the PDI and on scales of conviction, preoccupation and distress related to these beliefs. Ten per cent of the general population group had higher mean scores on the PDI than the psychiatric in-patient group. Peters *et al.* rightly emphasise the extent to which these data raise problems for any attempt to

3  The PDI asks questions such as 'Do you ever feel that electrical devices such as computers can influence the way you think?' and 'Do your thoughts ever feel alien to you in some way?'

make categorical or qualitative distinctions between 'normal' and 'deluded' beliefs. Unfortunately, however, there is still a tendency to essentialism: Peters *et al.* (1999b), for example, argue that what determines whether *a person will become overtly deluded* (my emphasis) rests on more than just having had some kind of experience or mental event, but will also partly depend on the strength of the interpretation, its emotional impact and how much one thinks about it (562). Similarly, it is claimed that it is where one is placed on these kinds of dimensions which 'make the belief pathological' (1999a: 93) and that 'it is imperative to incorporate dimensions of belief strength, preoccupation and distress in our psychometric measures because they are likely to determine *where individuals lie on the continuum from psychological health to mental illness*' (1999b: 555; my emphasis). Thus, where one is placed on these dimensions is assumed to provide insights into inherent characteristics of the individual (whether they are mentally ill) or of their beliefs (whether they are pathological). An alternative conceptualisation, using very different language, would focus on the complex social processes which produce what we have chosen to call conviction, preoccupation and distress, how these are 'acted out' in a way which disturbs the person themselves and/or others, and how an initial belief claim is transformed into the official judgement of delusion and to psychiatric patienthood (see Greenberg *et al.*, 1992; and Johnstone, 2000, for further discussion of this latter process).

## CONSTRUCTING A PATHOLOGICAL 'DELUDED' SUBJECT

In discussing hallucinations, I mentioned the very negative language used in some research on hearing voices. The same tendency is unfortunately evident in the literature on 'delusions'. For example, as I said earlier, research participants are routinely referred to as 'the deluded group' as if this were a straightforward aspect of their identity; they are also said to have pathological beliefs, to make excessively external attributions for negative events; to have an abnormal self-serving bias; to show hastiness in decision-making and to jump to conclusions. In addition, and similarly to research on hearing voices, there is a tendency to use aggregated group data on task performance as if it applied to every 'deluded' individual. (Exceptionally, Peters and her colleagues have consistently emphasised the extensive overlap in scores between groups said to be deluded and non-psychiatric groups.)

These practices help create the impression of a naturally separate, homogeneous group, objectively identified as deluded and afflicted with additional deviant tendencies redolent of the irrationality so strongly associated with modern views of madness. But what standards are being used here? Who has established, and how, what is a sufficient (non-excessive) amount of external attribution or what is a normal attribution? The problem is highlighted by data from the probabilistic reasoning task I described earlier, where participants have to decide from which of two sources a sequence of beads/names, etc.

is being drawn. 'Deluded' participants have been said to 'jump to conclusions' on this task; that is, to name the source after being shown fewer beads, names, etc., than non-psychiatric controls. But as Maher (1992) has pointed out, this practice leads to very few errors *and* may represent more optimal statistical reasoning; one of the reasons for group differences in this task is that many 'normal' people take more trials to reach a decision than is actually statistically necessary. Several researchers have noted this point but it does not seem to prevent those called 'deluded' from being depicted more negatively than 'normal' research participants, who are said to be conservative or over-cautious, rather than, say, slow or sluggish or indecisive. Garety and Freeman (1999) claim that people with delusions have a data-gathering bias, but so too do 'normal' controls although their bias is never described in quite the same negative way.

It is not a matter here of criticising researchers, who often also provide more neutral accounts of their work. But the fact that negative evaluative language so often accompanies more neutral accounts emphasises the power of the implicit, medically derived model which underlies the research. This model routinely uses negative evaluative language to refer to 'symptoms' and the bodily processes associated with them. This is arguably of no great concern when virtually everyone, including the afflicted person, agrees that a bodily process associated with their symptoms has been identified, that it and the symptoms are negative and that they wish to be rid of them. But the language may matter a great deal when there is no such agreed identification of an 'underlying process' or agreement on how it should be evaluated (*Do* we have an 'attribution style'? *Do* 'deluded' people make 'excessively' external attributions? Is it obvious what should be done about the 'symptoms'?). Such language, which interprets difference from an unstated standard as deficiency, obscures the judgemental aspects of the research process and the power relationships involved – researchers have far more power to create negative identities for their participants than vice versa. And by appearing to refer to inherently negative internal processes when it is actually talking about behaviour which deviates from an implicit standard, such language creates the impression that researchers have discovered something more fundamentally deviant about an already deviant person. It also creates the impression that research progress will be made by focusing on the person, their abnormalities and biases, rather than on the conditions of their lives. And constructing a pathological subject obscures the possibility that progress in understanding what we think of as delusions might lie not only in the study of those called 'deluded' but also in the study of those who impose such judgements.

## THE FUNCTIONS OF 'DELUSIONS'

Because the framework which underlies much psychological research on delusions was developed for the study of bodily processes, it cannot deal well with the possible social and psychological functions of 'delusions' or with the ways such beliefs may be seen as coherent, if obscure, systems of meaning. But if we move away from this framework, and see belief claims which come to be called 'delusions' as something a person *does* or constructs, rather than something they have, then the issues of function and meaning become as important as for any other form of behaviour.

One exception to the neglect of function is the work of Bentall and colleagues, based on the hypothesis that persecutory delusions function to protect covert low self-esteem. As I mentioned earlier, however, the results of often ingenious attempts to test this hypothesis have been inconsistent. But I would argue that this may have much to do with trying to squeeze the study of functions into a framework not well equipped to accommodate it and with the assumption that we possess a discrete measurable attribute called 'self-esteem', rather than with deficiencies in the idea of 'delusions' serving psychological functions. It would be unfortunate if the demands of an inappropriate framework led to the abandonment of a potentially valuable idea which focuses our attention on the active, purposive nature of belief claims.

Roberts (1991) has adopted a rather different approach to the study of the possible functions of 'delusional' beliefs. Using the 'Purpose in Life' test and the 'Life Regard Index', he reported no significant differences between a psychiatric group judged to have long-standing delusions (of more than two years), and a group of Anglican ordinands. There were, however, significant differences in the scores of the group said to be deluded and a psychiatric group who had previously expressed 'delusional' beliefs but were now said to be in remission, with the 'still deluded' group scoring more highly (i.e. positively). We must, of course, be careful about reifying ideas like meaning and purpose in life; Roberts also found, however, that the 'remitted' group scored significantly higher than the 'still deluded' group on an item asking about suicide intent, as well as on the Beck Depression Inventory. Even if we take these data only descriptively, they are intriguing and disturbing, suggesting as they do that a group judged to be chronically deluded are in some ways better off, psychological speaking, than a group said to be in remission. There may, of course, be many reasons for this, including reduced professional support or social contact, or increased social demands for the 'remitted' group. Interviews with the 'still deluded' group, however, suggest that at least one reason for the difference could lie in the positive functions potentially served by 'delusional' beliefs in the context of particular life circumstances. For example, each of the group gave very negative responses to the question 'What was your life like before you had these beliefs?' with themes of loneliness, inferiority, hopelessness, purposelessness and broken relationships. By contrast, responses to the question 'What is life like with these beliefs?' were overwhelmingly positive, including alleviation from fear and worry, freedom and protection from past hurts and a new sense of identity. But when asked to imagine life without their (deluded) beliefs, the group again gave strongly negative responses, envisaging an empty, futile and bleak existence. One man who had believed himself to be the Messiah, 'recovered' during the study and described the contrast:

> I liked to imagine [being the Messiah] because I felt so useless without it . . . I still feel inadequate now – it's as though I don't know anything. I always felt everything I said was worthless, but as Jesus everything I said was important – it came from God . . . I just want to hide away, I don't feel able to cope with people . . . I always feel lonely, I don't know what to say.
>
> (Roberts, 1991: 26)

Roberts has suggested that what we call delusions may be an adaptive response to whatever initiates the 'psychotic breakdown', a process 'of attributing meaning to experience through which order and security are gained' (1991: 20). Jackson and Fulford (1997a) have put forward a similar argument: that 'psychotic symptoms' may be seen as providing highly personal insights or solutions to life problems at a time of intense stress; it is the extent to which the person, and those around them, are able to use the 'insight' constructively which may partly determine whether they become a psychiatric patient. Roberts's study, however, also raises serious questions about the goals of intervention for psychosis as well as the question of why, if 'delusional' beliefs serve such important functions, they are ever abandoned, at least before alternative sources of reward are available. But before we invoke 'recovery from illness', it is worth noting that the phenomenon of 'unwilled' loss of important and cherished beliefs (loss of faith) has long been a subject of religious writings.

It is exceptionally difficult to incorporate this kind of analysis into a framework which seeks internal abnormalities to explain surface 'symptoms'. But an analysis involving function and life circumstances is not incompatible in principle with research on attribution and reasoning, providing the research is not seen as a neutral search for 'abnormal' stable and general underlying structures and intra-psychic processes. This point leads directly to the final problem or limitation I want to discuss, which faces much psychological research on 'delusions': the neglect of social context.

## DE-EMPHASISING AND EMPHASISING SOCIAL CONTEXT

Researchers de-emphasise the role of social context in 'delusions' in several ways, including providing little or no information on participants' backgrounds or circumstances and by using 'neutral' tasks which are not specifically related to the person's belief systems, in order to demonstrate that any bias or difference is 'generalized and pervasive' (Dudley et al., 1997b: 576). Social context is also minimised in the limited choice of variables suggested as important in accounting for 'delusions'. Garety and Freeman (1999), for example, suggest that 'delusions' probably develop against a background of 'a person's existing personality and beliefs and as a result of a combination of alterations or biases in perception, affect and judgement' (150).

The resulting focus on the individual and their assumed internal attributes at the expense of their life circumstances and relationships, raises a number of issues. One involves the possible social consequences of this research bias. If we study the individual in order to discover 'generalised and pervasive' differences from others, and these are interpreted negatively, then we make it easier to construct a pathological subject in the way I discussed earlier. But this then makes it seem more reasonable to continue studying the 'abnormal' individual in order to gain a better understanding of their 'abnormalities'. It is not inevitable that we do this, but it is an extremely strong tradition within psychology (Albee, 1986; Fox and Prilleltensky, 1997); the point is that the focus on the individual is made to seem reasonable by certain research assumptions and linguistic practices, rather than because it has been shown to be the most useful way of understanding behaviour. But such a focus has social consequences, one of which may be to protect from scrutiny the harmful actions of more powerful or privileged others. Birchwood (1999), for example, reminds us that many people called 'psychotic' have been sexually abused; as we saw in the section on hallucinations, other forms of abuse and neglect may also be implicated in 'psychotic symptoms'. Similarly, demographic research suggests that those said to have paranoid delusions are more likely than those given other psychiatric diagnoses to be of low social class, to have had limited education or to be immigrants (Harper, 1999); it is worth noting that the direction of effect, often assumed to be from psychosis to low social status, is by no means settled (Link et al., 1986; Muntaner et al., 1991).

The lack of attention to social context also raises questions about the interpretation of research data. For example, the probabilistic reasoning tasks described earlier also have a social element in that they require interaction between research and participant. Not only that, but in the version of the task claimed to show 'jumping to conclusions' by 'deluded' people, the sooner the participant reaches a conclusion, the sooner the test and the interaction is likely to end. Because researchers in this area rarely discuss the social aspects of their experimental tasks or provide information on social anxiety, it is difficult to know how relevant this is. Milton et al. (1978), however, reported an extremely high mean score on a social anxiety questionnaire for a psychiatric group said to be deluded. Garety et al. (1991) also reported that an anxious control group did not differ from a group with a diagnosis of delusional disorder in terms of 'jumping to conclusions' in a reasoning task. It has also been noted that both psychiatric and non-psychiatric research groups reach conclusions more quickly in these tasks when dealing with emotionally salient and self-referential material. But rather than seeing this as indicating that 'the delusional system may predispose [deluded] people to find personal significance in even neutral stimuli' (Dudley et al., 1997b: 583), we could see it as a reminder that even tasks which researchers call neutral involve social elements which might be more threatening or upsetting for those with the most serious psychiatric diagnoses.

But as well as raising questions about the social consequences of theories and the interpretation of research data, the neglect of social context potentially limits our understanding of 'delusional' beliefs. We have already seen this in relation to the ideas of conviction, preoccupation and distress and in relation to the possible functions of 'delusions'; the possibility that people called 'deluded' may have serious social difficulties also draws our attention to context. Roberts (1991) has made a crucial point which may be true by definition, but whose significance may be overlooked: that the person committed to a delusional world-view is strikingly alone. As Roberts puts it, 'delusions' involve seemingly ignoring the 'facts and reality of [your] neighbour and build[ing] for [yourself] a private world more conducive to [your] security and satisfaction' (21). Very aversive experiences with other people or the lack of social, psychological or economic resources to build a satisfying shared 'reality' could make this outcome more likely. But social isolation could also foster 'reasoning biases' which all of us show, especially when, it could be argued, we are anxious or under threat (and see Birchwood, 1999), but which may be 'corrected' or at least challenged when we share our beliefs and conclusions with others. Johnson (1988) has also suggested that the less time we spend in social interaction, the more time we spend with self-generated processes, perhaps with thinking repeatedly about particular events. This could lead to overestimating the frequency or significance of an event or make the event readily available for recall so that it exerts special influence over the interpretation of future events. Alternatively, particular interpretations of events may seem more true (carry more conviction) the more often they are rehearsed. Any of these processes could lead to or maintain idiosyncratic beliefs. It is not, then, a question of whether reasoning or attribution processes are implicated in the development of 'delusions', but of how we conceptualise these processes and whether it is helpful to talk of 'pervasive reasoning biases' or 'abnormal attributions' as if they were free-standing attributes of the individual capable of being studied or understood separately from either the content or context of belief claims.

In the final section, I want to take the issue of social context a little further and look at 'attribution' as a cultural rather than an individual phenomenon. I shall also return to the crucial point that 'delusions' can only exist officially as the outcome of a social interaction between two people of unequal power.

Kinderman and Bentall (1997) have provided preliminary evidence that, in comparison with a non-patient sample, a 'paranoid' group made more external-person (as distinct from external-circumstance) causal attributions for vignettes of negative social events. We might see this as indicating a particular kind of attribution or reasoning bias 'in' the group said to be deluded. Looked at in another way, however, the practice of making external-personal or 'other-blaming' attributions for negative events is a pervasive and important aspect of hierarchically organised societies and is systematically used by dominant groups to retain status and to discredit subordinate groups. Feminist scholars (e.g. French, 1986; Lerner, 1986) have documented the myriad ways this 'attribution bias' has been used in patriarchal societies against women – who have themselves been encouraged to adopt the opposite, internal bias – in contexts as diverse as Greek mythology, the Judaeo-Christian creation story, witchcraft trials and in modern 'rape myths'. It is, of course, not only women who may be the objects of this 'attribution bias'; disadvantaged groups throughout history have found themselves targets of blame by dominant groups for important negative outcomes; and, as Billig (1991) has noted, other-blaming stances are often used to help mobilise political and military groups.

An individual preference for external-person attributions in the face of negative outcomes, as measured by an attributions questionnaire, might therefore be conceptualised not so much as a psychological abnormality, or as a tendency to make excessively external attributions, or as an inherent attribute of people diagnosed as having paranoid delusions; instead, such attributions can be seen as reflecting a widely available aspect of our social accounting repertoire, more likely to be used under threat, and more readily accessible by dominant groups. But individuals or groups in positions of great power can adopt a persistent other-blaming stance without being called 'deluded', at least, as Harper (1999) has noted, by those who matter, or, he might have added, without appearing as participants in a study of 'delusions'. Indeed, social power may be gained by persistently making external attributions, provided these are of value to others. We might argue, then, that it is not a matter of those with (paranoid) 'delusions' having reasoning or attributional biases which differentiate them from the rest of us, but that when people with little social power persistently draw on a widely available and systematically used repertoire of accounting for negative outcomes, *and reach implausible conclusions which have no social value and which they cannot impose on others*, then they run the risk of being called 'deluded'.

Looking at attribution as a cultural as well as an individual phenomenon could help clarify a little-commented-on but quite striking feature of psychological research on 'delusions' – the consistent bias to male participants. An unselected sample of twelve papers (the first to hand), showed 135 male psychiatric participants with 'delusions' and forty-seven female, with all papers showing a bias to males. Interestingly, only one paper commented on the bias but could offer no explanation; two further papers did not mention the sex distribution of their participants, and none of the papers gave the distribution in the abstract, suggesting that it was not seen as important. Of course, it may not be meaningful other than in reflecting idiosyncratic recruitment practices or willingness to volunteer. But the male bias is very consistent and is not found in research on hallucinations: an unselected sample of twelve papers showed 178 male and 189 female voice-hearers in psychiatric groups; adding those few studies which use non-psychiatric voice-hearers produced 204 males and 258 females.

Let us assume for the moment that the discrepancy is meaningful and recall that it has arisen from research biased to the study of persecutory 'delusions' with which 'other blaming' may be associated. Such attributions may be more readily accessible by men in male-dominated cultures, even when otherwise they have little social power. This does not necessarily imply a sex difference on performance on 'neutral' attribution tasks; as Birchwood (1999) points out, it is when people are under stress or threat that such 'biases' may become apparent. Alternatively, the higher proportion of men in 'delusions' research may be related to Roberts's (1991) point that the 'deluded' person is strikingly alone. In Western culture at least, personal independence, autonomy and lack of connection to others are far more strongly associated with males than females. Thus the isolation which may both foster and result from beliefs which are not shared by others, represents less of a deviation from social norms, and therefore a more likely occurrence, for males than for females.

Another way of looking at the male–female discrepancy in the research literature on 'delusions', and again bearing in mind the research focus on paranoid beliefs, returns us to the issue of 'delusion' as a social judgement. Harper (1999) has emphasised the close links in the public mind between paranoia, violence and maleness, to the point where the sex of a 'paranoid schizophrenic' is not directly mentioned unless she is female. Harper has also emphasised the role of the perceived likelihood of acting on a belief claim in professional judgements of delusion; if men are seen as more likely to be violent then this could contribute to an excess of males said to have paranoid delusions. To complicate matters further, however, Harper also noted that at least some men's size and strength appeared to be used as one factor in constructing their persecutory fears as implausible and, therefore, delusional.

These arguments are speculative but they remind us that 'delusion' is a social construct and not an inherent property of a belief. They also emphasise again the potential pitfalls of attempting to demarcate a group which has enduringly different cognitive characteristics from 'normal' people and which can be studied independently of social context.

### The development and maintenance of delusions: an overview

The study of 'delusional' beliefs as attempts to explain events and experiences, involving 'ordinary' reasoning processes, represents very significant progress from their conceptualisation as meaningless symptoms of schizophrenia or mental illness. Much of the research, however, has retained major elements of the traditional model but without explicit acknowledgement or justification. These elements include a continued reliance on psychiatric diagnosis to define people as 'deluded', a practice which reinforces a view of delusions as a natural and not a socially constructed category; they also include an intense focus on the individual with little reference to their life experiences or context and, with the exception of Bentall and colleagues, a neglect of the content and function of 'delusional' beliefs. And, by focusing so strongly on the individual, psychological and psychiatric research have neglected the other half of the 'delusion' equation – the processes and people by which belief claims are transformed to 'delusions'.

A reconceptualisation which emphasises the social nature of 'delusions' also suggests a wider range of research questions and participants. For example:

1   How do people develop, maintain and discard whatever are thought of as implausible or bizarre beliefs? (In which case we need to cast the net wider than psychiatric groups and the devoutly religious and consider who should have the power to define 'implausible'.)
2   How do people develop and maintain highly personalised beliefs which are not shared by and are of no value to others? (In which case we need to ask questions about social relationships, social isolation and the personal functions of belief claims.)
3   How do people's reasoning and attribution processes change under stress or threat? (In which case we need to study the nature of the stress or threat in order to understand its links to particular belief claims.)
4   How are belief claims 'officially' transformed to delusions and patienthood? (In which case we need to study how the claim is acted out, how it is judged and assessed, how it is associated with distress and with disruption to social and personal behaviour and how others participate in these processes.)

## Psychological interventions for 'delusions' and voice-hearing

Attempts to alter 'delusions' and hallucinations, or, simply, madness, by psychological means have a long history (see, e.g., Chapter 2 of this book; Beck, 1952; Ayllon and Azrin, 1968; Ullman and Krasner, 1969; Falloon *et al.*, 1984; Slade and Bentall, 1988; Hingley, 1997a, 1997b; Haddock *et al.*, 1998b; Liberman *et al.*, 1998; Leudar and Thomas, 2000). The focus here, however, will be on interventions which have come to be known as cognitive-behavioural therapy (CBT). This is partly because a detailed discussion of all non-medical interventions is beyond the scope of this chapter; but there are several other reasons for this focus. First, CBT is now the most popular mainstream non-medical approach and has produced an extensive literature including several randomised controlled trials. Second, the results of this approach are of particular interest because, in common with psychodynamic approaches (Hingley, 1997a, 1997b), they reverse traditional psychiatric thinking on the wisdom and utility of encouraging 'psychotic' people to talk directly about their experiences and beliefs; third, CBT raises important issues of theory and practice which arguably have not been adequately addressed in the literature. Finally, the present popularity of CBT recalls earlier moments in the history of psychological interventions for madness. It is therefore important to place this approach in a historical and social context, not least to ask what lessons might be learned from the history of psychological approaches to the treatment of madness.

### Cognitive-behavioural therapy: descriptions and outcomes

The term 'CBT' covers a very wide range of interventions; Wykes *et al.* (1998) suggested that there were at least fifteen possible options. The relationship of these procedures to theory is also varied. Chadwick *et al.* (1996) suggest that the only common attribute of different forms of cognitive therapy may be a commitment to cognitive mediation, or the assumption that our responses to events are mediated by thoughts, images and beliefs. This, of course, only covers the 'cognitive' side of therapy; the 'behavioural' aspect may involve rather different and possibly conflicting assumptions (e.g. Coyne, 1982; Haage *et al.*, 1991) and the precise ways in which the two parts co-exist have yet to be fully addressed. Researchers/practitioners also appear not fully to agree about the basis of cognitive or cognitive-behavioural therapy. For example, Alford and Beck (1994) claim that 'cognitive therapy is guided by the cognitive *theory* of psychopathology rather than the application of techniques' (378), while Kingdon *et al.* (1994) claim that 'cognitive-behavioural *techniques* used in schizophrenia have generally been developed *pragmatically*, in clinical settings' (581; my emphasis). Haddock *et al.* (1998b) point out, further, that some procedures are derived from general psychological theory and note that there is 'considerable blurring and overlap about the putative psychological processes and treatment procedures involved [in the CBT of hallucinations]' (831).

We might see this variety of procedures and theoretical bases as a rich mix of ideas which will not benefit from being prematurely pushed under one label; I am also less concerned here with general theoretical issues of CBT than with specific issues relating to the concept of schizophrenia. For the moment, then, I will simply describe briefly some of the major procedures associated with the terms 'cognitive' and 'cognitive-behavioural therapy', as applied to 'delusions' and hearing voices, before discussing some specific issues raised by them. For hallucinations, the procedures may include the following: (1) Enhancing or adding to strategies already used by people to lessen voice-hearing or its aversiveness (e.g. distraction); modifying environmental stimulation; interfering with sub-vocalisation; activity scheduling and relaxation. (2) Focusing on the experience of voice-hearing (e.g. on the characteristics of voices); identifying antecedents of voice-hearing and developing constructive ways to manage or ameliorate them; relating voice content to the person's thoughts and worries, particularly those which are difficult to discuss; encouraging the person to accept voices as self-generated; linking voices to past aversive experiences. (3) Examining and questioning potentially distressing beliefs associated with voices (e.g. that the voice is all-powerful, or cannot be controlled or must be obeyed).

For 'delusions', cognitive-behavioural interventions may include the following: (1) Identification of events and experiences associated with 'delusional' inferences. (2) Reviewing evidence for beliefs, allowing the person to voice and explore their own doubts. (3) Suggesting consideration of alternative interpretations of events and experiences. (4) 'Testing' interpretations against outcomes using an agreed 'test'. For both voice-hearing and 'delusions', interventions may also involve examination of more general negative beliefs about the self (e.g. 'I deserve to be punished'), as well as discussion of the 'normality' of the person's experience in terms of their physical and psychological state, and circumstances. In addition, three elements have been emphasised: first, the importance of a collaborative, trusting relationship between therapist and client; second, the need for flexibility – sessions of varying lengths, perhaps conducted in different places and possibly over a long period of time; and, third, the need for a graded approach (e.g. discussing, first, less strongly held beliefs or less threatening voices) (see, e.g., Kingdon and Turkington, 1994; Fowler et al., 1995; Chadwick et al., 1996; Haddock and Slade, 1996; Nelson, 1997, Morrison, in press, for detailed accounts).

Much of the research on outcomes of CBT is in the form of case studies with small numbers of people (e.g. Alford, 1986; Fowler and Morley, 1989; Haddock et al., 1993; Chadwick and Birchwood, 1994; Chadwick and Lowe, 1994; Morrison, 1994). Such research often has the advantage of providing detailed information about participants, which helps make the outcomes understandable, as well as details of individual outcomes, which highlight both variability and regularities in ways which can be lost in group data. The disadvantages of case studies include the lack of comparison groups and the small numbers involved. In addition to case studies, there are a small number of group comparison studies in which two different psychological interventions are compared. Tarrier et al. (1993), for example, compared 'coping strategy enhancement' with 'problem-solving', while Haddock et al. (1998a) compared 'distraction' and 'focusing' with participants who heard voices. More recently, Kuipers et al. (1997, 1998); Tarrier et al. (1998, 2000) and Sensky et al. (2000) have reported the results of randomised controlled studies of CBT, using larger numbers of participants.

Taken together, these studies have used a wide variety of outcome measures, including psychiatric ratings of 'symptoms', assessments of loudness and frequency of voices, ratings of the conviction with which 'delusional' beliefs are held and of the distress associated with voices and beliefs, assessment of social functioning and measures of time spent in hospital during intervention and follow-up periods. The results, though in many ways very encouraging, are also mixed. On the positive side, there are consistent reports of statistically significant reductions in ratings of 'symptoms', mainly 'delusions' and hallucinations; there are somewhat less consistent, but still notable, reductions in 'delusional' conviction and in the distress associated with voices and 'delusions'. Tarrier *et al.* (1998) also reported that while their 'routine care' group spent a total of 204 days in hospital in the three-month before–after treatment period, participants in the CBT group spent only one day. There is also some indication that gains made during the intervention period may be maintained or strengthened during a follow-up period (Kuipers *et al.*, 1998; Sensky *et al.*, 2000).

On the less positive side, it is possible that the changes achieved, though statistically significant, are rather modest, particularly when a reasonable follow-up period – say 9–24 months – is included. Kuipers *et al.* (1998), for example, reported that 65 per cent of participants in the CBT group showed a 'reliable clinical change' on the Brief Psychiatric Rating Scale (BPRS), compared with 17 per cent in the 'standard treatment' group. But this change is not large, amounting to 5–10 points, where five points is the average variability in BPRS scores in the standard treatment group. No CBT participant showed a 'large clinical change' at eighteen-month follow-up (ten or more points on the BPRS), although 21 per cent had achieved this – compared with 3 per cent of the control group – just after the treatment period. Kuipers *et al.* also reported no significant difference in the number of days spent in hospital during the follow-up period between the CBT and the standard care groups, although only thirty-two people could be included in this analysis. Similarly, in Tarrier *et al.*'s (2000) comparison of CBT, supportive counselling and routine care, the time to relapse for the (combined) groups who had received either CBT or supportive counselling was not significantly different from that in the group receiving only routine care. As well as this, CBT does not appear to have a reliably positive effect on other important aspects of people's lives. For example, Kuipers *et al.* (1997, 1998) found no significant difference between CBT and standard treatment groups in assessments of depression, negative symptoms or social functioning. Tarrier *et al.* (1993) also found no evidence that specific gains from CBT generalised to 'negative symptoms' (although such gains were found by Tarrier *et al.*, 2000) or to social functioning. It appears, too, that quite a large proportion of people do not benefit from CBT: Kuipers *et al.* (1997) noted that only 50 per cent of their participants were 'treatment responders', although this may have risen to 65 per cent in the follow-up period. And Sensky *et al.* (2000) claimed that, depending on the assumed rate of improvement without CBT, the number of people who would need to be treated to show one 'success' is between two and six. There is the further important consideration of what CBT is compared to, given that it involves sometimes intense one-to-one contact with people over a relatively long period. Most studies offer no comparison, comparison with standard practice or comparison between two kinds of psychological interventions.

Tarrier et al. (1998, 2000) and Sensky et al. (2000), however, offer important comparisons between CBT and, respectively, 'supportive counselling' and 'befriending'. These interventions provided the same amount of individual contact as CBT but were not intended to offer any of its specific elements. The results are striking: Tarrier et al. found no significant difference between CBT and supportive counselling in reductions in the number and severity of 'positive symptoms' over a three-month period (about two weeks post-treatment). Participants from both groups also spent equally small amounts of time in hospital – one day – during the three-month period, compared with 204 days for the standard treatment group. Only CBT, however, made a statistically significant contribution to a regression analysis where the dependent variable was a 50 per cent or more improvement in ratings of 'symptoms'. In a 24-month follow-up (Tarrier et al., 2000) there were no significant differences between the groups receiving CBT or supportive counselling on 'symptomatic' changes, clinically significant changes (i.e. 20 per cent or greater improvement since pre-treatment on 'symptom' ratings) or time to relapse. Sensky et al. (2000) similarly found no significant difference between CBT and the befriending groups on any outcome measure at the end of the intervention period. At nine-month follow-up, however, while the CBT group had enhanced their improvement, the befriending group had deteriorated, resulting in a significant difference on all outcome measures (Comprehensive Psychiatric Rating Scale; Schizophrenia Change Score; Montgomery–Äsberg Depression Rating Scale; Scale for the Assessment of Negative Symptoms).

Researchers themselves have identified a number of methodological problems with studies involving CBT. Obviously these do not apply to all studies – indeed later research has tried to take account of some of them – but across the research literature problems identified include: publication of positive and not negative results; small sample sizes; heterogeneous samples; possible biases in recruitment; variable psychometric properties of assessment instruments; clinicians and assessors not blind to treatment conditions; lack of agreed outcome measures; participants withdrawing during the study; inadequate control or comparison groups; use of a very wide range of treatment elements; an emphasis on statistical rather than clinical significance and lack of control of variations in medication (e.g. Bouchard et al., 1996; Haddock et al., 1998b; Wykes et al., 1998; Sensky et al., 2000).

These issues are indeed problematic within the medically derived research framework which has been implicitly adopted in much of the CBT literature – and certainly in the randomised controlled trials – in which the aims are control of all factors thought to be extraneous to the intervention and precise specification of relationships between participant characteristics, treatment elements and measured outcomes. There are, however, other issues which are equally relevant to CBT interventions but which are less likely to be highlighted within this research model; these will be discussed in the next sections. But it is worth placing this discussion, and researchers' own concerns, in the following context. First, the very few accounts of CBT from *clients* suggest that for them it represented their first experience of having their 'psychotic' experiences discussed in detail and taken seriously; second, although some therapeutic results may be modest, most statistical comparisons with other treatments, across a range of outcome measures, favour CBT. This result alone would justify much more detailed study of CBT. Third, these results have usually been obtained with people whom professionals have not been able to help in other ways, including medication. Finally, the results have been obtained without the risk of physical damage which accompanies neuroleptic drugs.

### The conflicting models of CBT – I: Schizophrenia, symptoms and illness

One notable element of the CBT literature is the varied and ambiguous position of 'schizophrenia' within it. Some researchers/practitioners seem to distance themselves from the concept of schizophrenia and present their subject matter as 'individual symptoms', but without explaining how or why 'symptom' is being used in this context. As I noted earlier, 'symptom' is not a neutral term, but gains its meaning from a particular theoretical framework and carries the unspoken, if misguided, question, symptom of what? And, as I also noted, focusing on symptoms is theoretically regressive within a medical framework, only to be tolerated until researchers can make progress in understanding the relationships between symptoms and signs, and understand the biological processes which hold these clusters together. These biological processes then become the targets for intervention, rather than individual symptoms. Thus invoking 'symptoms' as the target of CBT simply muddies the conceptual waters rather than providing a solution to the problems of 'schizophrenia'.

For others, however, the issue is clearer, if no less problematic: their subject matter is still schizophrenia and the symptoms it causes. In justifying the use of CBT, for example, Sensky *et al.* (2000) claim that 'schizophrenia causes persistent and recurrent symptoms that are often distressing and socially disabling' (165), while Haddock *et al.* (1998b) argue that CBT may be applied to the 'symptoms that result from schizophrenia' (823). The use of 'schizophrenia' here involves as least three major problems. The first, obviously, is the lack of evidence for the validity of 'schizophrenia', so that to talk of the symptoms it causes makes no sense. Second, even if we accept the diagnosis of schizophrenia, then focusing on its symptoms must again be seen as a provisional and regrettable necessity resulting from lack of knowledge, rather like focusing on coughing in tuberculosis. Finally, a diagnosis of schizophrenia is supposedly given only if the person's behaviour cannot be explained in terms of their context. As we saw in Chapter 7, this assumption is crucial to the traditional psychiatric claim that 'schizophrenia' is a pathological brain disorder, understandable within a medical framework. But at least some CBT procedures aim to make the person's experience understandable in terms of their past and present circumstances. We thus have the curious situation where someone may be given a diagnosis which depends on the assumption of non-understandability, and then referred for an intervention which, at least for some of its practitioners, depends on the assumption of understandability.

These dilemmas have been circumvented in several ways. One is through invoking the idea of schizophrenia as a description so that its use appears to have no particular implications nor pose any theoretical problems. Turkington and Kingdon (1996), for example, claim that formulations derived from their 'normalising rationale' – i.e. from making 'symptoms' understandable – can be used to 'decatastrophise the term schizophrenia which is a descriptive term for those patients suffering from certain of those symptoms' (107). As we saw in the previous chapter, however, 'schizophrenia' is far from a descriptive term; on the contrary, it is not only an assumption-laden term, but its presentation as a description has been used strategically to obscure the lack of evidence to support its assumptions, while allowing practitioners to continue behaving as if the assumptions were true. The problem is compounded by the fact that Turkington and Kingdon provide no way of differentiating 'patients suffering from certain of these symptoms' (i.e. schizophrenics) from the 'many people who do not have schizophrenia [but who] hear voices' (107).

A second way of circumventing at least the understandability dilemma is to make 'symptoms' understandable within a vulnerability–stress model which appears to take account of biological, psychological and environmental factors in explaining 'symptoms' and 'illness'. Kingdon et al. (1994), for example, describe their 'normalising rationale' as one in which 'the illness has developed because of some vulnerability which has made them sensitive to specific stressors, life events and circumstances at that particular point in their life. Such stresses might be exacerbated by sleep and sensory deprivation, caused by, for example, overwork and isolation' (586). This vulnerability, however, is claimed to be at least 'genetic and neuropathological' (584) and to pre-dispose the person to stressors which, by implication, the rest of us might find benign (see also Wykes et al., 1998 and Brenner and Pfammatter, 1998). But the assumed vulnerability has never been identified or even properly articulated; instead, it remains a vague but exceptionally convenient idea which allows 'symptoms' to be normalised or made apparently understandable for that abnormal person but without the symptoms being made to look culturally understandable or expectable. Thus the idea of 'schizophrenia' as a biological disorder which produces incomprehensible behaviour *and* the use of a normalising rationale for its 'symptoms', are both made to seem reasonable.

Finally, the dilemmas produced by using 'schizophrenia' in the context of CBT have been avoided by reverting to the less specific term 'illness'; this term is widely used in the CBT literature whether or not researchers use the term 'schizophrenia'. But there is little discussion of what 'illness' might mean in this context; it is as if its meaning were both self-evident and self-evidently appropriate. The idea of illness, of course, carries the same problems as the idea of schizophrenia in terms of the understandability criterion for inferring mental illness or mental disorder. It is also worth noting that the attribution of illness is clearly a sensitive and contested area within the therapist–client relationship in CBT. Fowler *et al.* (1995), for example, claim that part of their role is to 'assist' patients to understand their problem in terms of illness, while Nelson (1997) talks of a CBT client 'accepting' that her psychotic experiences were a result of illness. The implication here is that clients are guided towards this view; that is, it is not one they spontaneously adopt. Similarly, Kuipers *et al.* (1996) state that '[i]nitially the implications for an alternative explanation of symptoms within a general illness model are not forced' (119), suggesting both client resistance and that the illness model might be more vigorously advocated by the therapist at a later stage. And Tarrier *et al.* offered their CBT clients a stark dichotomy which again emphasises the contested nature of the idea of illness:

> If the patient did not accept that the experiences were illness based then it was suggested that although the therapist and patient might hold different causal explanations of the patient's experience (*i.e. illness-v-reality based*) these differing explanations could be put to the test.
>
> (1993, 526; my emphasis)

### The conflicting models of CBT – 2: The therapist–client relationship

A second source of ambiguity in the CBT literature is the presentation of the relationship between therapist and client. Much emphasis has been placed on the importance of an open and collaborative relationship, with the phrase 'collaborative empiricism' used to describe the therapist's and client's joint exploration of 'delusional' beliefs. Similarly, Fowler *et al.* (1995), talk of client and therapist working together to achieve goals set by the client. There is, however, another language which runs parallel and gives a rather less collaborative impression: beliefs are 'disputed', 'challenged' and 'undermined'; 'faulty' cognitions are identified and 'corrected'; therapists' and clients' different views are 'put to the test'. Indeed, at times the language becomes openly militaristic, with therapists engaging in 'tactical withdrawal'; making forays of attack and retreat; 'closing off escape routes' or trying to show that cognitive approaches have potential in the therapeutic 'armamentarium' (Tarrier *et al.*, 1993; Chadwick and Birchwood, 1994; Chadwick and Lowe, 1994; Kingdon *et al.*, 1994; Nelson, 1997; Wykes *et al.*, 1998; Spaulding *et al.*, 1998).

This rather adversarial language may not match therapists' intentions, or what actually happens in CBT or clients' perception of it. But it cannot be dismissed as insignificant because it has the potential to create very different positions for client and therapist from those presented in the collaborative account; it is also part of a larger linguistic picture. Bowers (1990), for example, has analysed the 'affinities' between the vocabularies of cognitive theory and militarism, while, as Stein (1990) and Lupton (1994) have shown, militaristic metaphors are an integral part of the language of modern medicine in which diseases and disease-causing agents are presented as enemies to be conquered and destroyed. Such metaphors obviously raise important issues for doctor–patient relationships and for medical practice, but at least doctor and patient are assumed, rightly or wrongly, to be on the same side facing a common enemy. But when, as in CBT, the conflict appears to be over clients' *beliefs* then more complex and potentially adversarial positions are set up. These positions are further emphasised by the assumption of the client's (or their beliefs') irrationality and, by implication, of the therapist's rationality. Kingdon *et al.* (1994), for example, talk of tracing a delusion to its underlying irrational belief; Kuipers *et al.* (1998) see part of the therapist's role as helping the client to list rational alternatives to their 'delusional' beliefs; Fowler *et al.* (1995) refer to the therapist's 'objectivity', while Nelson (1997) talks of the 'chain of logical reasoning' which is constructed by the therapist. This language tends to be used as if 'rationality' were a straightforward technical term to whose meaning and practice the therapist has objective access. Yet it appears that clients' rationality may at times be judged by whether they accept a particular theoretical view, as Kingdon and Turkington's comment shows: 'The use of rational responses for voices, *i.e. treating voices as classical Beckian automatic thoughts*' (1998: 65; my emphasis). The problems of 'rationality' in this context are also illustrated by Alford and Beck's (1994) claim that they enhance patients' freedom to 'have their own thoughts' by emphasising to the patient 'that reason and observed evidence (rather than therapist opinion) should determine whether a belief is held or relinquished' (373). There is no acknowledgement that this prescription on holding beliefs is itself a statement of therapist opinion; nor is it acknowledged that if it were to be implemented then many of us – including therapists – might have to relinquish some cherished beliefs.

### CBT and the problem of individualism

CBT's focus is the individual, both their assumed psychological processes (beliefs, appraisals, assumptions, attributions, biases, etc.) *and* the individual as the target of change. This focus is not surprising, given that CBT brings together two strongly individualistic frameworks – cognitive theory and psychiatry. Psychiatry defines its assumed subject matter, mental disorder, as a 'syndrome . . . *in an individual* . . . considered to be a manifestation of a dysfunction *in the individual*' (APA, 1994: xxi–xxii), while cognitive theory has been described as focusing on the thinking and reasoning of the 'individual knower' (Sampson, 1981) and on humans as 'lone thinkers, making sense of their world through their cognitive reasoning abilities' (Riatt and Zeedyk, 2000: 54).

But it may be argued that CBT's focus on the individual is entirely appropriate; after all, it is individuals who are troubled or distressed, who are asking for (or seem in need of) help. And offering someone the chance to talk about and understand their experiences, to consider less distressing interpretations of events, and to explore ways of managing their problems, may be enormously helpful. It could also be argued that although CBT does concern itself mainly with the 'individual knower' it also offers opportunities for more contextual accounts. Certainly, a number of writers have invoked context as a way of making sense of 'psychotic' behaviour and experiences. Chadwick and Birchwood (1996), for example, 'try to explore possible connections or personal significance, between the voice content and the individual's history' (79), while Yusupoff and Tarrier (1996) talk of 'relegitimating' the person's psychotic experiences by 'enabling the patient to appreciate that he or she was not in a position to choose their earlier history and other factors which may have contributed to the development and maintenance of the psychosis' (92). There are, however, a number of reasons to be concerned about CBT's (largely) individualistic focus and to be cautious about the extent to which it will contribute to the provision of more contextual accounts of the development and amelioration of psychosis. To take the second point first, CBT's potential to foster an understanding of the possible relationships between life experiences, social conditions and psychosis, is limited by the fact that such understandings are 'privatised' either by remaining within the therapy relationship or by being published in the relatively unprestigious form of single case studies. The most prestigious form of therapy evaluation – randomised controlled trials – tends to be stripped of context, while one of the few attempts to identify predictors of response to CBT (Garety et al., 1997) looked mainly at the potential contribution of individual factors such as 'symptoms' and cognitive attributes, rather than at aspects of someone's relationships, life experiences or social status. It is perhaps not surprising, then, that case-study reports, valuable though they are, do not yet amount to a systematic analysis of the possible relationships between people's social worlds and hallucinations and 'delusions'. It is notable that there is little acknowledgement in the CBT literature of factors such as power, ethnicity, gender, class or poverty, far less systematic analysis of their possible significance in shaping or giving meaning to 'psychotic' experiences or of their role in fostering or restricting change. Birchwood et al.'s (2000) analysis of the similarities between voice-hearers' perceptions of the power relationships between them and their voices, and between them and significant others in their lives, is an important starting point of such an analysis, albeit one which still focuses on the 'individual knower'.

The assumptions of cognitive theory itself also place limitations on the development of non-individualistic analysis. The basic assumption of CBT is that people's reactions to events are mediated by their beliefs, assumptions and interpretations. It is certainly difficult to argue that we do not make assumptions about, or interpretations of, events; the issue is how best to conceptualise this process. Chadwick *et al.* (1996), for example, argue that it is the '*personal* meaning events have for people which determines if they are distressed and disturbed' (8–9; my emphasis). This could be interpreted positively as giving primacy to the client's experience and not to professionals' assumptions; and, as a counter to traditional assumptions about the meaninglessness of 'delusions', the idea has proved very valuable in practice (Chadwick *et al.*, 1996). But looked at in another way, an emphasis on *personal* meaning without reference to the social structures, power relations and linguistic practices which shape what we have come to think of as 'personal' meaning, could provide a route back to the 'lone thinkers' or 'individual knowers' of contemporary psychology (see, e.g., Billig, 1976; Vygotsky, 1978; Foucault, 1979; Henriques *et al.*, 1997).

There are two major reasons why we should be concerned about these issues. First, individualistic assumptions have the potential to limit our understanding of psychosis and the scope for its amelioration. For example, it is difficult to understand a black man's belief that he was really born of white parents, without reference to social hierarchies based on 'race' and the meanings of 'blackness' in a white-dominated society. Similarly, and as I noted earlier, in their descriptive study of voice-hearing in a psychiatric group, Nayani and David (1996) reported that the content of abusive voices (the majority) divided along gender lines, with women reporting 'words of abuse conventionally directed at women (e.g. slut) [while men] similarly described "male" insults such as those imputing homosexuality' (182). The majority of voices were also male. Again, our understanding of the content of these voices, their meaning to and impact on the individual and the gender relationship between voice and voice-hearer, may be restricted without reference to the conflation of masculinity and heterosexuality in our culture or without reference to the pervasive denigration of women through their sexuality and appearance (the content of women's voices also included 'fat cow' and 'ugly bitch'). In the same way, Chadwick *et al.*'s discussion of 'psychosis' in terms of individuals' needs for and assumptions about, attachment and autonomy and in terms of threats to the self, could arguably be extended by considering the dramatically different ways in which attachment and autonomy have been socially constructed for males and females (e.g. Gilligan, 1993). What constitutes a threat to the self is therefore likely – in the same way as the content of hallucinated voices – to be at least partially shaped by gender.

The second reason for concern is that there is a very important difference between offering help to individuals and constructing theories which make it look as if the individual is the natural target for intervention, rather than a target constructed by language and through research and clinical practice. At worst, a therapeutic focus on the individual, backed by research which separates people from their context, which searches for assumed cognitive operations and structures and in which the researcher decides what participants' responses mean, can make it look as if the individual's cognitive operations and their transformation in therapy are of greater importance than events, relationships or practices in the social world; in our concern with the person's appraisal of events, we may neglect to ask, to paraphrase Sampson (1981), how these 'events' came to enter the person's life in the first place. As I suggested earlier, such an approach has the potential to protect from scrutiny the harmful actions of individuals and groups more powerful and privileged than the psychiatric 'patient'.

## What are the goals of CBT?

The goal of medical treatment for 'schizophrenia' was straightforward: since a cure was not possible (or, more accurately, since no one knew what should be modified to effect a cure), then 'symptom' reduction was sought. Secondary outcomes, such as social and employment functioning, were also usually reported in outcome research, but 'symptom' reduction remained the major goal. The situation with CBT is much more complex. This is partly because psychological interventions for any problem are less likely to have standard, pre-set goals; but it is also because, as I noted earlier, CBT stands in an ambiguous relationship to the concept of schizophrenia and to the medically derived model on which it is based. As we might expect, then, CBT has been associated with a variety of goals. These include reducing the frequency and intensity of hallucinations; reducing the conviction of 'delusional' beliefs; reducing the distress associated with hallucinations and 'delusions'; teaching 'coping strategies' and encouraging clients to engage in 'self-management' of their experiences.

This variety of goals, and the equally varied ways they may be achieved, can be seen as a strength of psychological interventions. But it also raises some potentially problematic issues. The first is an apparent disagreement over 'symptom' reduction as a therapeutic goal. Haddock *et al.* (1996), for example, reported that one aim of their 'focusing' intervention was to reduce the frequency of hallucinated voices; Tarrier *et al.* similarly claimed that the aim of 'coping strategy enhancement' was to 'decrease symptoms' (1993: 525). By contrast, Kuipers *et al.* (1997) do not explicitly mention 'symptom' reduction as a goal; nor do Sensky *et al.* (2000). Indeed, Chadwick *et al.* (1996) are emphatic that the goal of their cognitive interventions is to 'ease the [client's] distress and disturbance. Working merely to change beliefs is not an end in itself' (170). They argue also that '[i]f, following a careful assessment, the therapist concludes that the client is not experiencing any distress or disturbance [from voices or "delusional" beliefs] then in our opinion cognitive therapy is not indicated' (170). In fact, cognitive interventions aimed at reducing distress associated with voice-hearing *did* reduce the frequency and duration of voice activity, a result which Chadwick and Birchwood (1994) described as 'unexpected, because this was not an objective' (199).

But it is notable that even when 'symptom' reduction is not explicitly stated as a goal, it is still reported as an outcome, based on psychiatric rating scales; indeed, it may be the first outcome reported (see Kuipers *et al.*, 1997; Sensky *et al.*, 2000). This situation can be explained partly by CBT's ambiguous relationship to traditional medical frameworks. 'Symptom' reduction may simply be taken for granted as a desirable outcome; the continued use of the medical term 'symptom' may also obscure the complex issues involved in goal-setting – who, after all, would *not* want the symptoms of their illness to be reduced? But in this context, reporting 'symptom' reduction can also function rhetorically. Not only does it suggest that the desirability of 'symptom' reduction is taken for granted, it tells us something of the anticipated (medical) audience for the research reports, i.e. the audience who need to be convinced of the worth of these 'new' therapies.

But if there is some disagreement or ambiguity over 'symptom' reduction as a goal of CBT, there is virtually complete agreement over the goal of reducing the distress associated with 'psychotic' experiences. Again, this may be seen as a strength of CBT, but the goal may not be without problems, as can be seen by considering what might be called the hidden or at least initially unagreed goals of CBT. This issue is particularly important given the emphasis on a collaborative approach with shared goal-setting, in the CBT literature. One such hidden goal, at least for some practitioners, is compliance with medication and acceptance of one's 'illness'. I noted earlier that this latter goal may be contested; that it is not necessarily the client's initial goal is clear from Turkington and Kingdon's comments that 'with the patient "on board" [following a normalising rationale] a variety of techniques can then be used to decrease distress and improve compliance' and that 'patients are often loath to accept biological rationales early on although they may accept them later in treatment' (1996: 103, 107). A lack of explicitness over the goal of medication compliance is also suggested by Kuipers *et al.*'s complex wording of one of their goals as 'to promote the active participation of the individual in the regulation of their risk of relapse and social disability' (1997: 320). That this could mean encouraging medication use is suggested by the authors' mention of 'increasing medication' as a 'coping strategy'. The possible tension which this lack of explicitness could create between therapist and client is suggested by the rather hesitant account of a CBT practitioner in Messari's (2000) study, talking of acceptance of illness and medication compliance as goals of CBT: 'in some ways it's a, it's a, it's a supplied goal by us, you know because er it's not [pause] it's not necessarily the sort of thing that you would want, the conclusion that they want to reach when they come along'. The point here is not that taking prescribed drugs should never be a therapeutic goal, nor is it to underestimate the difficulties faced by therapists in 'engaging' clients in CBT. The point is that the seemingly non-problematic goal of reducing distress can be used to justify therapy with less explicit and possibly more problematic, or at least contentious, goals within a therapeutic system which presents itself as open and collaborative. But it is precisely because distress reduction is so widely accepted as a therapeutic goal that it can be used in this strategic way.

It is not, then, that it is inappropriate as a goal – far from it – so much as that it allows the issue of the appropriateness of other goals to be obscured.

### Evaluating CBT

I noted earlier that much of the literature which evaluates CBT was in the form of case studies or uncontrolled trials with relatively small numbers of participants. Such research tends to be devalued in medicine, being (not unreasonably) seen as subject to unwanted bias. For this reason, randomised controlled trials (RCTs) have come to be seen as the most desirable of designs for investigating the efficacy of medical treatments; as I discussed earlier, several such trials have been reported for CBT.

But although RCTs have clear methodological benefits, they also have serious limitations, both ethical and methodological (Faulder, 1985). Ethically, they raise issues about the meaning of informed consent which have not yet been addressed in the CBT literature. Methodologically, RCTs can reach their answer only by reducing, or appearing to reduce, the influence of as many variables as possible and by minimising the number of questions posed. We might argue that RCTs are particularly limited in research on psychological interventions where the number of potentially important variables is so large, where there is great variability in participants, interventions and outcomes, and where contextual information may be crucial in interpreting the results. This is not to suggest that RCTs have no role in outcome research; they may be an important step in establishing that 'something is happening'. My concern is that they may limit the questions we ask, obscure the potential of psychological interventions for psychosis and, through their claims to a particular kind of scientific rigour, lead us to devalue alternative research methods. It is interesting, then, to note Tarrier et al.'s (1998) inclusion of 'two clinical anecdotes' at the end of their report of a randomised controlled trial of CBT for psychosis. The choice of language (not uncommon in medicine) is striking: an anecdote (*OED*: a short account of an entertaining or interesting incident) is clearly separate from and of inferior status to, a highly technical RCT report, yet the contextual information conveyed in Tarrier et al.'s 'anecdotes' is arguably crucial to our understanding of some of the therapy outcomes; it certainly illustrates the impossibility of trying to separate people's 'symptoms' from their lives and the problems of adopting 'symptom reduction' as an outcome measure. I am not suggesting that the authors saw this material in a light-hearted manner; my point is that the conventions of doing and reporting RCTs, with all the prestige that surrounds them, have the power to produce language which potentially devalues and marginalises important information which lies outside the limited framework of the RCT itself.

RCTs usually compare at least two interventions; in CBT research, the potential limitations of the design are also highlighted by researchers' interpretations of the results of comparison interventions. Kuipers et al. (1997)

compared CBT with standard treatment for psychosis; Tarrier *et al.* (1998, 2000) and Sensky *et al.* (2000), however, included a comparison with 'supportive counselling' and 'befriending' respectively. As I noted earlier, Tarrier *et al.* (1998) and Tarrier *et al.* (2000) found no significant difference between CBT and supportive counselling on most of their outcome analyses, while Sensky *et al.* reported no significant difference between CBT and befriending on any outcome measure just after the intervention, but significant differences on all measures at follow-up. The ways in which these important results have been received can again be seen as at least partly shaped by the assumptions which underlie RCTs in which a comparison intervention is assumed to contain all the elements of the 'trial' intervention except the active ones; this research design is often said, rather dismissively, to control for the 'nonspecific' effects of intervention. Thus the results of Tarrier *et al.* and Sensky *et al.* have been described as 'puzzling', 'surprising', 'a great surprise' and 'unexpected', while Sensky *et al.* have commented – also rather dismissively – that 'it remains likely that [the result] is another example of benefits to patients that are attributable to participating in a research trial' (2000: 171). But what constitutes the 'active' ingredients of the intervention is defined here by the researchers and not by those who receive the intervention. This may be appropriate for drug and other physical treatments where previous research has established the effects of certain chemicals on the body. In psychological and interpersonal interventions, however, the client may be as well or better placed than the researcher to decide what has or has not been helpful. This problem of researchers deciding what is 'active' in therapy is compounded by the fact that, as we have seen, psychological and psychiatric theory have tended to focus on a relatively narrow range of factors assumed to be important in 'schizophrenia' or psychosis. Thus, when *researchers* decide what is 'active' in therapy, they may be choosing from a limited range of variables, a range, moreover, which is systematically limited by the theoretical traditions of psychology and psychiatry. This suggests not only that the range of factors considered in the evaluation of CBT could be broadened, but also that a detailed analysis of *clients'* views should form part of CBT's evaluation and development.

### Evaluating CBT from the client's perspective

Kuiper's *et al.* (1997) and Sensky *et al.* (2000) asked their clients to complete satisfaction questionnaires. The mean rating reported by Sensky *et al.* for CBT was fifty, with seventy the maximum possible. While this is very encouraging, it is notable that the mean for the befriending group was forty-three, and not significantly different from CBT. Kuipers *et al.*, however, reported that of twenty CBT clients, 25 per cent were 'very satisfied'; 55 per cent were 'satisfied'; 15 per cent were neither satisfied nor dissatisfied and 5 per cent were dissatisfied. (Satisfaction data for the standard treatment comparison were not reported.) Although these data provide a good overview of some clients' ratings of CBT, they obviously do not allow any analysis of what was satisfying or dis-satisfying about the intervention. There is very little detailed information available on clients' views of CBT, but exploratory studies by Gill (2000) and Messari (2000)[4] suggest that clients' accounts can increase our understanding of why many find CBT a positive experience and of why 'non-specific' interventions such as supportive counselling might also have positive outcomes.

A major theme in clients' accounts is the importance of their relationship with the therapist:

> That was the main thing I got out of the therapy, simply the chance to talk about the problem.
>
> (Gill, 2000)

> He listens to it . . . whereas some possibly wouldn't allow you to, to, he listens to it.
>
> (Messari, 2000)

> It's [a] sympathetic ear, I suppose. He is listening to my belief system, he is taking it seriously.
>
> (ibid.)

> The most obvious answer [to what the therapist is trying to convey to me] is that you're human . . . it's as though they're responding to the human being that's in his own dilemma.
>
> (ibid.)

Clients' portrayals of CBT tend to conflict with its presentation in the litera-ture as an 'adjunct' treatment or as a procedure which can be integrated into standard clinical practice. On the contrary, the potential opposition between CBT and routine practice, which is implied in the previous statements, is highlighted in the following quotes:

> [CBT's] our only outlet . . . the rest of it is pure rehab, isn't it? Medication, vocation, you know, drama and gym, em, art, computer, nothing really. I mean, [CBT's] serious, isn't it?
>
> (Messari, 2000)

> But [the medical approach] just seems like a really crude approach because it just does nothing to understand why I, in the first place, have these beliefs.
>
> (ibid.)

4  Clients quoted here were seen by several therapists in different service settings. All therapists are referred to as 'he' to protect confidentiality.

I thought I was just stuck in this world where nobody would actually give you the time of day basically. Cause I thought that when I was, you know, ill, people really didn't have the time for you.

(Gill, 2000)

I don't have to feel that I'm stupid or just crazy or irrational.

(Messari, 2000)

As well as casting doubt on the status of CBT as an 'adjunct' intervention, these statements suggest that clients' satisfaction ratings are at least partly influenced by the contrast between CBT and what they had experienced before, as well as by specific aspects of CBT.

But although many clients spoke positively about their experience of CBT they still tended to portray themselves as passive recipients of 'treatment' from people who were part of the medical system; as one of Messari's participant's commented, 'It was just part of the hospital treatment.' Messari noted that most of her interviewees seemed not to know how or why they had initially come to receive CBT; Gill similarly noted that her participants understood coming to see the therapist in terms of the *therapist's* job, goals and techniques, but that no participant spontaneously stated what *their* tasks or goals were. The ways in which CBT is seen as simultaneously embedded in, and contrasting to, the existing system are highlighted by some of the responses to Messari's direct question about what her participants had hoped to achieve from CBT:

I hope it helps me get discharged . . . it's part of the programme and, I mean, a lot of patients here don't bother talking to their psychologist.
Int: How do you hope this would help you get discharged?
Well, er, because I'm doing the things I'm supposed to do.

(Messari, 2000)

It just makes you hopeful that you'll get, you'll be able to get discharged . . .

(ibid.)

Finally, and perhaps not surprisingly, clients' accounts of CBT were often dominated by the issue of the reality or truth of their experiences and beliefs. But the meaning of this issue varied widely across clients. For example, at least some were well aware that the therapist, like other staff, did not 'believe' them:

[He] would actually look at my side of things and humour me a little. I'm sure he thought I was as ridiculous as the doctors did, but he would humour me for a while and go along with what I said.

(Gill, 2000)

> [Y]ou know, he's going to try everything [to convince me it's not real] . . .
> I will probably [end] feeling that, yes, it's real probably, and alternatively
> he might convince me that it's unreal.

(Messari, 2000)

While for some clients 'not being believed' was a challenge, for others it was reassuring (perhaps things were not really as bad as they seemed), or even a pretence by the therapist so as not to upset the client by facing the full import of their beliefs being true. But clients also made a sharp distinction between their previous experience of not being believed and their experience of CBT in which they were listened to and taken seriously. As Messari points out, therapists' acknowledgement that the experiences or beliefs were real or true for the client seemed to be the important meeting point.

But this position was not entirely satisfactory because it left unresolved the question of how clients came to have their experiences or beliefs. Messari noted that, throughout the interviews, clients 'juggled' two conflicting accounts: 'this is true' and 'I am ill', at times invoking both within one short utterance in ways which raise questions about the meaning of ratings of 'belief conviction'. Seeing themselves as ill, however, was not an identity which gave clients any satisfaction, except perhaps of a negative kind (e.g. you were either really threatened all the time or you were ill); as we saw earlier, accepting oneself as ill may be an unnegotiated goal of CBT and this, together with the perception of CBT as part of the medical system, might contribute to the relatively small number of clients who expressed very high levels of satisfaction with CBT in Kuipers *et al.*'s and Sensky *et al.*'s studies. The following quote illustrates not only how clients might distance themselves from 'illness' but also the conflict inherent in medical and psychological accounts of psychosis:

> The one thing I *don't* know maybe is the fact that if you are . . . unwell,
> I'm getting well now, yeah? But let's just say you *were* unwell, would *you*
> respond to psychologist though?

(Messari, 2000)

These brief accounts highlight at least three points. First, clients (and therapists) are 'caught' between varied and often conflicting accounts of psychotic experiences and how they should be 'managed'. And, since these conflicts are certainly not resolved in the literature or in services, we should not be surprised if clients' accounts can at times seem hesitant, confused and contradictory. Second, clients' experience of CBT cannot be separated from their previous and ongoing experience of other forms of intervention. Finally, the collaborative approach which is said to characterise CBT could usefully be extended to collaboration over its evaluation.

## The future of CBT

As I noted earlier, CBT is not the first attempt to apply non-medical ideas to madness on a relatively large scale. Moral management or moral therapy attempted this in the eighteenth and nineteenth centuries (see Chapter 2); more recently, in the 1960s–80s, the token economy and other learning-theory-based systems were promoted and widely implemented in Britain and the US. Both of these systems (which were in some ways similar) have largely disappeared as identifiable sets of grand ideas on which to base the management of madness, although traces of moral therapy remain in today's occupational therapy, while aspects of learning theory inform some 'rehabilitation' programmes. Yet both moral therapy and learning theory systems attracted widespread support and made strong claims for their effectiveness; both produced evidence of their success and, while some might argue that the demise of token economy systems was hastened by the widespread use of neuroleptic drugs and by ethical concerns, the same arguments certainly cannot be advanced for the demise of moral therapy. It may therefore be timely to consider the future of CBT as the now-dominant psychological alternative to medical approaches to psychosis (at least in the UK). Such a discussion is particularly appropriate when we consider that at least three of the elements associated with the development and demise of moral therapy and, to a lesser extent of learning theory systems, are in place now: a high level of critical scrutiny of traditional approaches to madness; professional tensions over status and, third, suggestions that the 'new' ideas should be applied on a larger scale. A very detailed analysis of historical parallels and their implications for the future of CBT is beyond the scope of this chapter. My discussion will therefore focus mainly on moral therapy and CBT, partly for brevity but also because the similarities in their situations are so striking and because such comparisons emphasise the importance of a historical perspective in an area so dominated by appeals to scientific progress.

There are a number of similarities in ideas between moral therapy and CBT: both offered a radical alternative to dominant views of madness; both suggested that there may be no qualitative difference between the mad and the sane; both espoused the goal, sometimes implicit in CBT, of restoring the mad person to rationality and both sought to do this by non-medical means; both emphasised the importance of respectful and positive relationships between the mad and those who sought to change them; both adopted an educational approach (again often implicit in CBT) where the mad were brought gradually and respectfully to a different view of 'reality'.

Such ideas clearly challenge a view of the mad as suffering from a physical disease, to be understood and treated within a medical framework or, indeed, the earlier idea of the mad as bestial. We can argue that at least three possible responses can be made to such radical challenges to a dominant system of thought: the challenge may be ignored, but this is difficult to achieve if it has strong support and the dominant system is theoretically or empirically weak; or the challenge can entirely replace the 'old' system (a paradigm shift in Kuhn's terms) but, for all the reasons discussed in previous chapters, such a response was and is highly unlikely in the case of challenges to medical theories of madness. Finally, the challenge maybe assimilated and neutralised, so that it both ceases to be a challenge and, transformed, actually strengthens the dominant system by confirming its openness to new ideas. It can be argued that this third process of assimilation and neutralisation is exactly what happened in the case of moral therapy – to the point where what remained was an emphasis on engaging patients in activity, the forerunner of today's albeit more sophisticated occupational therapy. I have already mentioned some of the similarities in context between today's CBT and the nineteenth century's moral therapy. Without wishing to take an overly pessimistic approach or to predict the future, it is difficult not to note that several additional factors which I argued in Chapter 2 helped foster the assimilation and eventual demise of moral therapy, also appear to apply to CBT.

Moral therapy presented itself as a practical, pragmatic set of practices, rather than an approach arising from a coherent and unifying theory. And, although there seems to be some disagreement about this, CBT is also claimed to have developed pragmatically; there is certainly no one theory from which its very varied practices could be said to have emerged. In one sense, this is a strength in an area beset by premature theorising far beyond its data, but it also means that CBT could become fragmented, with greater use gradually being made only of those aspects which offer least challenge to dominant theory and practice.

A second commonality is in the use of medical language. Moral therapists spoke of afflictions, diseases and treatments; as we have seen, researchers and practitioners of CBT also make extensive use of medical language – schizophrenia, symptoms, illness, treatment, relapse – and exist in a highly ambiguous theoretical relationship to medicine. In addition, both approaches are characterised by a focus on the individual and their 'deficits' or 'abnormal attributes', rather than on the environments in which the madness developed. Thus, the conceptual distance between moral therapy/CBT and medical theories of madness is rapidly covered or obscured via the use of a shared language. The linguistic similarity of both CBT and moral therapy to medical theories of madness is strongly related to the presentation of CBT as an *adjunct* treatment (*OED*: a subordinate or incidental thing); or as a complementary treatment or a treatment for residual psychotic symptoms (Tarrier *et al.*, 1993, 1998, 2000; Haddock *et al.*, 1998b). Kuipers *et al.* (1998) have similarly suggested that new neuroleptics and CBT may be a particularly useful *combination* for treating previously medication-resistant schizophrenic symptoms, while Sensky *et al.* (2000) talk of integrating CBT into standard clinical practice. These statements privilege traditional medical approaches, either explicitly in choice of words or implicitly in word order (note that it is the new approach which has to be integrated into standard clinical practice, not the other way round). Such a presentation is greatly facilitated by CBT's use of medical language and by its ambiguous relationship to medical theory. But there is an interesting irony here. Scull (1979) highlighted the important role of the 'combination treatment' argument in the assimilation and demise of moral therapy. In the nineteenth century, however, the argument that a combination of medical and moral treatment was superior to either alone was advanced by the beleaguered medical profession as a means of improving their status in relation to the management of madness. Scull has called the argument a 'harmless concession' to the moral managers because, while doctors could administer both medical and moral treatment, non-medical practitioners could not. But, almost two centuries later, the 'combination' argument is advanced largely under the first authorship of non-medical CBT researchers. While this situation itself merits analysis, the point here is that the combination argument facilitates assimilation and neutralisation by retaining medicine's primary role in a taken-for-granted way and by leaving the way open for the idea that CBT is only a temporary necessity (a treatment for *residual* or *medication-resistant* symptoms), until better medical treatments and, ultimately, cures, are available.

A third aspect of commonality between CBT and moral therapy, or at least between their contexts, is the availability of theoretical ideas which facilitate the assimilation of challenges to dominant systems of thought. In the nineteenth century it was argued that psychological (moral) versions of madness were problematic because only the *brain* and not the mind (an immaterial essence) could be diseased; it was also argued that the only alternative to madness as a brain disorder was to see it as a spiritual malady. Our thinking may have changed since then, but as I noted in the previous chapter this nineteenth-century dichotomy is still very much part of both lay and professional presentations of madness: mad or bad; evil or ill; madness as disease versus madness caused by blameworthy others. Just as in the nineteenth century, such dichotomies create difficulties for alternative ideas which involve neither disease/illness nor guilt/blame, and make their assimilation or rejection more likely. The problem is compounded by the fact that there is now a wider range of theoretical ideas which can facilitate the assimilation and neutralisation of non-medical approaches. The vulnerability–stress model which is used in some versions of CBT is particularly powerful in this respect: it retains the primacy of biological disorder or weakness (whose nature or relationship to psychosis is never clearly specified) while simultaneously emphasising and de-emphasising context by suggesting that 'life events' may be made stressful by the person's prior 'vulnerability'. The intervention approach known as 'cognitive remediation' offers another potential route to the assimilation of CBT: while it shares CBT's focus on cognitive processes, its stated aim of 'directly treating the cognitive and neuropsychological impairments of schizophrenia' (Spaulding *et al.*, 1998) is much closer to a medical approach than are many versions of CBT. Nevertheless, the shared focus on an *individual's* cognitive processes, together with CBT's apparent reluctance to abandon a 'discourse of deficit', could facilitate CBT's gradual transformation into a narrower set of ideas and practices more closely resembling 'remediation'.

Finally, the variety of goals associated with CBT, which we might see as a strength, could also foster its assimilation, through a gradual emphasis on those goals most compatible with traditional medical approaches. For example, the aims of 'focusing' interventions for voice-hearing – to encourage the person to accept voices as thoughts; to relate these thoughts to their worries and pre-occupations and to provide alternative ways of dealing with these – are not easily assimilated into an illness model. By contrast, the goals of 'coping with symptoms', or 'reducing distress caused by symptoms', *are*. I am not suggest-ing that such goals are inappropriate; indeed, Chadwick *et al.* (1996) have discussed the latter goal in a way which takes it well beyond an illness model, while Tarrier *et al.*'s (1993) 'coping strategy enhancement' includes a functional analysis of voice-hearing. Nevertheless, unless strong and persistent efforts are made to place these goals within an explicitly non-illness framework, they will continue to provide a potential route to the assimilation of CBT. At the very least, these goals invite us to believe that psychological interventions to 'manage symptoms' or 'reduce distress' will only be needed until a cure for these same symptoms is found.

The assimilation and neutralisation of CBT is not, of course, inevitable. But these processes have a long and persistent history in the area of madness, from which valuable lessons on the construction and presentation of alternative ideas might be learned.

## 'Schizophrenia' and 'race'

The final set of ideas I shall discuss which offer potential alternatives to 'schiz-ophrenia' are perhaps most explicitly concerned with the relationship between psychotic experiences and social context; they also focus on the relationship between psychosis and membership of minority and subordinate ethnic groups (Littlewood, 1980; Littlewood and Lipsedge, 1982, 1989, 1997).

The starting point of Littlewood and Lipsedge's (1982) discussion was their 'realisation' that diagnoses of schizophrenia, when made about immigrant groups, 'often conveyed the doctor's lack of understanding rather than the pres-ence of the "key symptoms" by which this reaction is conventionally recognised by British psychiatrists. Patients appeared to be regarded as unintelligible because of their cultural background' (7); the emphasis here is on the important role of perceptions of irrationality in judgements of insanity. With this in mind, Littlewood and Lipsedge developed two major themes. First, that '[w]ith a sympathetic knowledge of another's culture and of their personal experience it is possible to understand much of what otherwise appears as inexplicable irra-tionality' and, second, that 'there is always an interrelation between personal experience and cultural preoccupations which is not haphazard, which is related to the interests of the group as a whole (or certain dominant sections of it) and which can be understood historically' (1982: 208–209). These themes have been illustrated by descriptions and analyses of the behaviour and backgrounds of a number of immigrant people – of West Indian, Cypriot, Jewish and Irish extraction – referred to the authors. The major aim of the analyses is to show how apparently incomprehensible behaviour, which might lead to a diagnosis of schizophrenia, can be rendered comprehensible by close examination of cultural beliefs and practices (e.g. about the behaviour of spirits; ways of warding off threat, etc.) and of personal experiences (racial discrimination; family disputes; conflict between the values of the old and new cultures, etc.).

Littlewood and Lipsedge's analyses have made an extremely valuable contribution to our understanding of possible links between psychosis and context; unfortunately, the assumption I discussed earlier for 'delusions' – that an observer's understanding of another's behaviour can serve as one criterion for inferring schizophrenia – seems to have been retained: Littlewood and Lipsedge use the diagnosis of schizophrenia for those people who, even after all their efforts, they still cannot understand. In other words, they assume that they are discussing *misdiagnosis*, and that it is possible 'properly' to diagnose schizophrenia:

> Nor is the diagnosis of schizophrenia merely futile labelling . . . If we say that patients like CJ or MO are schizophrenic when they are not, we are subjecting them to unnecessary long-term medication, the stigma of mental illness and a self-perception as an invalid. If, on the other hand, we fail to recognize schizophrenia, we have again misinterpreted our patient's experience and possibly condemned him to a gradual process of emotional deterioration, with its harmful effect on his personality, family and livelihood . . . It is essential for the psychiatrist to be able to distinguish between serious mental illnesses which, although they may have social precipitants, are not self-limiting and situational reactions which can be explained best in social and political terms.
>
> (1997: 108–109)

As well as implying that a diagnosis of schizophrenia is necessary if constructive help is to be offered to some people, Littlewood and Lipsedge provide no evidence for the validity of the distinction between 'serious mental illness' and 'situational reactions', nor for the concept of schizophrenia. Rather, and as with decisions about 'delusions', it is assumed that schizophrenics can be distinguished from pseudo-schizophrenics by the idiosyncrasy of their belief systems and their behaviour:

> EW uses acceptable symbols in her own rather unusual way, but EA, who is schizophrenic employs a much more personal and less accessible type of symbol . . . mentally ill individuals do not always invent their own system

> of symbolic communication; they often employ the dominant system
> which others use – but they are likely to do so in a way which to others
> seems inconvenient and clumsy. They use the system inflexibly.
>
> (1997: 220)

Again we are left with a diagnosis of schizophrenia which depends on the social perspective of a more powerful other. Littlewood and Lipsedge evade this problem simply by arguing that 'to symbolize is a cognitive process and schizophrenic patients have been found to have unusual cognitive patterns (whether biological or social in origin)' (1997: 220).

A second problem, or at least potential for misunderstanding, in Littlewood and Lipsedge's discussion is the implication that the cultural and personal background of white natives, and its relationship to their 'deviant' behaviour, can be readily understood by white psychiatrists and that it is only the cultures of certain minority immigrant groups which require special study. Certainly, Littlewood and Lipsedge's (1997) statement that 'we believe that even the mentally ill are making meaningful statements' (243) does not amount to a discussion of the ways in which their theoretical framework could apply across all groups or of the fact that subordination, discrimination, conflict and harassment are part of the everyday realities of non-immigrant and non-minority groups. To use an earlier example, it is difficult to understand (hallucinated) voice content reported in Nayani and David's (1996) study without reference to the social subordination of women and homosexuals. One implication of applying Littlewood and Lipsedge's analysis only to minority ethnic groups is the assumption that we need different explanations for psychosis when displayed by, say, a native Londoner or a West Indian immigrant:

> We felt that the causes of mental illness in ethnic minorities were the same
> as for members of the majority culture and the problem was simply one of
> understanding the background so as to make a conventional diagnosis . . .
> We began increasingly to question this assumption. The experiences of
> migration and of discrimination in housing, employment and everyday life
> were frequently expressed by patients, not as conscious complaints but
> symbolically in the actual structure of their illness.
>
> (1982: 7)

It is a short step from this to the position adopted by a recent news report (BBC HEALTH, 14 July 2000) that 'poor social conditions are causing black people to develop the symptoms of mental illness' and that 'although 75% of white patients with schizophrenia had some biological reason for their illness, in black patients it was only 25%'. These claims were apparently based on three types of research: (1) studies reporting a lower incidence of schizophrenia diagnoses in the Caribbean itself than in African-Caribbean immigrants to Britain (e.g. Mahy et al., 1999); (2) research reporting a lower prevalence of pregnancy and birth complications amongst 'psychotic patients' of African-Caribbean origin than amongst 'white psychotic patients' (Hutchinson *et al.*, 1997); (3) research (unpublished at the time of writing) claiming a higher rate of (unspecified) brain abnormality in white than black psychotic patients. The implication that black and white people have different reasons (biological v. social) for their 'symptoms' is very contentious but is made credible by the public's willingness to accept both a medical framework for bizarre behaviour and experiences and the conceptual simplification and sleight of hand involved in moving from birth complications or brain scan data to 'biological reasons for their illness'. Such claims, however, have three important advantages. First, they appear to address concerns about racism in both psychiatry and society; second, they preserve the concept of schizophrenia, at least for white people, by suggesting that the issue is whether 'the diagnosis of schizophrenia is as valid in the African-Caribbean community as it is in the white community'. Finally, these claims protect from scrutiny non-racial aspects of Western society which might be involved in the development of psychosis.

Reports like these illustrate the ways in which potentially radical analyses such as Littlewood and Lipsedge's, may be assimilated without disturbing the mainstream except in ways which may act to its advantage. The scope for assimilation in relation to 'race', however, is much greater than this. A search of recent literature on 'race', ethnicity and 'schizophrenia' revealed very few studies in which 'race' was analysed as a social construct which mediates psychological experience. By contrast, much research focused on biology and genetics (e.g. race differences in neuroleptic response; genetic linkage and schizophrenia in southern African families). In support of this trend, and public funding of it, Lewine and Caudle (1999) have argued that 'despite [National Institute of Mental Health] efforts to facilitate the study of women and minorities in federally funded schizophrenia research, there is a significant lack of information about race differences in brain morphology and neuropsychological function in schizophrenia'. They also argued that such data are necessary 'to prevent inappropriate generalization of research results across racial groups' (1). Littlewood and Lipsedge's (1997) comment that little of substance has been achieved since the publication of the first edition of their book in 1982, that minority ethnic patients and their families remain objects of study from one perspective, may be rather optimistic; if we are to return to the study of racial differences in the brain, then in this respect at least we are perhaps going backwards.

## 'Schizophrenia' and its alternatives: overview and conclusions

The development and use of 'schizophrenia' is characterised by intellectual and professional practices virtually guaranteed to produce and maintain invalid concepts and problematic research data. These practices include assuming that behaviour and experience can be understood using the conceptual tools of medicine; claiming patterns in behaviour by fiat rather than demonstrating them empirically; begging important questions; passing inferences off as observations; failing to make explicit the 'rules' governing 'schizophrenia's' validity, thus encouraging conceptual confusion and allowing inappropriate validating criteria to seem reasonable; accepting low standards of research practice, including questionable interpretation and misrepresentation of data; squeezing data into existing belief systems rather than changing theory in line with data and, finally, expecting scientific or supposedly scientific concepts to solve complex moral and social problems. Of course, no research area is perfect and some of these practices will be found at times in all research areas. But it is their sheer extent and pervasiveness which mark out 'schizophrenia'; it is these practices which have produced the concept and its surrounding assumptions and on which they depend for their maintenance. They are maintained too, of course, by their social desirability which, together with the complex and technical arguments which surround them, inhibit public questioning.

That we need alternatives to all of this is hardly in question, but it is asking a great deal of alternative accounts that they should overcome all of these problems; we should not be surprised if they have not done so. Rather than assuming that the answer lies in time and increasing research effort, however, I have tried to highlight areas of concern in the development of alternatives which, if we are not careful, could result in our repeating past mistakes. There is, first, a striking lack of a reflective approach to the production of knowledge about psychotic behaviour and experience. It is still implicitly and at times explicitly assumed that knowledge will automatically accrue through the ever more precise efforts of objective researchers. The contexts and belief systems which shape the behaviour of researchers and practitioners – often the same contexts which produced and maintain 'schizophrenia' – are rarely discussed. One consequence of this is that the extent of overlap between the assumptive frameworks of psychology (from where a good deal of the 'alternatives' have come) and those of medicine and psychiatry has been obscured. The dominant tradition in psychology involves focusing on the individual, with the assumption, shared by medicine and psychiatry, that 'surface' phenomena can best be understood as manifestations of structures and processes within the individual; psychology, like psychiatry, tends to essentialise social constructions such as delusions or mental disorder; all three disciplines show a preference for, or grant more prestige to, research methods which treat research 'subjects' as objects of study whose admissible responses are strictly controlled by the researcher and whose own interpretations of their behaviour in research settings may not be deemed relevant. Partly as a result of this assumptive framework, there is still a reluctance to consider fully the idea that psychotic behaviours and experiences are *relational*, that they arise in social and interpersonal contexts, that their form and content are given meaning by those contexts and that such behaviours are officially transformed to 'pathology' only through a relationship of unequal power. Context has been consistently marginalised or made secondary by traditional theory through, for example, the vulnerability–stress model which privileges an assumed inherent weakness or defect; through family research which insists on the family's influence only on the 'course of the illness' and through the claim that poverty or low social class are consequences and not antecedents of psychotic experiences. With some notable exceptions, there is little sign that context is becoming more central in alternative accounts.

Finally, there is a danger that we will seek an alternative account of 'schizophrenic' behaviours and experiences which will (seem) to do all of the administrative, social and moral work we have required of 'schizophrenia': we will demand that an alternative account will somehow show us how to discriminate between the 'pathological' who require or deserve action from authority and the 'non-pathological' who do not, *and* that it will tell us what action ought to be taken or what outcomes ought to be sought. We are so used to assuming that 'schizophrenia' has solved these problems that there is likely to be strong public and professional reluctance to acknowledge not only that it has not but that alternative accounts cannot either, although they may contribute constructively to policy debates.

The situation in research and practice is in many ways much more positive than it was a decade ago; but the tendency to remain within traditional systems of thought means that the cautionary conclusion of the first edition still stands: it is unlikely that constructive alternatives to 'schizophrenia' (as distinct from its replacement with equally problematic concepts) will develop *and persist* unless we face not only the deficiencies of the concept but also the social and intellectual habits which have allowed it to flourish.

# Bibliography

Abrams, R. and Taylor, M.A. (1977) 'Catatonia: prediction of response to somatic treatments', *American Journal of Psychiatry* 134: 78–80.

Albee, G.W. (1986) 'Towards a just society: lessons from observations on the primary prevention of psychopathology', *American Psychologist* 41: 891–898.

Alford, B.A. (1986) 'Behavioral treatment of schizophrenic delusions: a single-case experimental analysis', *Behavior Therapy* 17: 637–644.

Alford, B.A. and Beck, A.T. (1994) 'Cognitive therapy of delusional beliefs', *Behaviour Research and Therapy* 32: 369–380.

Al-Issa, I. (1977) 'Social and cultural aspects of hallucinations', *Psychological Bulletin* 84: 570–587.

Allen, G., Harvald, B. and Shields, J. (1967) 'Measurement of twin concordance', *Acta Genetica* (Basel) 17: 475–481.

Allen, M.G., Cohen, S. and Pollin, W. (1972) 'Schizophrenia in veteran twins: a diagnostic review', *American Journal of Psychiatry* 128: 939–945.

Alpert, M. (1985) 'The signs and symptoms of schizophrenia', *Comprehensive Psychiatry* 26: 103–112.

Alpert, M. and Silvers, K.N. (1970) 'Perceptual characteristics distinguishing auditory hallucinations in schizophrenics and acute alcoholic psychosis', *American Journal of Psychiatry* 127: 298–302.

American Psychiatric Association (1952) *Diagnostic and Statistical Manual of Mental Disorders* (1st edn, revised), Washington, DC: APA.

American Psychiatric Association (1968) *Diagnostic and Statistical Manual of Mental Disorders* (2nd edn), Washington, DC: APA.

American Psychiatric Association (1980) *Diagnostic and Statistical Manual of Mental Disorders* (3rd edn), Washington, DC: APA.

American Psychiatric Association (1987) *Diagnostic and Statistical Manual of Mental Disorders* (3rd edn, revised), Washington, DC: APA.

American Psychiatric Association (1994) *Diagnostic and Statistical Manual of Mental Disorders* (4th edn), Washington, DC: APA.

American Psychiatric Association (2000) *Diagnostic and Statistical Manual of Mental Disorders: Text Revision*, Washington, DC: APA.

Anderson, C.A., Lepper, M.A. and Ross, L. (1980) 'Perseverance of social theories: the role of explanation in the persistence of discredited information', *Journal of Personality and Social Psychology* 39: 1037–1049.

Andreasen, N.C. (1991) 'Schizophrenia and related disorders in DSM-IV: editor's introduction', *Schizophrenia Bulletin* 17: 25–26.

Andreasen, N.C. and Carpenter, W.T. (1993) 'Diagnosis and classification of schizophrenia', *Schizophrenia Bulletin* 19: 199–214.

Andreasen, N.C. and Flaum, M.A. (1990) 'Schizophrenia and related psychotic disorders', *Hospital and Community Psychiatry* 41: 954–956.

Andreasen, N.C. and Flaum, M. (1991) 'Schizophrenia: the characteristic symptoms', *Schizophrenia Bulletin* 17: 27–49.

Andreasen, N.C., Flaum, M., Swayze, V.W., Tyrrell, G. and Arndt, S. (1990a) 'Positive and negative symptoms in schizophrenia: a critical re-appraisal', *Archives of General Psychiatry* 47: 615–621.

Andreasen, N.C., Swayze, V.W., Flaum, M., Yates, W.R., Arndt, S. and McChesney, C. (1990b) 'Ventricular enlargement in schizophrenia evaluated with computed tomographic scanning. Effects of gender, age and stage of illness', *Archives of General Psychiatry* 47: 1008–1015.

Antonarakis, S.E., Blouin, J.L., Lasseter, V.K., Gehrig, C., Radhakrishna, U., Nestadt, G., Housman, D.E., Kazazian, H.H., Kalman, K., Gutman, G., Fantino, E., Chandy, K.G., Gargus, J.J. and Pulver, A.E. (1999) 'Lack of linkage or association between schizophrenia and the polymorphic trinucleotide repeat within the KCNN3 gene on chromosome 1q21', *American Journal of Medical Genetics* 88: 348–351.

Antrobus, J.S., Singer, J.L. and Greenberg, S. (1966) 'Studies in the stream of consciousness: experimental enhancement and suppression of spontaneous cognitive processes', *Perceptual and Motor Skills* 23: 399–417.

Astrachan, B.M., Harrow, M., Adler, D., Brauer, L., Schwartz, A., Schwartz, C. and Tucker, G.A. (1972) 'A checklist for the diagnosis of schizophrenia', *British Journal of Psychiatry* 121: 529–539.

Astrup, C. and Noreik, K. (1966) *Functional Psychosis: Diagnostic and Prognostic Models*, Springfield, Ill.: Charles C. Thomas.

Ayllon, T. and Azrin, N. (1968) *The Token Economy: A Motivational System for Therapy and Rehabilitation*, New York: Appleton Century Crofts.

Barr, C., Kennedy, K.L., Pakstis, A.J., Castiglione, C.M., Kidd, J.R., Wetterberg, L. and Kidd, K.K. (1994) 'Linkage study of a susceptibility locus for schizophrenia in the pseudoautosomal region', *Schizophrenia Bulletin* 20: 277–286.

Barrett, T.R. and Etheridge, J.B. (1992) 'Verbal hallucinations in normals: 1. People who hear "voices"', *Applied Cognitive Psychology* 6: 379–387.

Beck, A.T. (1952) 'Successful outpatient psychotherapy of a chronic schizophrenic with a delusion based on borrowed guilt', *Psychiatry* 15: 305–312.

Beck, A.T. (1962) 'Reliability of psychiatric diagnoses: a critique of systematic studies', *American Journal of Psychiatry* 119: 210–216.

Beck, A.T., Ward, C., Mendelson, M., Mock, J. and Erbaugh, J. (1962) 'Reliability of psychiatric diagnosis: 2. A study of consistency of clinical judgements and ratings', *American Journal of Psychiatry* 119: 351–357.

Beck, J.C. and van der Kolk, B. (1987) 'Reports of childhood incest and current behaviour of chronically hospitalized psychotic women', *American Journal of Psychiatry* 144: 1474–1476.

Beck, L.W. (1953) 'Constructions and inferred entities', in H. Feigl and M. Brodbeck (eds) *Readings in the Philosophy of Science*, New York: Appleton Century Crofts.

Behrendt, R.P. (1998) 'Underconstrained perception: a theoretical approach to the nature and functions of verbal hallucinations', *Comprehensive Psychiatry* 39: 236–248.

Benjamin, A.C. (1937) *An Introduction to the Philosophy of Science*, New York: Macmillan.

Benjamin, L.S. (1976) 'A reconsideration of the Kety and associates' study of genetic factors in the transmission of schizophrenia', *American Journal of Psychiatry* 113: 1129–1133.

Bennett, E. (1983) 'The biasing effect of possession of information on clinicians' subsequent recognition of client information', unpublished Masters thesis, North East London Polytechnic.

Bentall, R.P. (1990a) 'The illusion of reality: a review and integration of psychological research on hallucinations', *Psychological Bulletin* 107: 82–95.

Bentall, R.P. (1990b) 'The syndromes and symptoms of psychosis: or why you can't play "twenty questions" with the concept of schizophrenia and hope to win', in R.P. Bentall (ed.) *Reconstructing Schizophrenia*, London: Routledge.

Bentall, R.P. (1995) 'Brains, biases, deficits and disorders', *British Journal of Psychiatry* 167: 153–155.

Bentall, R.P. (1999) 'Commentary on Garety and Freeman – III: three psychological investigators and an elephant', *British Journal of Clinical Psychology* 38: 323–327.

Bentall, R.P., Haddock, G. and Slade, P.D. (1994) 'Cognitive behaviour therapy for persistent auditory hallucinations: from theory to therapy', *Behavior Therapy* 25: 51–66.

Bentall, R.P. and Kaney, S. (1996) 'Abnormalities of self-representation and persecutory delusions: a test of a cognitive model of paranoia', *Psychological Medicine* 26: 1231–1237.

Bentall, R.P., Kaney, S. and Dewey, M.E. (1991) 'Persecutory delusions: an attribution theory analysis', *British Journal of Clinical Psychology* 30: 13–23.

Bentall, R.P., Kinderman, P. and Kaney, S. (1994) 'The self, attributional processes and abnormal beliefs: towards a model of persecutory delusions', *Behaviour Research and Therapy* 32: 331–341.

Bentall, R.P. and Slade, P.D. (1985) 'Reality testing and auditory hallucinations: a signal-detection analysis', *British Journal of Clinical Psychology* 24: 159–169.

Bentall, R.P. and Slade, P.D. (1986) 'Verbal hallucinations, unintendedness and the validity of the schizophrenia diagnosis', *The Behavioral and Brain Sciences* 9: 519–520.

Bentall, R.P. and Young, H.F. (1996) 'Sensible hypothesis testing in deluded, depressed and normal subjects', *British Journal of Psychiatry* 168: 372–375.

Berrios, G.E. (1991) 'Delusions as "wrong beliefs": a conceptual history', *British Journal of Psychiatry* 159 (Suppl. 14): 6–13.

Billig, M. (1976) *Social Psychology and Intergroup Relations*, London: Academic Press.

Billig, M. (1990) 'Rhetoric of social psychology', in I. Parker and J. Shotter (eds) *Deconstructing Social Psychology*, London: Routledge.

Billig, M. (1991) *Ideology and Opinions: Studies in Rhetorical Psychology*, London: Sage.

Birchwood, M. (1999) 'Commentary on Garety & Freeman – I: "Cognitive approaches to delusions – a critical review of theories and evidence"', *British Journal of Clinical Psychology* 38: 315–318.

Birchwood, M. and Chadwick, P. (1997) 'The omnipotence of voices: testing the validity of a cognitive model', *Psychological Medicine* 27: 1345–1353.

Birchwood, M., Meaden, A., Trower, P., Gilbert, P. and Plaistow, J. (2000) 'The power and omnipotence of voices: subordination and entrapment by voices and significant others', *Psychological Medicine* 30: 337–344.

Blakemore, C. (1988) *The Mind Machine*, BBC2, 18 October.

Blashfield, R.K. and Draguns, J.G. (1976) 'Evaluative criteria for psychiatric classification', *Journal of Abnormal Psychology* 85: 140–150.

Bleuler, E. ([1911] 1950) *Dementia Praecox or the Group of Schizophrenias* (trans. J. Zitkin), New York: International Universities Press.

Bleuler, M. (1991) 'The concept of schizophrenia in Europe during the past one hundred years', in W.F. Flack Jr, D.R. Miller and M. Weiner (eds) *What is Schizophrenia?*, New York: Springer-Verlag.

Bockoven, J.S. (1956a) 'Moral treatment in American psychiatry', *Journal of Nervous and Mental Disease* 124: 167–194.

Bockoven, J.S. (1956b) 'Moral treatment in American psychiatry', *Journal of Nervous and Mental Disease* 124: 292–321.

Bouchard, S., Vallières, A., Roy, M.-A. and Maziade, M. (1996) 'Cognitive restructuring in the treatment of psychotic symptoms in schizophrenia: a critical analysis', *Behavior Therapy* 27: 257–277.

Bowers, J. (1990) 'All hail the great abstraction: star wars and the politics of cognitive psychology', in I. Parker and J. Shotter (eds) *Deconstructing Social Psychology*, London: Routledge.

Boyle, M. (1994) 'Schizophrenia and the art of the soluble', *The Psychologist* 7: 399–404.

Boyle, M. (1996a) 'Schizophrenia re-evaluated', in T. Heller, J. Reynolds, R. Gomm, R. Muston and S. Pattison (eds) *Mental Health Matters*, London: Macmillan.

Boyle, M. (1996b) Review of C.D. Frith 'Cognitive Neuropsychology of Schizophrenia', *British Journal of Psychology* 87: 164–165.

Boyle, M. (1997) *Re-thinking Abortion: Psychology, Gender, Power and the Law*, London: Routledge.

Breggin, P. (1990) 'Brain damage, dementia and persistent cognitive dysfunction associated with neuroleptic drugs: evidence, etiology and implications', *Journal of Mind and Behaviour* 11: 425–464.

Breggin, P. (1993) *Toxic Psychiatry*, London: Fontana.

Brenner, H.D. and Pfammatter, M. (1998) 'Outcome and costs of psychological therapies in schizophrenia', in T. Wykes, N. Tarrier and S. Lewis (eds) *Outcome and Innovation in Psychological Treatments for Schizophrenia*, Chichester: Wiley.

Brewin, J., Cantwell, R., Dalkin, T., Fox, R., Medley, I., Glazebrook, C., Kwiecinski, R. and Harrison, G. (1997) 'Incidence of schizophrenia in Nottingham', *British Journal of Psychiatry* 177: 140–144.

Bridgman, P.W. (1927) *The Logic of Modern Physics*, New York: Macmillan.

Brill, H. (1974) 'Classification and nomenclature of psychiatric conditions', in S. Arieti (ed.) *American Handbook of Psychiatry*, Vol. 1 (2nd edn), New York: Basic Books.

British Psychological Society (2000) *Recent Advances in Understanding Mental Illness and Psychotic Experiences*, Leicester: British Psychological Society.

Brockington, I.F., Kendell, R.E. and Leff, J.P. (1978) 'Definitions of schizophrenia: concordance and prediction of outcome', *Psychological Medicine* 8: 387–398.

Brown, G.W., Birley, J.L.T. and Wing, J.K. (1972) 'Influence of family life on the course of schizophrenic disorders: a replication', *British Journal of Psychiatry* 121: 241–258.

Bryer, J.B., Nelson, B.A., Miller, J.B. and Krol, P.A. (1987) 'Childhood sexual and physical abuse as factors in adult psychiatric illness', *American Journal of Psychiatry* 144: 1426–1430.

Butler, R.W. and Braff, D.L. (1991) 'Delusions: a review and integration', *Schizophrenia Bulletin* 17: 633–647.

Bynum, W.F. (1964) 'Rationales for therapy in British psychiatry: 1780–1835', *Medical History* 18: 317–335.

Campbell, P. (1999) 'The service user/survivor movement', in C. Newnes, G. Holmes and C. Dunn (eds) *This is Madness: A Critical look at Psychiatry and the Future of Mental Health Services*, Ross-on-Wye: PCCS Books.

Cancro, R. (1976) 'Some diagnostic and therapeutic considerations of the schizophrenic syndrome', in R. Cancro (ed.) *Annual Review of the Schizophrenic Syndrome*, Vol. 5, New York: Bruner Mazel.

Cannon, T.D., Kaprio, J., Lönnqvist, J., Huttunen, M. and Koskenvuo, M. (1998) 'The genetic epidemiology of schizophrenia in a Finnish twin cohort', *Archives of General Psychiatry* 55: 67–74.

Cantor, N. and Mischel, W. (1977) 'Traits as prototypes: effects on recognition memory', *Journal of Personality and Social Psychology* 35: 38–48.

Cantor, N., Smith, E.E., de Sales French, R. and Mezzich, J. (1980) 'Psychiatric diagnosis as prototype categorization', *Journal of Abnormal Psychology* 89: 181–193.

Cardno, A.G., Marshall, E.J., Coid, B., Macdonald, A.M., Ribchester, T.R., Davies, N.J., Venturi, P., Jones, L.A., Lewis, S.W., Sham, P.C., Gottesman, I.I., Farmer, A.E., McGuffin, P., Reveley, A. and Murray, R.M. (1999) 'Heritability estimates for psychotic disorders', *Archives of General Psychiatry* 56: 162–168.

Carnap, R. (1937) 'Testability and meaning. Part IV', *Philosophy of Science* 4: 1–40.

Carnap, R. (1974) *An Introduction to the Philosophy of Science* (ed. Martin Gardner), New York: Basic Books.

Carpenter, W., Bartko, J. and Strauss, J. (1978) 'Signs and symptoms as predictors of outcome: a report from the International Pilot Study of Schizophrenia', *American Journal of Psychiatry* 135: 940–945.

Carpenter, W.T., Strauss, J.S. and Bartko, J. (1973a) 'Flexible system for the diagnosis of schizophrenia: report from the International Pilot Study of Schizophrenia', *Science* 182: 1275–1278.

Carpenter, W.T., Strauss, J.S. and Salvatore, M. (1973b) 'Are there pathognomic symptoms in schizophrenia: an empiric investigation of Schneider's first-rank symptoms', *Archives of General Psychiatry* 28: 847–852.

Castel, R. (1994) '"Problematization" as a mode of reading history', in J Goldstein (ed.) *Foucault and the Writing of History*, Oxford: Blackwell.

Castel, R., Castel, F. and Lovell, A. (1982) *The Psychiatric Society*, New York: Columbia University Press.

Cerasi, E. and Luft, R. (1967) 'Insulin response to glucose infusion in diabetic and non-diabetic monozygotic twin pairs: genetic control of insulin response?', *Acta Endocrinologica* 55: 330–345.

Chadwick, P. and Birchwood, M. (1994) 'The omnipotence of voices: a cognitive approach to auditory hallucinations', *British Journal of Psychiatry* 164: 190–201.

Chadwick, P. and Birchwood, M. (1996) 'Cognitive therapy for voices', in G. Haddock and P.D. Slade (eds) *Cognitive-behavioural Interventions with Psychotic Disorders*, London: Routledge.

Chadwick, P., Birchwood, M. and Trower, P. (1996) *Cognitive Therapy for Delusions, Voices and Paranoia*, Chichester: Wiley.

Chadwick, P. and Trower, P. (1996) 'Cognitive therapy for punishment paranoia: a single case experiment', *Behaviour Research and Therapy* 34: 351–356.

Chadwick, P.D.J. and Lowe, C.F. (1990) 'Measurement and modification of delusional beliefs', *Journal of Consulting and Clinical Psychology* 58: 225–232.

Chadwick, P.D.J. and Lowe, C.F. (1994) 'A cognitive approach to measuring and modifying delusions', *Behaviour Research and Therapy* 32: 355–367.

Chalmers, A. (1990) *Science and its Fabrication*, Milton Keynes: Open University Press.

Chapman, L.J. and Chapman, J.P. (1967) 'The genesis of popular but erroneous psychodiagnostic observations', *Journal of Abnormal Psychology* 72: 193–204.

Chapman, L.J. and Chapman, J.P. (1982) 'Test results are what you think they are', in D. Kahneman, P. Slovic and A. Tversky (eds) *Judgement Under Uncertainty: Heuristics and Biases*, Cambridge: Cambridge University Press.

Chua, S.E. and McKenna, P.J. (1995) 'Schizophrenia – a brain disease?', *British Journal of Psychiatry* 166: 563–582.

Clare, A. (1976) *Psychiatry in Dissent: Controversial Issues in Thought and Practice* (2nd edn 1980), London: Tavistock.

Claridge, G.S. (1994) 'Single indicator of risk for schizophrenia: probable fact or likely myth?', *Schizophrenia Bulletin* 20: 151–168.

Cooper, J.E., Kendell, R.E., Gurland, B.J., Sharpe, L., Copeland, J.R.M. and Simon, R. (1972) *Psychiatric Diagnosis in New York and London. A Comparative Study of Mental Hospital Admissions*, Institute of Psychiatry and Maudsley Monographs No. 20, London: Oxford University Press.

Corcoran, R., Cahill, C. and Frith, C.D. (1997) 'The appreciation of visual jokes in people with schizophrenia: a study of mentalizing ability', *Schizophrenia Research* 24: 319–327.

Corcoran, R., Mercer, G. and Frith, C.D. (1995) 'Schizophrenia, symptomatology and social inference: investigating "theory of mind" in people with schizophrenia', *Schizophrenia Research* 17: 5–13.

Costello, C.G. (1992) 'Research on symptoms versus research on syndromes: arguments in favour of allocating more research time to the study of symptoms', *British Journal of Psychiatry* 160: 304–308.

Coyne, J.C. (1982) 'A critique of cognitions as causal entities', *Cognitive Therapy and Research* 6: 3–13.

Crocker, J. (1981) 'Judgement of covariation by social perceivers', *Psychological Bulletin* 90: 272–292.

Cronbach, L.J. and Meehl, P.E. (1955) 'Construct validity in psychological tests', *Psychological Bulletin* 52: 281–302.

Crookshank, F.G. (1956) 'The importance of a theory of signs and a critique of language in the study of medicine', a supplement to C.K. Ogden and I.A. Richards (eds) *The Meaning of Meaning* (10th edn), London: Routledge and Kegan Paul.

Crow, T.J. (1980) 'Molecular pathology of schizophrenia: more than one disease process?', *British Medical Journal* 280: 66–68.

Crow, T.J. (1984) 'A re-evaluation of the viral hypothesis: is psychosis the result of retroviral integration at a site close to the cerebral dominance gene?', *British Journal of Psychiatry* 145: 243–253.

Crowe, R.R. (1982) 'Recent genetic research in schizophrenia', in F. Henn and H. Nasrallah (eds) *Schizophrenia as a Brain Disease*, New York: Oxford University Press.

Crowe, R.R., Black, D.W., Wesner, R., Andreasen, N.C., Cookman, A., and Roby, J. (1991) 'Lack of linkage to chromosome 5q11–q13 markers in six schizophrenia pedigrees', *Archives of General Psychiatry* 48: 357–361.

Curtis, L., Blouin, J.L., Radhakrishna, U., Gehrig, C., Lasseter, V.K., Wolyniec, P., Nestadt, G., Dombroski, B., Kazazian, H.H., Pulver, A.E., Housman, D., Bertrand, D. and Antonarakis, S.E. (1999) 'No evidence for linkage between schizophrenia markers at chromosome 15q13–14', *American Journal of Medical Genetics* 88: 109–112.

Cutting, J. (1985) *The Psychology of Schizophrenia*, Edinburgh: Churchill Livingstone.

Davey, B. (1993) 'Psychosis', in M. Romme and S. Escher, *Accepting Voices*, London: Mind Publications.

David, A. (1994) 'The neuropsychological origin of auditory hallucinations', in A. David and J. Cutting (eds) *The Neuropsychology of Schizophrenia*, Hove: Erlbaum.

Davidson, L. and McGlashan, T. (1997) 'The varied outcomes of schizophrenia', *Canadian Journal of Psychiatry* 42: 34–43.

Davies, B. and Harré, R. (1990) 'Positioning: the discursive production of selves', *Journal for the Theory of Social Behaviour* 20: 43–63.

Davison, G.C. and Neale, J.M. (eds) (2001) *Abnormal Psychology*, New York: Wiley.

Day, J.C. and Bentall, R.P. (1996) 'Neuroleptic medication and the psychosocial treatment of psychotic symptoms: some neglected issues', in G. Haddock and P.D. Slade (eds) *Cognitive-behavioural Interventions with Psychotic Disorders*, London: Routledge.

de Leon, J., Simpson, G.M. and Peralta, V. (1992) 'Positive and negative symptoms in schizophrenia: where are the data?', *Biological Psychiatry* 31: 431–434.

DeLisi, L.E. (1997) 'The genetics of schizophrenia: past, present, and future concepts', *Schizophrenia Research* 28: 163–175.

Der, G., Gupta, S. and Murray, R. (1990) 'Is schizophrenia disappearing?', *The Lancet* 335: 513–516.

Doane, J.A., West, K.L., Goldstein, M.J., Rodnick, E.H. and Jones, J.E. (1981) 'Parental communication deviance and affective style', *Archives of General Psychiatry* 38: 679–715.

Dudley, R.E.J., John, C.H., Young, A.W. and Over, D.E. (1997a) 'Normal and abnormal reasoning in people with delusions', *British Journal of Clinical Psychology* 36: 243–258.

Dudley, R.E.J., John, C.H., Young, A.W. and Over, D.E. (1997b) 'The effect of self-referent material on the reasoning of people with delusions', *British Journal of Clinical Psychology* 36: 575–584.

Dunton, W.R. (1944) 'The American Journal of Psychiatry 1844–1944', *American Journal of Psychiatry* 100: 45–60.

Earnst, K.S. and Kring, A.M. (1997) 'Construct validity of negative symptoms: an empirical and conceptual review', *Clinical Psychology Review* 17: 167–189.

Edwards, D. (1997) *Discourse and Cognition*, London and Beverly Hills, Calif.: Sage.

Emmet, E.R. (1968) *Learning to Philosophise* (2nd edn), Harmondsworth: Penguin Books.

Endicott, J., Nee, J., Fleiss, J., Cohen, J., Williams, J.B. and Simon, R. (1982) 'Diagnostic criteria for schizophrenia: reliabilities and agreement between systems', *Archives of General Psychiatry* 39: 884–889.

Engel, G.L. (1977) 'The need for a new medical model: a challenge for biomedicine', *Science* 196: 129–136.

Engel, G.L. (1980) 'Clinical applications of the biosocial model', *American Journal of Psychiatry* 137: 535–544.

Engle, R.L. (1963) 'Medical diagnosis: past, present and future. II. Philosophical foundations and historical development of our concepts of health, disease and diagnosis', *Archives of Internal Medicine* 112: 520–529.

Engle, R.L. and Davis, B.J. (1963) 'Medical diagnosis: past, present and future. 1. Present concepts of the meaning and limitations of medical diagnosis', *Archives of Internal Medicine* 112: 512–519.

Ensink, B. (1993) 'Trauma: a study of child abuse and hallucinations', in M. Romme and S. Escher (eds) *Accepting Voices*, London: Mind Publications.

Essen-Möller, E. (1941) 'Psychiatrishe Untersuchungen an einer Serie von Zwillingen', *Acta Psychiatrica et Neurologica Scandinavica* (Suppl. 23).

Falloon, I.R.H., Boyd, J.L. and McGill, C.W. (1984) *Family Care of Schizophrenia*, New York: The Guilford Press.

Farran-Ridge, C. (1926) 'Some symptoms referable to the basal ganglia and occurring in dementia praecox and epidemic encephalitis', *Journal of Mental Science* 72: 513–523.

Faulder, C. (1985) *Whose Body Is It? The Troubling Issue of Informed Consent*, London: Virago.

Fear, C.F. and Healy, D. (1997) 'Probabilistic reasoning in obsessive-compulsive and delusional disorders', *Psychological Medicine* 27: 199–208.

Fear, C., Sharp, H. and Healy, D. (1996) 'Cognitive processes in delusional disorders', *British Journal of Psychiatry* 168: 61–67.

Feighner, J.P., Robins, E., Guze, S.B., Woodruff, R.A., Winokur, G. and Muñoz, R. (1972) 'Diagnostic criteria for use in psychiatric research', *Archives of General Psychiatry* 26: 57–63.

Fenton, W.S., Mosher, L.R. and Matthews, S.M. (1981) 'Diagnosis of schizophrenia: a critical review of current diagnostic systems', *Schizophrenia Bulletin* 7: 452–476.

Fernando, S. (1993) 'Psychiatry and racism', *Changes: An International Journal of Psychology and Psychotherapy* 11: 46–58.

First, M.B., Frances, A.J., Pincus, H.A., Vettorello, N. and Davis, W.W. (1994) 'DSM-IV in progress: changes in substance related, schizophrenic and other primarily adult disorders', *Hospital and Community Psychiatry* 45: 18–20.

Fischer, M. (1973) 'Genetic and environmental factors in schizophrenia', *Acta Psychiatrica Scandinavica* (Suppl. 238).

Flaum, M. and Andreasen, N.C. (1991) 'Diagnostic criteria for schizophrenia and related disorders: options for DSM-IV', *Schizophrenia Bulletin* 17: 133–156.

Flaum, M. and Andreasen, N.C. (1995) 'The reliability of distinguishing primary v secondary negative symptoms', *Comprehensive Psychiatry* 36: 421–427.

Flaum, M., Arndt, S. and Andreasen, N.C. (1991) 'The reliability of "bizarre" delusions', *Comprehensive Psychiatry* 32: 59–65.

Foucault, M. (1971) *Madness and Civilisation: A History of Insanity in the Age of Reason*, London: Tavistock.

Foucault, M. (1972) *The Archaeology of Knowledge*, London: Tavistock.

Foucault, M. (1976) *The Birth of the Clinic*, London: Tavistock.

Foucault, M. (1979) *The History of Sexuality: Vol. 1 An Introduction*, London: Allen Lane.

Fowler, D., Garety, P. and Kuipers, E. (1995) *Cognitive Behaviour Therapy for Psychosis: Theory and Practice*, Chichester: Wiley

Fowler, D. and Morley, S. (1989) 'The cognitive-behavioural treatment of hallucinations and delusions: a preliminary study', *Behavioural Psychotherapy* 17: 267–282.

Fox, D. and Prilleltensky, I. (1997) *Critical Psychology: An Introduction*, London: Sage.

Frances, A., Mack, A.H., First, M.B., Widiger, T.A., Ross, R. and Forman, L. (1994) 'DSM-IV meets philosophy', *Journal of Medicine and Philosophy* 19: 207–218.

Franzek, E. and Beckmann, H. (1998) 'Different genetic background of schizophrenia spectrum psychosis: a twin study', *American Journal of Psychiatry* 155: 76–83.

Freidson, E. (1970) *The Profession of Medicine: A Study of the Sociology of Applied Knowledge*, New York: Harper and Row.

French, M. (1986) *Beyond Power: On Women, Men and Morals*, London: Sphere Books.

Frith, C.D. (1992) *The Cognitive Neuropsychology of Schizophrenia*, Hillsdale, N.J.: Erlbaum.

Frith, C.D. (1999) 'Commentary on Garety & Freeman II: "Cognitive approaches to delusions – a critical review of theories and evidence"', *British Journal of Clinical Psychology* 38: 319–321.

Gaines, A.D. (1995) 'Culture specific delusions: sense and nonsense in cultural context', *The Psychiatric Clinics of North America* 18: 281–301.

Garety, P.A. (1991) 'Reasoning and delusions', *British Journal of Psychiatry* 159 (Suppl. 14): 14–18.

Garety, P.A., Fowler, D., Kuipers, E., Freeman, D., Dunn, G., Bebbington, P., Hadley, C. and Jones, S. (1997) 'London–East Anglia randomised controlled trial of cognitive-behavioural therapy for psychosis. II: Predictors of outcome', *British Journal of Psychiatry* 171: 420–426.

Garety, P.A. and Freeman, D. (1999) 'Cognitive approaches to delusions: a critical review of theories and evidence', *British Journal of Clinical Psychology* 38: 113–154.

Garety, P.A. and Hemsley, D.R. (1994) *Delusions: Investigations into the Psychology of Delusional Reasoning*, Hove: Psychology Press.

Garety, P.A., Hemsley, D.R. and Wessely, S. (1991) 'Reasoning in deluded schizophrenic and paranoid patients: biases in performance on a probabilistic inference task', *Journal of Nervous and Mental Disease* 179: 194–201.

Garety, P.A., Kuipers, E., Fowler, D., Chamberlain, F. and Dunn, G. (1994) 'Cognitive behaviour therapy for drug-resistant psychosis', *British Journal of Medical Psychology* 67: 259–271.

Georgaca, E. (2000) 'Reality and discourse: a critical analysis of the category of "delusions"', *British Journal of Medical Psychology* 73: 227–242.

Gergen, K. (1999) *An Invitation to Social Construction*, London and Beverly Hills, Calif.: Sage.

Gergen, K.J. (1990) 'Therapeutic professions and the diffusion of deficit', *The Journal of Mind and Behaviour* 11: 353–368.

Gershon, E.S., Badner, J.A., Goldin, L.R., Sanders, A.R., Cravchik, A. and Detera-Wadleigh, S.D. (1998) 'Closing in on genes for manic-depressive illness and schizophrenia', *Neuropsychopharmacology* 18: 233–242.

Gift, T.E., Strauss, J.S., Kokes, R.F., Harder, D.W. and Ritzler, B.A. (1980) 'Schizophrenia: affect and outcome', *American Journal of Psychiatry* 137: 580–585.

Gilbert, G.N. and Mulkay, M. (1984) *Opening Pandora's Box: A Sociological Analysis of Scientists' Discourse*, Cambridge: Cambridge University Press.

Gill, E. (2000) 'Clients' understanding and experiences of cognitive-behavioural therapy for "delusions"', Unpublished report, University of East London.

Gill, R. (1993) 'Justifying injustice: broadcasters' accounts of inequality in radio', in E. Burman and I. Parker (eds) *Discourse Analytic Research: Repertoires and Readings of Texts in Action*, London: Routledge.

Gilligan, C. (1993) *In a Different Voice: Psychological Theory and Women's Development* (2nd edn), Cambridge, Mass.: Harvard University Press.

Goldberg, D.M. (2000) 'Predictions for psychiatry', *Journal of the Royal Society of Medicine* 93 (December): 649–651.

Goldstein, M.J. (1987) 'The UCLA high-risk project', *Schizophrenia Bulletin* 13: 505–514.

Gottesman, I.I. and Moldin, S.O. (1997) 'Schizophrenia genetics at the millennium: cautious optimism', *Clinical Genetics* 52: 404–407.

Gottesman, I.I. and Shields, J. (1972) *Schizophrenia and Genetics: A Twin Study Vantage Point*, London: Academic Press.

Gottesman, I.I. and Shields, J. (1976) 'A critical review of recent adoption, twin and family studies of schizophrenia: behavioural genetics perspectives', *Schizophrenia Bulletin* 2: 360–401.

Gottesman, I.I. and Shields, J. (1982) *Schizophrenia: The Epigenic Puzzle*, Cambridge: Cambridge University Press.

Gould, L.N. (1949) 'Auditory hallucinations and subvocal speech', *Journal of Nervous and Mental Disease* 109: 418–427.

Gould, L.N. (1950) 'Verbal hallucinations as automatic speech: the reactivation of a dormant speech habit', *American Journal of Psychiatry* 107: 110–119.

Gould, S.J. (1981) *The Mismeasure of Man*, New York: W.W. Norton.

Grange, K. (1962) 'The ship symbol as a key to former theories of the emotions', *Bulletin of the History of Medicine* 36: 512–523.

Greenberg, D., Witztum, E. and Buchbinder, J.T. (1992) 'Mysticism and psychosis: the fate of Ben Zoma', *British Journal of Medical Psychology* 65: 223–235.

Greenfield, S.F., Strakowski, S.M., Tohen, M., Batson, S.C. and Kolbrener, M.L. (1994) 'Childhood abuse in first episode psychosis', *British Journal of Psychiatry* 164: 831–834.

Gurling, H. (1989) Letter, *The Lancet*, 14 February: 277.

Haage, D.A.F., Dyck, M.J. and Ernst, D. (1991) 'Empirical status of cognitive theory of depression', *Psychological Bulletin* 110: 215–236.

Haddock, G., Bentall, R.P. and Slade, P.D. (1993) 'Psychological treatment of auditory hallucinations: two case studies', *Behavioural and Cognitive Psychotherapy* 21: 335–346.

Haddock, G., Bentall, R.P. and Slade, P.D. (1996) 'Psychological treatment of auditory hallucinations: focusing or distraction?', in G. Haddock and P.D. Slade (eds) *Cognitive-behavioural Interventions with Psychotic Disorders*, London: Routledge.

Haddock, G. and Slade, P.D. (eds) (1996) *Cognitive-behavioural Interventions with Psychotic Disorders*, London: Routledge.

Haddock G., Slade, P.D., Bentall, R.P., Reid, D. and Faragher, E.B. (1998a) 'A comparison of the long-term effectiveness of distraction and focusing in the treatment of auditory hallucinations', *British Journal of Medical Psychology* 71: 339–349.

Haddock, G., Tarrier, N., Spaulding, W., Yusupoff, L., Kinney, C. and McCarthy, E. (1998b) 'Individual cognitive-behavior therapy in the treatment of hallucinations and delusions: a review', *Clinical Psychology Review* 18: 821–838.

Haier, R.J., Rosenthal, D. and Wender, P.H. (1978) 'MMPI assessment of psychopathology in the adopted-away offspring of schizophrenics', *Archives of General Psychiatry* 35: 171–175.

Hallam, R.S. (1985a) *Anxiety: A Psychological Approach to Panic and Agoraphobia*, New York: Academic Press.

Hallam, R.S. (1985b) Letter, *Bulletin of the British Psychological Society* 38: 341.

Haller, M.M. (1963) *Eugenics*, New Brunswick, N.J.: Rutgers, The State University.

Hamilton, D.L. (ed.) (1981) *Cognitive Processes in Stereotyping and Intergroup Behaviour*, Hillsdale, N.J.: Lawrence Erlbaum Associates.

Harding, S. (1986) *The Science Question in Feminism*, Ithaca, N.Y.: Cornell University Press.

Harding, S. (1991) *Whose Science, Whose Knowledge? Thinking From Women's Lives*, Milton Keynes: Open University Press.

Hare, E.H. (1959) 'The origin and spread of dementia paralytica', *Journal of Mental Science* 105: 594–626.

Hare, E.H. (1973) 'A short note on pseudo-hallucinations', *British Journal of Psychiatry* 122: 469–476.

Hare, E.H. (1983) 'Was insanity on the increase?', *British Journal of Psychiatry* 142: 439–455.

Hare, E.H. (1986) 'Schizophrenia as an infectious disease', in A. Kerr and P. Snaith (eds) *Contemporary Issues in Schizophrenia*, London: Royal College of Psychiatrists/Gaskell.

Harper, D.J. (1999) 'Deconstructing paranoia: an analysis of the discourses associated with the concept of paranoid delusion', unpublished PhD thesis, Manchester Metropolitan University.

Harrison, G., Owens, D., Holton, A., Neilson, D. and Boot, D. (1988) 'A prospective study of severe mental disorder in Afro-Caribbean patients', *Psychological Medicine* 18: 643–657.

Harrop, C.E., Trower, P. and Mitchell, I.J. (1996) 'Does the biology go round the symptoms? A Copernican shift in schizophrenia paradigms', *Clinical Psychology Review* 16: 641–654.

Harrow, M., Yonan, C.A., Sands, J.R., and Marengo, J. (1994) 'Depression in schizophrenia: are neuroleptics, akinesia or ahedonia involved?', *Schizophrenia Bulletin* 20: 327–338.

Hatfield, A. (1987) 'The expressed emotion theory: why families object', *Hospital and Community Psychiatry* 38: 341.

Hawi, Z., Mynett-Johnson, L., Murphy, V., Straub, R.E., Kendler, K.S., Walsh, D., McKeon, P. and Gill, M. (1999) 'No evidence to support the association of the potassium channel gene hSKCa3 CAG repeat with schizophrenia or bipolar disorder in the Irish population', *Molecular Psychiatry* 4: 488–491.

Hawk, A.B., Carpenter, T. and Strauss, J.S. (1975) 'Diagnostic criteria and 5-year outcome in schizophrenia', *Archives of General Psychiatry* 32: 343–347.

Heery, M. (1993) 'Inner voice experiences: a study of 30 cases', in M. Romme and S. Escher (eds) *Accepting Voices*, London: Mind Publications.

Heise, D.R. (1988) 'Delusions and the construction of reality', in J.F. Oltmanns and B.A. Maher (eds) *Delusional Beliefs*, New York: Wiley.

Hempel, C.G. (1961) 'Introduction to the problems of taxonomy', in J. Zubin (ed.) *Field Studies in the Mental Disorders*, New York: Grune and Stratton.

Hemsley, D.R. and Garety, P.A. (1986) 'The formation of delusions: a Bayesian analysis', *British Journal of Psychiatry* 149: 51–56.

Hendrick, I. (1928) 'Encephalitis lethargica and the interpretation of mental disease', *American Journal of Psychiatry* 7: 989–1014.

Henriques, J., Hollway, W., Urwin, C., Venn, C. and Walkerdine, V. (1997) *Changing the Subject* (2nd edn), London: Routledge.

Hingley, S.M. (1997a) 'Psychodynamic perspectives on psychosis and psychotherapy I: Theory', *British Journal of Medical Psychology* 70: 301–312.

Hingley, S.M. (1997b) 'Psychodynamic perspectives on psychosis and psychotherapy II: Practice', *British Journal of Medical Psychology* 70: 313–324.

Hoffer, A. and Pollin, W. (1970) 'Schizophrenia in the NAS-NRC panel of 15,909 veteran twin pairs', *Archives of General Psychiatry* 23: 469–477.

Hoffman, R.E. (1986) 'Verbal hallucinations and language production processes in schizophrenia', *The Behavioral and Brain Sciences* 9: 503–517.

Hoffman, R.E. and Rapaport, J. (1994) 'A psycholinguistic study of auditory/verbal hallucinations: preliminary findings', in A. David and J. Cutting (eds) *The Neuropsychology of Schizophrenia*, Hove: Erlbaum.

Holt, R.R. (1964) 'Imagery: the return of the ostracized', *American Psychologist* 19: 254–264.

Honig, A., Romme, M.A.J., Ensink, B.J., Escher, S.D.M.A.C., Pennings, M.H.A. and Devries, M.W. (1998) 'Auditory hallucinations: a comparison between patients and nonpatients', *Journal of Nervous and Mental Disease* 186: 646–651.

Hoskins, R.G. (1933) 'Schizophrenia from the physiological point of view', *Annals of Internal Medicine* 7: 445–456.

Hoskins, R.G. and Sleeper, F.H. (1933) 'Organic factors in schizophrenia', *Archives of Neurology and Psychiatry* 30: 123–132.

Houts, A.C. and Follette, W.C. (1998) 'Mentalism, mechanisms and medical analogues: reply to Wakefield (1998)', *Journal of Consulting and Clinical Psychology* 66: 853–855.

Hovatta, I., Lichtermann, D., Juvonen, H., Suvisaari, J., Terwilliger, J.D., Arajarvi, R., Kokko-Sahin, M.L., Ekelund, J., Lonnqvist, J. and Peltonen, L. (1998) 'Linkage analysis of putative schizophrenia gene candidate regions on chromosomes 3p, 5q, 6p, 8p, 20p and 22q in a population-based sampled Finnish family set', *Molecular Psychiatry* 3: 452–457.

Huq, S.F., Garety, P.A. and Hemsley, D.R. (1988) 'Probabilistic judgements in deluded and non-deluded subjects', *Quarterly Journal of Experimental Psychology: Human Learning and Memory* 40A: 801–812.

Hutchinson, G., Takei, N., Bhugra, D., Fahy, T.A., Gilvarry, C., Mallett, R., Moran, P., Leff, J. and Murray, R.M. (1997) 'Increased rate of psychosis among African-Caribbeans in Britain is not due to an excess of pregnancy and birth complications', *British Journal of Psychiatry* 171: 145–147.

Hyman, S.E. (2000) 'The NIMH perspective: next steps in schizophrenia research', *Biological Psychiatry* 47: 1–7.

Ingraham, L.J. and Kety, S.S. (2000) 'Adoption studies of schizophrenia', *American Journal of Medical Genetics* 97: 18–22.

Inouye, T. and Shimizu, A. (1970) 'The electromyographic study of verbal hallucinations', *Journal of Nervous and Mental Disease* 151: 415–422.

Jablensky, A. (1986) An interview, *The Times*, 3 March.

Jackson, H.F. (1990) 'Are there biological markers of schizophrenia?', in R.P. Bentall (ed.) *Reconstructing Schizophrenia*, London: Routledge.

Jackson, M. and Fulford, K.W.M. (1997a) 'Spiritual experience and psychopathology', *Philosophy, Psychiatry and Psychology* 4: 41–65.

Jackson, M. and Fulford, K.W.M. (1997b) 'Response to commentaries', *Philosophy, Psychiatry and Psychology* 4: 87–90.

Jackson, M.C. (1991) 'A study of the relationship between psychotic and religious experience', unpublished PhD thesis, University of Oxford.

Jacobson, A. and Richardson, B. (1987) 'Assault experiences of 100 psychiatric inpatients: evidence of the need for routine inquiry', *American Journal of Psychiatry* 144: 908–913.

Jarvis, E. (1998) 'Schizophrenia in British immigrants: recent findings, issues and implications', *Transcultural Psychiatry* 35: 39–74.

Jaspers, K. (1963) *General Psychopathology*, Chicago: University of Chicago Press.

Jaynes, J. (1976) *The Origins of Consciousness in the Breakdown of the Bicameral Mind*, London: Allen Lane.

Jelliffe, S.E. (1927) 'The mental pictures in schizophrenia in epidemic encephalitis. Their alliances, differences and a point of view', *American Journal of Psychiatry* 6: 413–465.

Johnson, M.K. (1988) 'Discriminating the origin of information', in J.F. Oltmanns and B.A. Maher (eds) *Delusional Beliefs*, New York: Wiley.

Johnson, M.K., Hashtroudi, S. and Lindsay, D.S. (1993) 'Source monitoring', *Psychological Bulletin* 114: 3–28.

Johnson, W.G., Ross, J.M. and Mastia, M.A. (1977) 'Delusional behaviour: an attributional analysis of development and modification', *Journal of Abnormal Psychology* 86: 421–426.

Johnstone, L. (2000) *Users and Abusers of Psychiatry* (2nd edn), London: Routledge.

Jones, E. and Watson, J.P. (1997) 'Delusion, the overvalued idea and religious beliefs: a comparative analysis of their characteristics', *British Journal of Psychiatry* 170: 381–386.

Jones, K. (1972) *A History of the Mental Health Services*, London: Routledge and Kegan Paul.

Jones, P.B. (1999) 'Are there bullets in the smoking gun? Invited commentaries: A Jamaican psychiatrist evaluates diagnoses at a London psychiatric hospital', *British Journal of Psychiatry* 175: 286.

Kahneman, D., Slovic, P. and Tversky, A. (eds) (1982) *Judgement Under Uncertainty: Heuristics and Biases*, New York: Cambridge University Press.

Kallmann, F.J. (1938) *The Genetics of Schizophrenia*, Locust Valley, N.Y.: J.J. Augustin.

Kallmann, F.J. (1946) 'The genetic theory of schizophrenia: an analysis of 691 schizophrenic twin index families', *American Journal of Psychiatry* 103: 309–322.

Kaney, S. and Bentall, R.P. (1989) 'Persecutory delusions and attributional style', *British Journal of Medical Psychology* 62: 191–198.

Kaney, S., Bowen-Jones, K., Dewey, M.E. and Bentall, R.P. (1997) 'Two predictions about paranoid ideation: deluded, depressed and normal participants' subjective frequency and consensus judgements for positive, neutral and negative events', *British Journal of Clinical Psychology* 36: 349–364.

Kay, S.R. (1990) 'Significance of the negative/positive distinction in schizophrenia', *Schizophrenia Bulletin* 16: 635–652.

Keith, S.J. and Matthews, S.M. (1991) 'The diagnosis of schizophrenia: a review of onset and duration issues', *Schizophrenia Bulletin* 17: 51–67.

Kendell, R.E. (1972) 'Schizophrenia: the remedy for diagnostic confusion', *British Journal of Hospital Medicine* 8: 383–390.

Kendell, R.E. (1975a) 'The concept of disease and its implications for psychiatry', *British Journal of Psychiatry* 127: 305–315.

Kendell, R.E. (1975b) *The Role of Diagnosis in Psychiatry*, Oxford: Blackwell Scientific Publications.

Kendell, R.E. (1991) 'Schizophrenia: a medical view of a medical concept', in W.F. Flack Jr, D.R. Miller and M. Weiner (eds) *What is Schizophrenia?*, New York: Springer-Verlag.

Kendell, R.E., Brockington, I.F. and Leff, J.P. (1979) 'Prognostic implications of six alternative definitions of schizophrenia', *Archives of General Psychiatry* 36: 25–31.

Kendell, R.E., Everitt, B., Cooper, J.E., Sartorius, N. and David, M.E. (1968) 'The reliability of the "Present State Examination"', *Social Psychiatry* 3: 123–129.

Kendler, K.S. (1990) 'Toward a scientific psychiatric nosology: strengths and limitations', *Archives of General Psychiatry* 47: 969–973.

Kendler, K.S., Glazer, W.M. and Morgenstern, H. (1983) 'Dimensions of delusional experience', *American Journal of Psychiatry* 140: 466–469.

Kendler, K.S., Spitzer, R.L. and Williams, J.B.W. (1989) 'Psychotic disorders in DSM-III-R', *American Journal of Psychiatry* 146: 953–962.

Kennedy, J.L., Giuffra, L.A., Moises, H.W., Cavalli-Sforza, L.L., Pakstis, A.J., Kidd, J.R., Castiglione, C.M., Sjogren, B., Wetterberg, L. and Kidd, K.K. (1988) 'Evidence against linkage of schizophrenia to markers on chromosome 5 in a northern Swedish pedigree', *Nature* (10 November) 336: 167–169.

Kety, S.S. (1974) 'From rationalization to reason', *American Journal of Psychiatry* 131: 957–963.

Kety, S.S. (1978) 'Heredity and environment', in J.D. Shershaw (ed.) *Schizophrenia: Science and Practice*, Cambridge, Mass.: Harvard University Press.

Kety, S.S., Rosenthal, D. and Wender, P.H. (1978a) 'Genetic relationships within the schizophrenia spectrum: evidence from adoption studies', in R.L. Spitzer and D.F. Klein (eds) *Critical Issues in Psychiatric Diagnosis*, New York: Raven Press.

Kety, S.S., Rosenthal, D., Wender, P. and Schulsinger, F. (1968) 'The types and prevalence of mental illness in the biological and adoptive families of adopted schizophrenics', in D. Rosenthal and S.S. Kety (eds) *The Transmission of Schizophrenia*, Oxford: Pergamon.

Kety, S.S., Rosenthal, D., Wender, P. and Schulsinger, F. (1971) 'Mental illness in the biological and adoptive families of adopted schizophrenics', *American Journal of Psychiatry* 128: 302–306.

Kety, S.S., Rosenthal, D., Wender, P. and Schulsinger, F. (1976) 'Studies based on a total sample of adopted individuals and their relatives: why they were necessary, what they demonstrated and failed to demonstrate', *Schizophrenia Bulletin* 2: 413–428.

Kety, S.S., Rosenthal, D., Wender, P.H., Schulsinger, F. and Jacobsen, B. (1975) 'Mental illness in the biological and adoptive families of adopted individuals who have become schizophrenic. A preliminary report based on psychiatric interviews', in R. Fieve, D. Rosenthal and H. Brill (eds) *Genetic Research in Psychiatry*, London: Johns Hopkins University Press.

Kety, S.S., Rosenthal, D., Wender, P.H., Schulsinger, F. and Jacobsen, B. (1978b) 'The biologic and adoptive families of adopted individuals who became schizophrenic: prevalence of mental illness and other characteristics', in L.C. Wynne, R.L.

Cromwell and S. Matthysse (eds) *The Nature of Schizophrenia: New Approaches to Research and Treatment*, New York: Wiley.

Kety, S.S., Wender, P.H., Jacobsen, B., Ingraham, L.J., Jansson, L., Faber, B. and Kinney, D. (1994) 'Mental illness in the biological and adoptive relatives of schizophrenia adoptees', *Archives of General Psychiatry* 51: 442–455.

Kinderman, P. and Bentall, R.P. (1996) 'Self-discrepancies and persecutory delusions: evidence for a model of paranoid ideation', *Journal of Abnormal Psychology* 105: 106–113.

Kinderman, P. and Bentall, R.P. (1997) 'Causal attributions in paranoia and depression; internal, personal and situational attributions for negative events', *Journal of Abnormal Psychology* 106: 341–345.

King, D.J. and Cooper, S.J. (1989) 'Viruses, immunity and mental disorder', *British Journal of Psychiatry* 154: 1–7.

Kingdon, D. and Turkington, D. (1998) 'Cognitive behaviour therapy of schizophrenia', in T. Wykes, N. Tarrier and S. Lewis (eds) *Outcome and Innovation in Psychological Treatments for Schizophrenia*, Chichester: Wiley.

Kingdon, D., Turkington, D. and John, C. (1994) 'Cognitive behaviour therapy of schizophrenia: the amenability of delusions and hallucinations to reasoning', *British Journal of Psychiatry* 164: 581–587.

Kingdon, D.G. and Turkington, D. (1994) *Cognitive Behavioural Therapy of Schizophrenia*, New York: Guilford Press, and London: Lawrence Erlbaum.

Kirch, D.G. (1993) 'Infection and autoimmunity as etiologic factors in schizophrenia: a review and reappraisal', *Schizophrenia Bulletin* 19: 355–370.

Kirk, S.A. and Kutchins, H. (1992) *The Selling of DSM: The Rhetoric of Science in Psychiatry*, New York: Aldine de Gruyter.

Klein, D.F. (1978) 'A proposed definition of mental illness', in R.L. Spitzer and D.F. Klein (eds) *Critical Issues in Psychiatric Diagnosis*, New York: Raven Press.

Klosterkötter, J., Albers, M., Steinmeyer, E.M., Hensen, A. and Sass, H. (1995) 'Positive or negative symptoms: which are more appropriate as diagnostic criteria for schizophrenia?', *Acta Psychiatrica Scandinavica* 92: 321–326.

Kraepelin, E. (1896) *Psychiatrie* (5th edn), Leipzig: Barth.

Kraepelin, E. (1899) *Psychiatrie* (6th edn), Leipzig: Barth.

Kraepelin, E. (1905) *Lectures on Clinical Psychiatry*, London: Ballière Tindall.

Kraepelin, E. (1919) *Dementia Praecox and Paraphrenia* (trans. R.M. Barclay), Edinburgh: Livingstone. (Originally published in *Psychiatrie*, 8th edn, 1913.)

Kramer, M., Sartorius, N., Jablensky, A. and Gulbinat, W. (1979) 'The ICD-9 classification of mental disorders: a review of its development and contents', *Acta Psychiatrica Scandinavica* 59: 241–262.

Kräupl-Taylor, F. (1971) 'A logical analysis of the medico-psychological concept of disease', *Psychological Medicine* 1: 356–364.

Kräupl-Taylor, F. (1976) 'The medical model of the disease concept', *British Journal of Psychiatry* 129: 588–594.

Kräupl-Taylor, F. (1979) *The Concepts of Illness, Disease and Morbus*, Cambridge: Cambridge University Press.

Kräupl-Taylor, F. (1982) 'Sydenham's disease entities', *Psychological Medicine* 12: 243–250.

Kringlen, E. (1964) 'Schizophrenia in male monozygotic twins', *Acta Psychiatrica Scandinavica* (Suppl. 178).

Kringlen, E. (1966) 'Schizophrenia in twins: an epidemiological–clinical study', *Psychiatry* 29: 173–184.

Kringlen, E. (1968) 'An epidemiological–clinical twin study on schizophrenia', in D. Rosenthal and S.S. Kety (eds) *The Transmission of Schizophrenia*, Oxford: Pergamon.

Kringlen, E. (1976) 'Twins – still our best method', *Schizophrenia Bulletin* 2: 429–439.

Kuhn, T.S. (1970) *The Structure of Scientific Revolutions*, Vol. 2 of *International Encyclopaedia of Unified Science* (No. 2, 2nd edn), Chicago: Chicago University Press.

Kuipers, E. (1998) 'Working with carers: interventions for relative and staff carers of those who have psychosis', in T. Wykes, N. Tarrier and S. Lewis (eds) *Outcome and Innovation in Psychological Treatments for Schizophrenia*, Chichester: Wiley.

Kuipers, E., Fowler, D., Garety, P., Chisholm, D., Freeman, D., Dunn, G., Bebbington, P. and Hadley, C. (1998) 'London–East Anglia randomised controlled trial of cognitive-behaviour therapy for psychosis III: follow-up and economic evaluation at 18 months', *British Journal of Psychiatry* 173: 61–68.

Kuipers, E., Garety, P. and Fowler, D. (1996) 'An outcome study of cognitive-behavioural treatment for psychosis', in G. Haddock and P.D. Slade (eds) *Cognitive-behavioural Interventions with Psychotic Disorders*, London: Routledge.

Kuipers, E., Garety, P., Fowler, D., Dunn, G., Bebbington, P., Freeman, D. and Hadley, C. (1997) 'London–East Anglia randomised controlled trial of cognitive-behaviour therapy for psychosis I: Effects of the treatment phase', *British Journal of Psychiatry* 171: 319–327.

Kuipers, E., Leff, J. and Lam, D. (1992) *Family Work for Schizophrenia: A Practical Guide*, London: Gaskell.

Kutchins, H. and Kirk, S.A. (1997) *Making us Crazy: DSM: The Psychiatric Bible and the Creation of Mental Disorders*, New York: The Free Press.

Lader, M.H., Ron, M. and Petursson, H. (1984) 'Computed axial brain tomography in long-term benzodiazepine users', *Psychological Medicine* 14: 203–206.

Lakatos, I. (1978) 'History of science and its rational reconstruction', in J. Worrall and G. Currie (eds) *Imre Lakatos: Philosophical Papers* Vol. 1: *The Methodology of Scientific Research Programmes*, Cambridge: Cambridge University Press.

Lander, E.S. (1988) 'Splitting schizophrenia', *Nature* 336 (10 November): 105–106.

Langdon, R., Mitchie, P.T., Ward, P.B., McConaghy, N., Catts, S.V. and Coltheart, M. (1997) 'Defective self and/or other mentalising in schizophrenia: a cognitive neuropsychological approach', *Cognitive Neuropsychiatry* 2: 167–193.

Langfeldt, G. (1960) 'Diagnosis and prognosis of schizophrenia', *Proceedings of the Royal Society of Medicine* 53: 1047–1052.

Leff, J., Kuipers, L., Berkowitz, R., Eberlein Vries, R. and Sturgeon, D. (1982) 'A controlled trial of social intervention in the families of schizophrenic patients', *British Journal of Psychiatry* 141: 121–134.

Leff, J., Sartorius, N., Jablensky, A., Korten, A. and Emberg, G. (1992) 'The International Pilot Study of Schizophrenia: five-year follow-up findings', *Psychological Medicine* 22: 131–145.

Leff, J. and Vaughn, C. (1981) 'The role of maintenance therapy and relatives' expressed emotion in relapse of schizophrenia: a two-year follow-up', *British Journal of Psychiatry* 139: 102–104.

Leigh, D. (1961) *The Historical Development of British Psychiatry* Vol. 1: *18th and 19th Centuries*, Oxford: Pergamon.

Leon, C.A. (1989) 'Clinical course and outcome of schizophrenia in Cali, Columbia: a 10-year follow-up study', *Journal of Nervous and Mental Disease* 177: 593–606.

Leonhard, K. (1980) 'Contradictory issues in the origin of schizophrenia', *British Journal of Psychiatry* 136: 437–444.

Lerner, G. (1986) *The Creation of Patriarchy*, New York: Oxford University Press.

Lerner, M.J. (1980) *The Belief in a Just World: A Fundamental Delusion*, New York: Plenum.

Leudar, I. and Thomas, P. (2000) *Voices of Reason, Voices of Insanity: Studies of Verbal Hallucinations*, London: Routledge.

Leudar, I., Thomas, P., McNally, D. and Glinski, A. (1997) 'What voices can do with words: pragmatics of verbal hallucinations', *Psychological Medicine* 27: 885–898.

Lewine, R.R. and Caudle, J. (1999) 'Race in the "decade of the brain"', *Schizophrenia Bulletin* 25: 1–5.

Lewis, N.D.C. (1966) 'History of the nosology and the evolution of the concept of schizophrenia', in P.H. Hoch and J. Zubin (eds) *Pathology of Schizophrenia*, New York: Grune and Stratton.

Li, T., Breen, G., Brown, J., Liu, X., Murray, R.M., Shaw, D.J., Sham, P.C., St. Clair, D. and Collier, D.A. (1999) 'No evidence of linkage disequilibrium between a CAG repeat in the SCA1 gene and schizophrenia in Caucasian and Chinese schizophrenic subjects', *Psychiatric Genetics* 9: 123–127.

Liberman, R., Marder, S., Marshall, B.D., Mintz, J. and Kuehnel, T. (1998) 'Biobehavioural therapy: interactions between pharmacotherapy and behaviour therapy in schizophrenia', in T. Wykes, N. Tarrier and S. Lewis (eds) *Outcome and Innovation in Psychological Treatments for Schizophrenia*, Chichester: Wiley.

Lidz, T. and Blatt, S. (1983) 'Critique of the Danish–American studies of the biological and adoptive relatives of adoptees who became schizophrenic', *American Journal of Psychiatry* 140: 426–434.

Lidz, T., Blatt, S. and Cook, B. (1981) 'Critique of the Danish–American studies of the adopted away offspring of schizophrenic parents', *American Journal of Psychiatry* 138: 1063–1068.

Lilienfeld, S.O. and Marino, L. (1995) 'Mental disorder as a roschian concept: a critique of Wakefield's "harmful dysfunction" analysis', *Journal of Abnormal Psychology* 104: 411–420.

Link, B.G., Dohrenwend, B.P. and Skodol, A.E. (1986) 'Socio-economic status and schizophrenia: noisome occupational characteristics as a risk factor', *American Sociological Review* 51: 242–258.

Linney, Y.M., Peters, E.R. and Ayton, P. (1998) 'Reasoning biases in delusion-prone individuals', *British Journal of Clinical Psychology* 37: 285–302.

Littlewood, R. (1980) 'Anthropology and psychiatry: an alternative approach', *British Journal of Medical Psychology* 53: 213–225.

Littlewood, R. (1997) 'Commentary on "Spiritual experience and psychopathology"', *Philosophy, Psychiatry and Psychology* 4: 67–73.

Littlewood, R. and Lipsedge, M. (1982) *Aliens and Alienists: Ethnic Minorities and Psychiatry*, Harmondsworth: Penguin.

Littlewood, R. and Lipsedge, M. (1989) *Aliens and Alienists: Ethnic Minorities and Psychiatry* (2nd edn), London: Unwin Hyman.

Littlewood, R. and Lipsedge, M. (1997) *Aliens and Alienists: Ethnic Minorities and Psychiatry* (3rd edn), London: Routledge.

Lupton, D. (1994) *Medicine as Culture: Illness, Disease and the Body in Western Society*, London: Sage.

Luxenburger, H. (1928) 'Vorläufiger Bericht über psychiatrische Serienuntersuchungen an Zwillingen', *Zeitschrift für die gesamte Neurologie und Psychiatrie* 116: 297–326.

Lyon, H.M., Kaney, S. and Bentall, R.P. (1994) 'The defensive function of persecutory delusions. Evidence from attribution tasks', *British Journal of Psychiatry* 164: 637–646.

McCabe, M.S., Fowler, R.C., Cadoret, R.J. and Winokur, G. (1971) 'Familial differences in schizophrenia with good and poor prognosis', *Psychological Medicine* 1: 326–332.

MacCorquodale, K. and Meehl, P.E. (1948) 'On a distinction between hypothetical constructs and intervening variables', *Psychological Review* 55: 95–107.

McCowan, P.K. and Cook, L.C. (1928) 'The mental aspects of chronic epidemic encephalitis', *The Lancet*, 30 June: 1316–1320.

McCulloch, M.L. (1983) 'A testing time for the test of time', *Bulletin of the British Psychological Society* 36: 1–5.

McGlashan, T.H. and Fenton, W.S. (1991) 'Classical sub-types for schizophrenia: literature review for DSM-IV', *Schizophrenia Bulletin* 17: 609–632.

McGrath, J. and Emmerson, W.B. (1999) 'Treatment of schizophrenia', *British Medical Journal* 319 (16th October): 1045–1048.

McGuffin, P., Festenstein, H. and Murray, R. (1983) 'A family study of HLA antigens and other genetic markers in schizophrenia', *Psychological Medicine* 13: 31–43.

McGuire, P.K., Shah, G.M.S. and Murray, R.M. (1993) 'Increased blood flow in Broca's area during auditory hallucinations in schizophrenia', *The Lancet* 342: 703–706.

McKellar, P. (1968) *Experience and Behaviour*, Harmondsworth: Penguin.

Maher, B.A. (1988) 'Anomalous experience and delusional thinking: the logic of explanations', in J.F. Oltmanns and B.A. Maher (eds) *Delusional Beliefs*, New York: Wiley.

Maher, B.A. (1992) 'Delusions: contemporary etiological hypotheses', *Psychiatric Annals* 22: 260–268.

Maher, B.A. and Ross, J.S. (1984) 'Delusions', in H.E. Adams and P.B. Sutker (eds) *Comprehensive Handbook of Psychopathology*, New York: Plenum Press.

Mahy, G.E., Mallett, R., Leff, J. and Bhugra, D. (1999) 'First-contact incidence rate of schizophrenia on Barbados', *British Journal of Psychiatry* 175: 28–33.

Margo, A., Hemsley, D. and Slade, P.D. (1981) 'The effects of varying auditory input on schizophrenic hallucinations', *British Journal of Psychiatry* 139: 122–127.

Marks, R.C. and Luchins, D.J. (1990) 'Relationship between brain imaging findings in schizophrenia and psychopathology: a review of the literature relating to positive and negative symptoms', in N.C. Andreasen (ed.) *Modern Problems of Pharmacopsychiatry: Positive and Negative Symptoms and Syndromes*, Basel, Switzerland: S. Karger A.G.

Marshall, J.C. and Halligan, P.W. (1996) 'Towards a cognitive neuropsychiatry', in P.W. Halligan and J.C. Marshall (eds) *Method in Madness*, Hove: Psychology Press.

Marshall, J.R. (1984) 'The genetics of schizophrenia re-visited', *Bulletin of the British Psychological Society* 37: 177–181.

Marshall, J.R. (1985) 'Schizophrenia and the need for a critical analysis of information', in J.M. Brittain (ed.) *Consensus and Penalties for Ignorance in the Medical Sciences*, London: Taylor Graham.

Marshall, J.R. and Pettitt, A.N. (1985) 'Discordant concordant rates', *Bulletin of the British Psychological Society* 38: 6–9.

Mason, P., Harrison, G., Croudace, T., Glazebrook, C. and Medley, I. (1997) 'The predictive validity of a diagnosis of schizophrenia. A report from the International Study of Schizophrenia co-ordinated by the World Health Organization and the Department of Psychiatry, University of Nottingham', *British Journal of Psychiatry* 170: 321–327.

Maudsley, H. (1873) *Body and Mind*, London: Macmillan.

Maxmen, J. (1985) *The New Psychiatrists*, New York: New American Library.

Maxwell, A.E. (1961) *Analysing Qualitative Data*, London: Methuen.

Medawar, P. (1984) *Pluto's Republic*, Oxford: Oxford University Press.

Mednick, S.A. (1958) 'A learning theory approach to research in schizophrenia', *Psychological Bulletin* 55: 316–327.

Meehl, P.E. (1972) 'A critical afterword', in I.I. Gottesman and J. Shields, *Schizophrenia and Genetics: A Twin Study Vantage Point*, New York: Academic Press.

Mellor, C.S. (1970) 'First-rank symptoms of schizophrenia', *British Journal of Psychiatry* 117: 15–23.

Mercer, K. (1986) 'Racism and transcultural psychiatry', in P. Miller and N. Rose (eds) *The Power of Psychiatry*, Cambridge: Polity Press.

Messari, S. (2000) 'CBT for psychosis: a qualitative exploration of therapists' and clients' accounts', unpublished Clin Ps. D thesis, University of East London.

Miller, D.R. and Flack, W.F. (1991) 'Defining schizophrenia: a critique of the mechanistic framework', in W.F. Flack, D.R. Miller and M. Wiener (eds) *What is Schizophrenia?*, New York: Springer-Verlag.

Miller, J. (1986) 'Primitive thoughts', *Canadian Psychologist* 127: 155–157.

Miller, L.J., O'Conner, E. and Di Pasquale, T. ((1993) 'Patients' attitudes towards hallucinations', *American Journal of Psychiatry* 150: 584–588.

Miller, M.D., Johnson, R.L. and Richmond, L.H. (1965) 'Auditory hallucinations and descriptive language skills', *Journal of Psychiatric Research* 3: 43–56.

Milton, F., Patwa, V.K. and Hafner, R.J. (1978) 'Confrontation versus belief modification in persistently deluded patients', *British Journal of Medical Psychology* 51: 127–130.

Mitchley, N.J., Barber, J., Gray, J.M., Brooks, D.N. and Livingstone, M.G. (1998) 'Comprehension of irony in schizophrenia', *Cognitive Neuropsychiatry* 3: 127–138.

Mojtabai, R. and Nicholson, R.A. (1995) 'Inter-rater reliability of ratings of delusions and bizarre delusions', *American Journal of Psychiatry* 152: 1804–1806.

Moldin, S.O. and Gottesman, I.I. (1997) 'At issue: genes, experience and chance in schizophrenia – positioning for the 21st century', *Schizophrenia Bulletin* 23: 547–561.

Moncrieff, J. (2000) 'Psychiatric imperialism: the medicalisation of modern living', *Asylum Journal* 12: 24–26.

Morris, J.N. (1978) *The Uses of Epidemiology* (3rd edn), Edinburgh: Churchill Livingstone.

Morrison, A. (ed.) (in press) *A Casebook of Cognitive Therapy for Psychosis*, London: Brunner Routledge.

Morrison, A.P. (1994) 'Cognitive behaviour therapy for auditory hallucinations without concurrent medication: a single case', *Behavioural and Cognitive Psychotherapy* 22: 259–264.

Morrison, A.P. and Haddock, G. (1997) 'Cognitive factors in source monitoring and auditory hallucinations', *Psychological Medicine* 27: 669–679.

Morrison, A.P., Wells, A. and Sarah, N. (2000) 'Cognitive factors in predisposition to auditory and visual hallucinations', *British Journal of Clinical Psychology* 39: 67–78.

Muntaner, C., Tien, A.Y., Eaton, W.W. and Garrison, R. (1991) 'Occupational characteristics and the occurrence of psychotic disorders', *Social Psychiatry and Psychiatric Epidemiology* 26: 273–280.

Murphy, J.M. (1978) 'The recognition of psychoses in non-western societies', in R.L. Spitzer and D.F. Klein (eds) *Critical Issues in Psychiatric Diagnosis*, New York: Raven Press.

Nayani, T.H. and David, A.S. (1996) 'The auditory hallucination: a phenomenological survey', *Psychological Medicine* 26: 177–189.

Neale, J.M. and Oltmanns, T.F. (1980) *Schizophrenia*, New York: Wiley.

Nelson, H.E. (1997) *CBT with Schizophrenia: A Practice Manual*, Cheltenham: Stanley Thornes.

Neves-Pereira, M., Bassett, A.S., Honer, W.G., Lang, D., King, N.A. and Kennedy, J.L. (1998) 'No evidence for linkage of the CHRNA7 gene region in Canadian schizophrenia families', *American Journal of Medical Genetics* 81: 361–363.

Newnes, C., Holmes, G. and Dunn, C. (1999) *This is Madness: A Critical look at Psychiatry and the Future of Mental Health Services*, Ross-on-Wye: PCCS Books.

Nisbett, R.E. and Ross, L.D. (1980) *Human Inference: Strategies and Shortcomings of Social Judgement*, Englewood Cliffs, N.J.: Prentice Hall.

Nopoulos, P., Swayze, V., Flaum, M., Ehrhardt, J.C., Yuh, W.T. and Andreasen, N.C. (1997) 'Cavum septi pellucidi in normals and patients with schizophrenia as detected by magnetic resonance imaging', *Biological Psychiatry* 41: 1102–1108.

Ogden, C.K. and Richards, I.A. (eds) (1956) *The Meaning of Meaning: A Study of the Influence of Language on Thought and of the Science of Symbolism* (10th edn), London: Routledge and Kegan Paul.

Oltmanns, T.F. (1988) 'Approaches to the definition and study of delusions', in J.F. Oltmanns and B.A. Maher (eds) *Delusional Beliefs*, New York: Wiley.

Onstad, S., Skre, I., Torgensen, S. and Kringlen, E. (1991) 'Twin concordance for DSM-IIIR schizophrenia', *Acta Psychiatrica Scandinavica* 83: 395–401.

Paikin, H., Jacobsen, B., Schulsinger, F., Godtfredsen, K., Rosenthal, D., Wender, P. and Kety, S.S. (1974) 'Characteristics of people who refused to participate in a social and psychological study', in S.A. Mednick, F. Schulsinger, J. Higgins and B. Bell (eds) *Genetics, Environment and Psychopathology*, Amsterdam: North Holland Publishing Co.

Parker, I. (1992) *Discourse Dynamics: Critical Analysis for Social and Individual Psychology*, London: Routledge.

Parker, I., Georgaca, E., Harper, D., McLaughlin, T. and Stowell-Smith, M. (1995) *Deconstructing Psychopathology*, London: Sage.

Parsian, A., Suarez, B.K., Isenberg, K., Hampe, C.L., Fisher, L., Chakraverty, S., Meszaros, K., Lenzinger, E., Willinger, U., Fuchs, K., Aschauer, H.N. and Cloninger, C.R. (1997) 'No evidence for a schizophrenia susceptibility gene in the vicinity of IL2RB on chromosome 22', *American Journal of Medical Genetics* 74: 361–364.

Parsons, S. and Armstrong, A. (2000) 'Psychiatric power and authority: a scientific and moral defence', in P. Barker and C. Stevenson (eds) *The Construction of Power and Authority in Psychiatry*, Oxford: Butterworth Heinemann.

Paton-Saltzberg, R. (1982) Letter, *Bulletin of the British Psychological Society* 35: 397–398.

Peralta, V., de Leon, J. and Cuesta, M.J. (1992) 'Are there more than two syndromes in schizophrenia? A critique of the positive/negative dichotomy', *British Journal of Psychiatry* 161: 335–343.

Persico, A.M., Wang, Z.W., Black, D.W., Andreasen, N.C., Uhl, G.R. and Crowe, R.R. (1995a) 'Exclusion of close linkage between the synaptic vesicular monoamine transporter locus and schizophrenia spectrum disorders', *American Journal of Medical Genetics* 60: 563–565.

Persico, A.M., Wang, Z.W., Black, D.W., Andreasen, N.C., Uhl, G.R. and Crowe, R.R. (1995b) 'Exclusion of close linkage of the dopamine transporter gene with schizophrenia spectrum disorders', *American Journal of Psychiatry* 152: 134–136.

Peters, E., Day, S., McKenna, J. and Orbach, G. (1999a) 'Delusional ideation in religious and psychotic populations', *British Journal of Clinical Psychology* 38: 83–96.

Peters, E.R., Joseph, S.A. and Garety, P.A. (1999b) 'Measurement of delusional ideation in the normal population: introducing the PDI (Peters *et al.* Delusions Inventory)', *Schizophrenia Bulletin* 25: 553–576.

Phillips, L., Broverman, I.K. and Zigler, E. (1966) 'Social competence and psychiatric diagnosis', *Journal of Abnormal Psychology* 71: 209–214.

Pogue-Geile, M.F. (1989) 'The prognostic significance of negative symptoms in schizophrenia', *British Journal of Psychiatry* (Suppl. 7): 123–127.

Posey, T.B. and Losch, M. (1983) 'Auditory hallucinations of hearing voices in 375 normal subjects', *Imagery, Cognition and Personality* 3: 99–113.

Potter, J. and Reicher, S. (1987) 'Discourses of community and conflict: the organisation of social categories in accounts of a "riot"', *British Journal of Social Psychology* 26: 25–40.

Potter, J. and Wetherell, M. (1987) *Discourse and Social Psychology*, London: Sage.

Potter, J., Wetherell, M., Gill, R. and Edwards, D. (1990) 'Discourse: noun, verb or social practice?', *Philosophical Psychology* 3: 205–217.

Price, B. (1950) 'Primary biases in twin studies: a review of prenatal and natal difference-producing factors in monozygotic pairs', *American Journal of Human Genetics* 2: 293–352.

Prilleltensky, I. (1989) 'Psychology and the status quo', *American Psychologist* 44: 795–802.

Prilleltensky, I. (1994) 'Psychology and social ethics', *American Psychologist* 49: 966–967.

Pyke, D.A., Cassar, J., Todd, J. and Taylor, K.W. (1970) 'Glucose tolerance and serum insulin in identical twins of diabetics', *British Medical Journal* 4: 649–651.

Rankin, P. and O'Carroll, P. (1995) 'Reality monitoring and signal detection in individuals prone to hallucinations', *British Journal of Clinical Psychology* 34: 517–528.

Revely, A. and Murray, R.M. (1980) 'The genetic contribution to the functional psychoses', *British Journal of Hospital Medicine* 24: 166–171.

Riatt, F.E. and Zeedyk, M.S. (2000) *The Implicit Relation of Psychology and Law: Women and Syndrome Evidence*, London: Routledge.

Roberts, G. (1991) 'Delusional belief systems and meaning in life: a preferred reality?', *British Journal of Psychiatry* 159 (Suppl. 14): 19–28.

Robins, E. and Guze, S.B. (1970) 'Establishment of diagnostic validity in psychiatric illness: its application to schizophrenia', *American Journal of Psychiatry* 126: 983–987.

Romme, M. (1993) 'Social psychiatry', in M. Romme and S. Escher (eds) *Accepting Voices*, London: Mind Publications.

Romme, M. and Escher, S. (1993) *Accepting Voices*, London: Mind Publications.

Romme, M.A.J., Honig, A., Noorthoorn, E.O. and Escher, A.D.M.A.C. (1992) 'Coping with hearing voices: an emancipatory approach', *British Journal of Psychiatry* 161: 99–103.

Rosanoff, A.J., Handy, L.M., Plesset, I.R. and Brush, S. (1934) 'The etiology of so-called schizophrenic psychoses with special reference to their occurrence in twins', *American Journal of Psychiatry* 91: 247–286.

Rose, S., Kamin, L.J. and Lewontin, R.C. (1984) *Not in Our Genes*, Harmondsworth: Penguin.

Rosenthal, D. (1962a) 'Problems of sampling and diagnosis in the major twin studies of schizophrenia', *Psychiatric Research* 1: 116–134.

Rosenthal, D. (1962b) 'Familial concordance by sex with respect to schizophrenia', *Psychological Bulletin* 59: 401–421.

Rosenthal, D. (1970) *Genetic Theory and Abnormal Behavior*, New York: McGraw-Hill.

Rosenthal, D., Wender, P.H., Kety, S.S., Schulsinger, F., Welner, J. and Østergaard, L. (1968) 'Schizophrenics' offspring reared in adoptive homes', in D. Rosenthal and S.S. Kety (eds) *The Transmission of Schizophrenia*, Oxford: Pergamon.

Rosenthal, D., Wender, P.H., Kety, S.S., Welner, J. and Schulsinger, F. (1974) 'The adopted away offspring of schizophrenics', in S.A. Mednick, F. Schulsinger, J. Higgins and B. Bell (eds) *Genetics, Environment and Psychopathology*, Amsterdam: North Holland Publishing Co.

Ross, C.A. and Pam, A. (1995) *Pseudoscience in Biological Psychiatry: Blaming the Body*, New York: Wiley.

Roth, M. and Kroll, J. (1986) *The Reality of Mental Illness*, Cambridge: Cambridge University Press.

Rotter, J.B. (1954) *Social Learning and Clinical Psychology*, New York: Prentice Hall.

Rowe, J.T.W. (1906) 'Is dementia praecox the "new peril" in psychiatry?', *American Journal of Insanity* 63: 385–393.

Ryle, G. (1949) *The Concept of Mind*, New York: Harper and Row.

Sabshin, M. (1990) 'Turning points in twentieth-century American psychiatry', *American Journal of Psychiatry* 147: 1267–1274.

Sacks, O. (1971) 'Parkinsonism: a so-called new disease', *British Medical Journal* 3: 111.

Sacks, O. (1982) *Awakenings*, London: Pan Books.

Sadler, J.Z. and Agich, G.J. (1996) 'Diseases, functions, values and psychiatric classification', *Philosophy, Psychiatry and Psychology* 2: 219–231.

Sakheim, D.K. and Devine, S.E. (1995) 'Trauma-related syndromes', in C.A. Ross and A. Pam (eds) *Pseudoscience in Biological Psychiatry: Blaming The Body*, New York: Wiley.

Sampson, E.E. (1981) 'Cognitive psychology as ideology', *American Psychologist* 36: 730–743.

Sampson, E.E. (1989) 'The deconstruction of the self', in J. Shotter and K.J. Gergen (eds) *Texts of Identity*, London: Sage.

Sarason, S.B. (1981) *Psychology Misdirected*, New York: Free Press.

Sarbin, T.R. (1967) 'The concept of hallucination', *Journal of Personality* 35: 359–380.

Sarbin, T.R. (1968) 'Ontology recapitulates philology: the mythic nature of anxiety', *American Psychologist* 23: 411–418.

Sarbin, T.R. (1970) 'Towards a theory of imagination', *Journal of Personality* 38: 52–76.

Sarbin, T.R. and Juhasz, J.B. (1967) 'The historical background of the concept of hallucination', *Journal of the History of the Behavioral Sciences* 3: 339–358.

Sarbin, T.R. and Juhasz, J.B. (1978) 'The social psychology of hallucinations', *Journal of Mental Imagery* 2: 117–144.

Sarbin, T.R. and Mancuso, J.C. (1980) *Schizophrenia: Medical Diagnosis or Moral Verdict?*, New York: Pergamon.

Sartorius, N. (1994) *Foreword: Guide to the ICD-10 Classification of Mental and Behavioural Disorders*, Geneva: World Health Organization (American Psychiatric Press).

Sartorius, N. *et al.* (1993) 'Progress towards achieving a common language in psychiatry: results from the field trials of the clinical guidelines accompanying the WHO classification of mental and behavioural disorders in ICD-10', *Archives of General Psychiatry* 50: 115–124.

Sartorius, N., Jablensky, A. and Shapiro, R. (1978) 'Cross-cultural differences in the short-term prognosis of schizophrenic psychoses', *Schizophrenia Bulletin* 4: 102–112.

Scheibe, K.E. and Sarbin, T.R. (1965) 'Towards a theoretical conceptualization of superstition', *British Journal for the Philosophy of Science* 62: 143–158.

Schmauss, C. and Krieg, J.C. (1987) 'Enlargement of cerebrospinal fluid spaces in long-term benzodiazepine abusers', *Psychological Medicine* 17: 869–873.

Schneider, K. (1959) *Clinical Psychopathology* (5th edn), New York: Grune and Stratton.

Schneider, K. (1974) 'Primary and secondary symptoms in schizophrenia', in S.R. Hirsch and M. Shepherd (eds) *Themes and Variations in European Psychiatry*, Bristol: John Wright.

Schon, D.A. (1983) *The Reflective Practitioner: How Professionals Think in Action*, New York: Basic Books.

Schultz, D.P. (1965) *Sensory Restrictions: Effects on Behaviour*, New York: Academic Press.

Schultz, S.K. and Andreasen, N.C. (1999) 'Schizophrenia', *Lancet* 353 (24 April): 1425–1430.

Scull, A.T. (1975) 'From madness to mental illness: medical men as moral entrepreneurs', *Archives Europeenes de Sociologica* 16: 218–251.

Scull, A.T. (1979) *Museums of Madness: The Social Organisation of Insanity in Nineteenth Century England*, London: Allen Lane.

Sensky, T., Turkington, D., Kingdon, D., Scott, J.L., Scott, J., Siddle, R., O'Carroll, M. and Barnes, T.R.E. (2000) 'A randomized controlled trial of cognitive-behaviour therapy for persistent symptoms in schizophrenia resistant to medication', *Archives of General Psychiatry* 57: 165–172.

Serretti, A., Lilli, R., Di Bella, D., Bertelli, S., Nobile, M., Novelli, E., Catalano, M. and Smeraldi, E. (1999) 'Dopamine receptor D4 gene is not associated with major psychoses', *American Journal of Medical Genetics* 88: 486–491.

Sharp, H.M., Fear, C.F. and Healy, D. (1997) 'Attribution style and delusions: an investigation based on delusional content', *European Psychiatry* 12: 1–7.

Shastry, B.S. (1999) 'Recent developments in the genetics of schizophrenia', *Neurogenetics* 2: 149–154.

Shepherd, M. (1976) 'Definition, classification and nomenclature: a clinical overview', in D. Kemali, G. Bartholini and D. Richer (eds) *Schizophrenia Today*, Oxford: Pergamon.

Shergill, S.S., Murray, R.M. and McGuire, P.K. (1998) 'Auditory hallucinations: a review of psychological treatments', *Schizophrenia Research* 32: 137–150.

Sherrington, R., Brynjolfsson, J., Petursson, H., Potter, M., Dudleston, K., Barraclough, B., Wasmuth, J., Dobbs, M. and Gurling, H. (1988) 'Localization of a susceptibility locus for schizophrenia on chromosome 5', *Nature* 336 (10 November): 164–167.

Shields, J., Gottesman, I.I. and Slater, E. (1967) 'Kallmann's 1946 schizophrenic twin study in the light of new information', *Acta Psychiatrica Scandinavica* 43: 385–396.

Shweder, R.A. (1977) 'Likeness and likelihood in everyday thought: magical thinking in judgements about personality', *Current Anthropology* 18: 637–658.

Silberman, R.M. (1971) *CHAM: A Classification of Psychiatric States*, Amsterdam: Excerpta Medica.

Sims, A. (1997) 'Commentary on "spiritual experience and psychopathology"', *Philosophy, Psychiatry and Psychology* 4: 79–81.

Singh, M.M. (1987) 'Is the positive/negative distinction in schizophrenia valid?', *British Journal of Psychiatry* 150: 870–880.

Skinner, B.F. (1948) 'Superstition in the pigeon', *Journal of Experimental Psychology* 38: 168–172.

Skinner, B.F. (1953) *Science and Human Behavior*, New York: Macmillan.

Skinner, B.F. (1974) *About Behaviorism*, New York: Knopf.

Skultans, V. (1975) *Madness and Morals: Ideas on Insanity in the Nineteenth Century*, London: Routledge and Kegan Paul.

Skultans, V. (1979) *English Madness: Ideas on Insanity 1580–1890*, London: Routledge and Kegan Paul.

Slade, P.D. (1972) 'The effects of systematic desensitization on auditory hallucinations', *Behaviour Research and Therapy* 10: 85–91.

Slade, P.D. (1974) 'The external control of auditory hallucinations: an information theory analysis', *British Journal of Social and Clinical Psychology* 13: 73–79.

Slade, P.D. (1976) 'Towards a theory of auditory hallucinations: outline of a hypothetical four-factor model', *British Journal of Social and Clinical Psychology* 18: 309–317.

Slade, P.D. and Bentall, R.P. (1988) *Sensory Deception: A Scientific Analysis of Hallucinations*, London: Croom-Helm.

Slade, P.D. and Cooper, R. (1979) 'Some difficulties with the term "schizophrenia": an alternative model', *British Journal of Social and Clinical Psychology* 15: 415–423.

Slater, E. (1953) *Psychotic and Neurotic Illnesses in Twins*, London: HMSO.

Spaulding, W., Reed, D., Storzback, D., Sullivan, M., Weiler, M. and Richardson, C. (1998) 'The effects of a remediation approach to cognitive therapy for schizophrenia', in T. Wykes, N. Tarrier and S. Lewis (eds) *Outcome and Innovation in Psychological Treatments for Schizophrenia*, Chichester: Wiley.

Spitzer, R.L. (1975) 'On pseudoscience in science, logic in remission and psychiatric diagnosis: a critique of Rosenhan's "On being sane in insane places"', *Journal of Abnormal Psychology* 84: 442–452.

Spitzer, R.L., Andreasen, N.C. and Endicott, J. (1978a) 'Schizophrenia and other psychotic disorders in DSM-III', *Schizophrenia Bulletin* 4: 489–494.

Spitzer, R.L. and Endicott, J. (1978) 'Medical and mental disorder: proposed definition and criteria', in R.L. Spitzer and D.F. Klein (eds) *Critical Issues in Psychiatric Diagnosis*, New York: Raven Press.

Spitzer, R.L., Endicott, J. and Robins, E. (1978b) 'Research diagnostic criteria: rationale and reliability', *Archives of General Psychiatry* 35: 773–782.

Spitzer, R.L., First, M.B., Kendler, K.S. and Stein, D.J. (1993) 'The reliability of three definitions of bizarre delusions', *American Journal of Psychiatry* 150: 880–884.

Spitzer, R.L. and Fleiss, J.L. (1974) 'Reanalysis of the reliability of psychiatric diagnosis', *British Journal of Psychiatry* 125: 341–347.

Spitzer, R.L. and Williams J.B.N. (1988) 'Having a dream: a research strategy for DSM-IV', *Archives of General Psychiatry* 45: 871–874.

Spitzer, R.L. and Wilson, J.B.N. (1983) 'The revision of DSM-III', *Psychiatric Annals* 13: 808–811.

Spitzer, R.L. and Wilson, P.T. (1969) 'DSM-II revisited: a reply', *International Journal of Psychiatry* 7: 421–426.

St. Clair, D., Blackwood, D., Muir, W., Baillie, D., Hubbard, A., Wright, A., and Evans, H.J. (1989) 'No linkage of chromosome 5q11–q13 markers to schizophrenia in Scottish families', *Nature* (25 May) 339: 305–309.

Stampfer, H.G. (1990) '"Negative symptoms": a cumulative trauma stress disorder?', *Australian and New Zealand Journal of Psychiatry* 24: 516–528.

Startup, M. (1999) 'Schizotypy, dissociative experiences and childhood abuse: relationship among self-report measures', *British Journal of Clinical Psychology* 38: 333–344.

Stein, H.F. (1990) *American Medicine as Culture*, Boulder, Colo.: Westview.

Stengel, E. (1959) 'Classification of mental disorders', *Bulletin of the World Health Organisation* 21: 601–663.

Stephens, J.H. (1970) 'Long-term course and prognosis in schizophrenia', *Seminars in Psychiatry* 2: 464–485.

Stephens, J.H. (1978) 'Long-term prognosis and follow-up in schizophrenia', *Schizophrenia Bulletin* 4: 25–47.

Stoppard, J. (2000) *Understanding Depression: Feminist Social Constructionist Approaches*, London: Routledge.

Strachan, A.M. (1986) 'Family intervention for the rehabilitation of schizophrenia: towards protection and coping', *Schizophrenia Bulletin* 12: 678–698.

Strauss, J.S. (1969) 'Hallucinations and delusions as points on continua functions', *Archives of General Psychiatry* 21: 581–586.

Strauss, J.S. (1975) 'A comprehensive approach to psychiatric diagnosis', *American Journal of Psychiatry* 132: 1193–1197.

Strauss, J.S., Bartko, J.J. and Carpenter, W.T. (1973) 'The use of clustering techniques for the classification of psychiatric patients', *British Journal of Psychiatry* 122: 531–540.

Strauss, J.S. and Carpenter, W.T. (1974) 'The prediction of outcome in schizophrenia. II. The relationship between predictor and outcome variables', *Archives of General Psychiatry* 31: 37–42.

Strauss, J.S. and Carpenter, W.T. (1977) 'Prediction of outcome in schizophrenia: III. Five-year outcome and its predictors', *Archives of General Psychiatry* 34: 159–163.

Strauss, J.S. and Carpenter, W.T. (1978) 'The prognosis of schizophrenia: rationale for a multidimensional concept', *Schizophrenia Bulletin* 4: 56–66.

Strauss, J.S. and Carpenter, W.T. (1981) *Schizophrenia*, New York: Plenum Medical.

Strauss, J.S. and Gift, T.E. (1977) 'Choosing an approach for diagnosing schizophrenia', *Archives of General Psychiatry* 34: 1248–1253.

Swayze, V.W., Andreasen, N.C., Alliger, R.J., Ehrhardt, J.C. and Yuh, W.T. (1990) 'Structural brain abnormalities in bi-polar affective disorder. Ventricular enlargement and focal signal hyperintensities', *Archives of General Psychiatry* 47: 1054–1059.

Szasz, T. (1976) *Schizophrenia: The Sacred Symbol of Psychiatry*, Oxford: Oxford University Press.

Szasz, T. (1987) *Insanity: The Idea and its Consequences*, New York: Wiley.

Tarrier, N., Beckett, R., Harwood, S., Baker, A., Yusupoff, L. and Ugarteburu, I. (1993) 'A trial of two cognitive-behavioural methods of treating drug-resistant residual psychotic symptoms in schizophrenic patients: I. Outcome', *British Journal of Psychiatry* 162: 524–532.

Tarrier, N., Kinney, C., McCarthy, E., Humphreys, L., Wittkowski, A. and Morris, J. (2000) 'Two-year follow-up of cognitive-behavioral therapy and supportive counseling in the treatment of persistent symptoms in chronic schizophrenia', *Journal of Consulting and Clinical Psychology* 68: 917–922.

Tarrier, N., Yusupoff, L., Kinney, C., McCarthy, E., Gledhill, A., Haddock, G. and Morris, J. (1998) 'Randomised controlled trial of intensive cognitive behavioural therapy for patients with chronic schizophrenia', *British Medical Journal* 317 (1 August): 303–307.

Thouless, R.H. (1974) *Straight and Crooked Thinking*, London: Pan Books.

Tien, A.Y. (1991) 'Distributions of hallucinations in the population', *Social Psychiatry and Psychiatric Epidemiology* 26: 287–292.

Tienari, P. (1963) 'Psychiatric illness in identical twins', *Acta Psychiatrica Scandinavica* (Suppl. 171).

Tienari, P. (1975) 'Schizophrenia in Finnish male twins', in M.H. Lader (ed.) *Studies of Schizophrenia*, Ashford: Headley Brothers.

Tienari, P. (1991) 'Interaction between genetic vulnerability and family environment: the Finnish adoptive study of schizophrenia', *Acta Psychiatrica Scandinavica* 84: 460–465.

Tienari, P., Sorri, A., Lahti, I., Naarala, M., Wahlberg, K.E., Moring, J., Pohjola, J. and Wynne, L.C. (1987) 'Genetic and psychosocial factors in schizophrenia: the Finnish adoptive family study', *Schizophrenia Bulletin* 13: 477–484.

Tienari, P., Sorri, A., Lahti, I., Naarala, M., Wahlberg, K.E., Pohjola, J. and Moring, J. (1985a) 'Interaction of genetic and psychosocial factors in schizophrenia', *Acta Psychiatrica Scandinavica* 71 (Suppl. 319): 19–30.

Tienari, P., Sorri, A., Lahti, I., Naarala, M., Wahlberg, K.E., Rönkkö, T., Pohjola, J. and Moring, J. (1985b) 'The Finnish adoption study of schizophrenia', *The Yale Journal of Biology and Medicine* 58: 227–237.

Tienari, P. and Wynne, L.C. (1994) 'Adoption studies of schizophrenia', *Annals of Medicine* 26: 233–237.

Tienari, P., Wynne, L.C., Moring, I.L., Naarala, M., Sorri, A., Wahlberg, K.E., Saarento, O., Seitamaa, M., Kaleva, M. and Läksy, K. (1994) 'The Finnish adoptive study of schizophrenia: implications for family research', *British Journal of Psychiatry* 164 (Suppl. 23): 20–26.

Toon, P.D. (1976) Letter, *British Journal of Psychiatry* 128: 99.

Torrey, E.F. and Peterson, M.R. (1973) 'Slow and latent viruses in schizophrenia', *The Lancet* (7 July): 22–24.

Tsuang, M.T., Dempsey, M. and Raucher, F. (1976) 'A study of "atypical schizophrenia": a comparison with schizophrenia and affective disorder by sex, age of admission, precipitant, outcome and family history', *Archives of General Psychiatry* 33: 1157–1160.

Tsuang, M.T., Stone, W.S. and Faraone, S.V. (2001) 'Genes, environment and schizophrenia', *British Journal of Psychiatry* 178 (Suppl. 40): 18–24.

Tsuang, M.T., Stone, W.S. and Faraone, S.V. (1999) 'Schizophrenia: a review of genetic studies', *Harvard Review of Psychiatry* 7: 185–207.

Tuke, S. (1813) *A Description of the Retreat*, York: W. Alexander.

Turkington, D. and Kingdon, D. (1996) 'Using a normalising rationale in the treatment of schizophrenic patients', in G. Haddock and P.D. Slade (eds) *Cognitive-behavioural Interventions with Psychotic Disorders*, London: Routledge.

Turner, B.S. (1995) *Medical Power and Social Knowledge* (2nd edn), London: Sage.

Turner, W.J. (1979) 'Genetic markers for schizotaxia', *Biological Psychiatry* 14: 177–206.

Tyrrell, D.A.J., Crow, J.J., Parry, R.P., Johnstone, E. and Ferrier, I.N. (1979) 'Possible virus in schizophrenia and some neurological disorders', *Lancet* (21 April): 839–841.

Ullman, L.P. and Krasner, L. (1969) *A Psychological Approach to Abnormal Behavior*, Englewood Cliffs, N.J.: Prentice Hall.

Ussher, J.M. and Nicolson, P. (eds) (1992) *Gender Issues in Clinical Psychology*, London: Routledge.

Vaillant, G. (1978) 'A 10-year follow-up of remitting schizophrenics', *Schizophrenia Bulletin* 4: 78–84.

Vaillant, G.E. (1964) 'Prospective prediction of schizophrenic remission', *Archives of General Psychiatry* 11: 509–518.

van Marrelo, A. and van der Stap, T. (1993) 'Voices, religion and mysticism', in M. Romme and S. Escher (eds) *Accepting Voices*, London: Mind Publications.

Vaughn, C. and Leff, J. (1976) 'The measurement of expressed emotion in the families of psychiatric patients', *British Journal of Social and Clinical Psychology* 15: 157–165.

von Economo, C. (1931) *Encephalitis Lethargica: Its Sequelae and Treatment*, Oxford: Oxford University Press.

Vygotsky, L.S. (1978) *Mind in Society*, Cambridge, Mass.: Harvard University Press.

Wahlberg, K.E., Wynne, L.C., Oja, H., Keskitalo, P., Pykäläinen, L., Lahti, I., Moring, J., Naarala, M., Sorri, A., Seitamaa, M., Läksy, K., Kolassa, J. and Tienari, P. (1997) 'Gene–environment interaction in vulnerability to schizophrenia: findings from the Finnish adoptive family study of schizophrenia', *American Journal of Psychiatry* 154: 355–362.

Wakefield, J.C. (1992a) 'Disorder as harmful dysfunction: a conceptual critique of DSM-III-R's definition of mental disorder', *Psychological Review* 99: 232–247.

Wakefield, J.C. (1992b) 'The concept of mental disorder: on the boundary between biological facts and social values', *American Psychologist* 47: 373–388.

Wakefield, J.C. (1995) 'Dysfunction as a value-free concept: a reply to Sadler and Agich', *Philosophy, Psychiatry and Psychology* 2: 233–246.

Wakefield, J.C. (1997a) 'Diagnosing DSM-IV – Part I: DSM-IV and the concept of disorder', *Behaviour Research and Therapy* 35: 633–649.

Wakefield, J.C. (1997b) 'Diagnosing DSM-IV – Part II: Eysenck (1986) and the essentialist fallacy', *Behaviour Research and Therapy* 35: 651–665.

Wakefield, J.C. (1999a) 'Philosophy of science and the progressiveness of the DSM's theory-neutral nosology: response to Follette and Houts: Part 1', *Behaviour Research and Therapy* 37: 963–999.

Wakefield, J.C. (1999b) 'The concept of disorder as a foundation for the DSM's theory-neutral nosology: response to Follette and Houts: Part 2', *Behaviour Research and Therapy* 37: 1001–1027.

Wallace, A.F.C. (1959) 'Cultural determinants of response to hallucinatory experience', *Archives of General Psychiatry* 1: 58–69.

Warburton, D.M. (1985) 'Addiction, dependence and habitual substance use', *Bulletin of the British Psychological Society* 38: 285–288.

Ward, C.H., Beck, A.T., Mendelson, M., Mock, J.E. and Erbaugh, J.K. (1962) 'The psychiatric nomenclature', *Archives of General Psychiatry* 7: 198–205.

Warner, R. (1994) *Recovery from Schizophrenia* (2nd edn), London: Routledge.

Watt, A.D.C., Gillespie, C. and Chapel, H. (1987) 'A study of genetic linkage in schizophrenia', *Psychological Medicine* 17: 363–370.

Watts, F., Powell, G.E. and Austen, S.V. (1973) 'The modification of abnormal beliefs', *British Journal of Medical Psychology* 46: 359–363.

Wearden, A.J., Tarrier, N., Barrowclough, C., Zastowney, T.R. and Rahill, A.A. (2000) 'A review of expressed emotion research in health care', *Clinical Psychology Review* 20: 633–666.

Wender, P.H. (1963) 'Dementia praecox: the development of the concept', *American Journal of Psychiatry* 119: 1143–1151.

Wender, P.H., Rosenthal, D., Kety, S.S., Schulsinger, F. and Welner, J. (1973) 'Social class and psychopathology in adoptees: a natural experimental method for separating the roles of genetic and experimental factors', *Archives of General Psychiatry* 28: 318–325.

Wender, P.H., Rosenthal, D., Kety, S.S., Schulsinger, F. and Welner, J. (1974) 'Cross-fostering: a research strategy for clarifying the role of genetic and experiential factors in the etiology of schizophrenia', *Archives of General Psychiatry* 30: 121–128.

Wilson, M. (1993) 'DSM-III and the transformation of American Psychiatry', *American Journal of Psychiatry* 150: 399–410.

Wing, J.K. (1978a) 'Clinical concepts of schizophrenia', in J.K. Wing (ed.) *Schizophrenia: Toward a New Synthesis*, London: Academic Press.

Wing, J.K. (1978b) *Reasoning about Madness*, Oxford: Oxford University Press.

Wing, J.K. (1988) 'Abandoning what?', *British Journal of Clinical Psychology* 27: 325–328.

Wing, J.K., Cooper, J.E. and Sartorius, N. (1974) *Description and Classification of Psychiatric Symptoms*, Cambridge: Cambridge University Press.

Wing, L. (1970) 'Observations of the psychiatric section of the International Classification of Diseases and the British Glossary of Mental Disorders', *Psychological Medicine* 1: 79–85.

Witelson, S.F. (1986) 'Man's changing hypotheses of his internal universe', *Canadian Psychology* 27: 123–127.

Wong, D.F., Wagner, H.N., Tune, L.E., Dannals, R.F., Pearlson, G.D., Links, J.M., Tamminga, C.A., Broussolle, E.P., Ravert, H.T., Wilson, A.A., Toung, J.K.T., Malat, J., Williams, J.A., O'Tuama, L.A., Snyder, S.H., Kuhar, M.J. and Gjedde, A. (1986) 'Positron emission tomography reveals elevated D2 dopamine receptors in drug-naive schizophrenics', *Science* 234: 1558–1563.

World Health Organization (1948) *Manual of the International Statistical Classification of Diseases, Injuries and Causes of Death* (6th revision), Bulletin of The World Health Organization (Suppl. 1), Geneva: WHO.

World Health Organization (1965) *Report of the First Seminar on Psychiatric Diagnosis. Classification and Statistics. Functional Psychosis, with Emphasis on Schizophrenia*, London/Geneva: WHO.

World Health Organization (1967) *Manual of the International Statistical Classification of Diseases, Injuries and Causes of Death* (8th revision), Geneva: WHO.

World Health Organization (1973) *The International Pilot Study of Schizophrenia*, Geneva: WHO.

World Health Organization (1974) *Glossary of Mental Disorders and Guide to their Classification for Use in Conjunction with the ICD* (8th revision), Geneva: WHO.

World Health Organization (1977) *Manual of the International Statistical Classification of Diseases, Injuries and Causes of Death* (9th revision), Geneva: WHO.

World Health Organization (1978) *Mental Disorders: Glossary and Guide to their Classification in Accordance with the 9th Revision of the International Classification of Diseases*, Geneva: WHO.

World Health Organization (1979) *Schizophrenia: An International Follow-up Study*, Chichester: Wiley.

World Health Organization (1992–4) *International Classification of Diseases and Related Health Problems* (10th revision), Vol. 1: *Tabular List, 1992*; Vol. 2: *Instruction Manual, 1993*; Vol. 3: *Alphabetical Index, 1994*, Geneva: WHO.

World Health Organization (1993) *The ICD-10 Classification of Mental and Behavioural Disorders: Diagnostic Criteria for Research*, Geneva: WHO.

Wykes, T., Tarrier, N. and Lewis, S. (1998) 'Innovation and outcome in psychological treatments for schizophrenia: the way ahead?', in T. Wykes, N. Tarrier and S. Lewis (eds) *Outcome and Innovation in Psychological Treatments for Schizophrenia*, Chichester: Wiley.

Young, H.F. and Bentall, R.P. (1995) 'Hypothesis testing in patients with persecutory delusions: comparison with depressed and normal subjects', *British Journal of Clinical Psychology* 34: 353–369.

Young, H.F. and Bentall, R.P. (1997a) 'Probabilistic reasoning in deluded, depressed and normal subjects: effects of task difficulty and meaningful versus non-meaningful material', *Psychological Medicine* 27: 455–465.

Young, H.F. and Bentall, R.P. (1997b) 'Social reasoning in individuals with persecutory delusions: the effects of additional information on attributions for the observed behaviour of others', *British Journal of Clinical Psychology* 36: 569–573.

Young, H.F., Bentall, R.P., Slade, P.D. and Dewey, M.E. (1987) 'The role of brief instructions and suggestibility in the elicitation of auditory and visual hallucinations in normal and psychiatric subjects', *Journal of Nervous and Mental Disease* 175: 41–48.

Young, J.Z. (1951) *Doubt and Certainty in Science*, Oxford: Oxford University Press.

Yusupoff, L. and Tarrier, N. (1996) 'Coping strategy enhancement for persistent hallucinations and delusions', in G. Haddock and P.D. Slade (eds) *Cognitive-behavioural Interventions with Psychotic Disorders*, London: Routledge.

Zakzanis, K.K. and Hansen, K.T. (1998) 'Dopamine $D_2$ densities and the schizophrenic brain', *Schizophrenia Research* 32: 201–206.

Zigler, E. and Glick, M. (1988) 'Is paranoid schizophrenia really camouflaged depression?', *American Psychologist* 43: 284–290.

Zilboorg, G. (1941) *A History of Medical Psychology*, New York: Norton.

Zimmerman, M. (1988) 'Why are we rushing to publish DSM-IV?', *Archives of General Psychiatry* 45: 1135–1138.

Zimmerman, M. (1990) 'Is DSM-IV needed at all?', *Archives of General Psychiatry* 47: 974–976.

# Index

Note: page numbers in **bold** refer to information presented in tables.